High Definition Body Sculpting

Alfredo E. Hoyos • Peter M. Prendergast

High Definition Body Sculpting

Art and Advanced Lipoplasty Techniques

Springer

Alfredo E. Hoyos, MD
Elysium Aesthetics
Bogota
Colombia

Peter M. Prendergast, MB, BCh, MRCSI
Venus Medical
Dublin
Ireland

ISBN 978-3-642-54890-1 ISBN 978-3-642-54891-8 (eBook)
DOI 10.1007/978-3-642-54891-8
Springer Heidelberg New York Dordrecht London

Library of Congress Control Number: 2014941288

Printed on acid-free paper

Springer is part of Springer Science+Business Media (www.springer.com)

Foreword

> The Plastic Surgeon is undoubtedly the greatest of all contemporary artists. He paints on living canvas and sculpts in human flesh. C. H. Willi 1955

Charles H. Willi (1926) [1] was the first surgeon to inject small pieces of fat with a syringe for aesthetic purposes. Giorgio Fischer (1975) [2] was the first to describe the removal of fat through small incisions (5 mm) using a cannula with an internal cutting mechanism (to be used at the discretion of the surgeon) that was called the "planotome" that was attached to a suction machine. Syringe-assisted-, ultrasound-assisted-, laser-assisted-, water jet-assisted-, power-assisted-, and percussion massage-assisted liposuction techniques evolved. Bircoll (1982) [3] described the use of autologous fat from liposuction for syringe injection for contouring and filling defects. The addition of stem cells to the fat being transferred to improve fat survival is now coming to the fore. Thus it can be seen that cosmetic surgery is forever changing and improving through new instruments, new ideas, and modifications of old techniques.

Dr. Hoyos has developed procedures for dynamic definition of body areas and has published some of his techniques, while Dr. Prendergast, well published in cosmetic medicine and surgery, has become a proponent of those techniques. This book on high definition body sculpting involves refined techniques with newer ultrasonic-assisted and power-assisted liposuction to improve the sculpted appearance of the body. The addition of fat transfer allows a more complete method of defining the features of the body. The authors, working together on the content of the book, present a unique approach to body contouring for cosmetic surgeons interested in improving their results in liposuction and fat transfer. The techniques are presented in a comprehensive and understandable manner and include most areas of the body that may need improvement for a sculpted appearance. The chapters containing the techniques make use of "Warnings" to allow the reader to avoid dangerous maneuvers. Their results are excellent and cosmetic surgeons should take into consideration adding the authors' techniques to their own practices.

References

1. Will CH (1926) The face and its improvement by aesthetic plastic surgery. MacDonald & Evans Ltd, London
2. Fischer G (1975) Surgical treatment of cellulitis. Third International Congress of International Academy of Cosmetic Surgery, Rome
3. Bircoll M (1982) Autologous fat transplantation. The Asian Congress of Plastic Surgery, Singapore

Tustin, CA, USA Melvin A. Shiffman, MD

Preface

The evolution of fat removal techniques for the purpose of beautification has been characterized by incremental improvements and refinements over the years. Blunt and narrow cannulae replaced sharp, large-diameter ones. Wet and superwet techniques replaced aggressive, dry liposuction. Various energy or power-assisted technologies were introduced to facilitate fat removal, reduce trauma, or improve skin retraction. High-definition body sculpting represents a new concept in beautifying the human body through lipoplasty. The techniques employed in high-definition body sculpting are not merely improvements on older methods; they are significantly different.

This book represents the culmination of the pioneering work of Colombian plastic surgeon Alfredo Hoyos. The impetus for this work was the increasing demand from patients for body shape and form that appeared athletic, muscular, or sexy. As well as acquiring formal skills as an aesthetic surgeon, Hoyos's attributes as a sculptor and artist as well afforded him the unique ability to develop his passion for art through body contouring surgical techniques. His bold endeavors using novel techniques and painstakingly thorough liposuction yielded results that were hitherto unobtainable using conventional techniques. Since Hoyos published the results of his earlier experience with high-definition lipoplasty, he has refined the techniques, developed new instrumentation, and employed newer ultrasound and power-assisted devices to achieve optimum results. The results of total body sculpting are not just transformational; they are also reproducible.

In the following chapters, we provide to the liposuction surgeon an introduction to the advanced lipoplasty techniques employed in high-definition body sculpting. The book covers art and anatomy, concepts in human sculpting, ultrasound-assisted technology, instrumentation, and step-by-step techniques in all body applications for male and female patients. Numerous photographs and illustrations provide useful visual guides to the techniques, maneuvers, and results of high-definition body sculpting. The book is also intended as a manual to complement a formal preceptorship in high-definition lipoplasty.

High-definition body sculpting attempts to achieve aesthetically ideal human form by revealing underlying anatomical structures, rather than simply removing superfluous subcutaneous fat. The lipoplasty surgeon must work as a sculptor, manipulating light and shadows by adding or removing fat, and sculpting controlled irregularities to produce a convincing work of human art. This book provides a unique practical insight into these advanced lipoplasty techniques. To this end, we are confident that the book will interest body contouring surgeons who can use the information, advice, and guidelines to broaden their practice and expand their horizons in this exciting field of aesthetic surgery.

Bogota, Colombia Alfredo E. Hoyos, MD
Dublin, Ireland Peter M. Prendergast, MB, BCh, MRCSI

Acknowledgments

No book project can come to fruition without the help of the background team. Thank you to Ellen Blasig who embraced this project and to the rest of the Springer team, including Rosemarie Unger and Antonia von Saint Paul. Thank you to Daniel Glassberg and Joni Fraser for their patience and guidance during development of the project. A special thank you to David Guarin, Mauricio Perez, and Udalvis Bellido who spent time reviewing the manuscript and generously offering their expertise and advice.

Justin Craig, Elise Taylor, and Mary Kate Wright produced the illustrations and artwork. Without their beautiful contributions, the book would not exist.

We wish also to extend our gratitude to the real pioneers: the patients who rightfully asked for more. Now more is the new standard.

Contents

Part I

Art and Science

1 The Human Form as Art: Contours, Proportions, and Aesthetic Ideals

Introduction

Through the ages, the human form has been featured greatly in the artistic expression of artists and sculptors. In the fifth century BC, the Greek sculptor Polykleitos created *Doryphorus,* the bronze sculpture that exemplifies the perfectly harmonious and balanced proportions of the human body (Fig. 1.1). This muscular nude male exhibits athletic readiness in classic "contrapposto," or counterpose, where the arms and shoulders twist off axis to the legs and hips. There is minimal body fat and excellent muscular definition. His contemporary, Phidias, is regarded as one of the greatest sculptors of Classical Greece. Phidias' colossal chryselephantine and gold statue of Zeus at Olympia was regarded as one of the seven wonders of the ancient world.

No sculptor could carve such captivating and convincing works of art without having accurate knowledge of the human anatomy. The skin and subcutaneous fat is merely draped over the anatomical wonders beneath. If an artist or sculptor does not know all of the muscles, tendons, and bony landmarks, how can he display them through the skin in his masterpiece? He must also understand their functions and how they change with motion: a muscular body in action is characterized by concavities, convexities, and shadows that instantly portray the state of health. For millennia, the work of Claudius Galen dominated the understanding of anatomy in Europe. Galen (AD 129–201) dissected pigs and

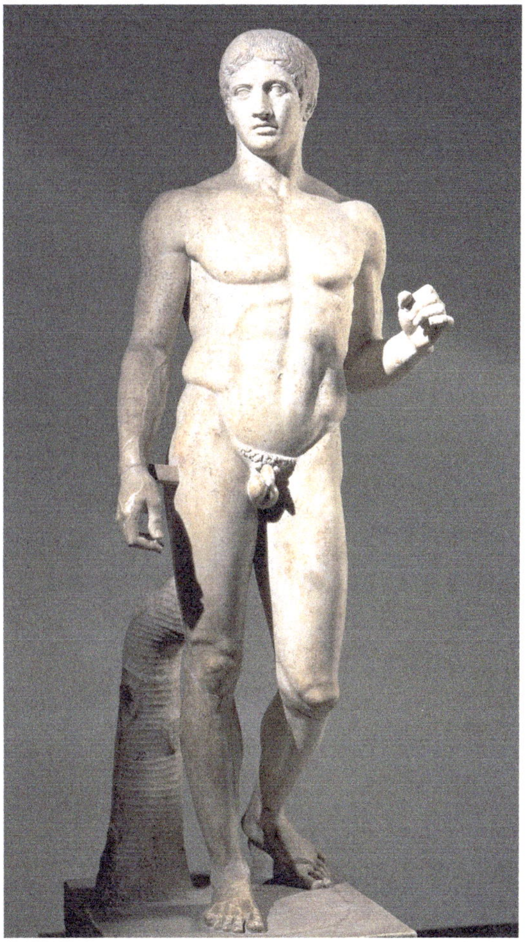

Fig. 1.1 The sculpture *Doryphorus*, detailing the male form in classic "contrapposto" (Courtesy of Bridgeman Art)

A.E. Hoyos, P.M. Prendergast, *High Definition Body Sculpting*,
DOI 10.1007/978-3-642-54891-8_1, © Springer-Verlag Berlin Heidelberg 2014

primates and demonstrated his findings in numerous texts and treatises. His teachings remained uncontested until 1543, when the influential work of Flemish anatomist Andreas Vesalius was published, entitled *De Humani Corporis Fabrica.*

Art and Anatomy

The merging of art and anatomy is perhaps most evident and glorious in the works of Leonardo da Vinci. His anatomical manuscripts are filled with detailed and intricate drawings that elegantly reveal muscular anatomy, symmetry, and human proportions (Fig. 1.2). His knowledge of anatomy was derived from his own independent dissections and research and is elegantly and beautifully portrayed in many of his renowned paintings. Michelangelo similarly celebrated human physicality through his work as an artist and sculptor. *David* represents one of the most recognized sculptures of the Renaissance and showcases the human body in all its strength, athleticism, and youthful beauty (Fig. 1.3). The muscular definition of deltoid, biceps, pectoralis major, rectus abdominis, and

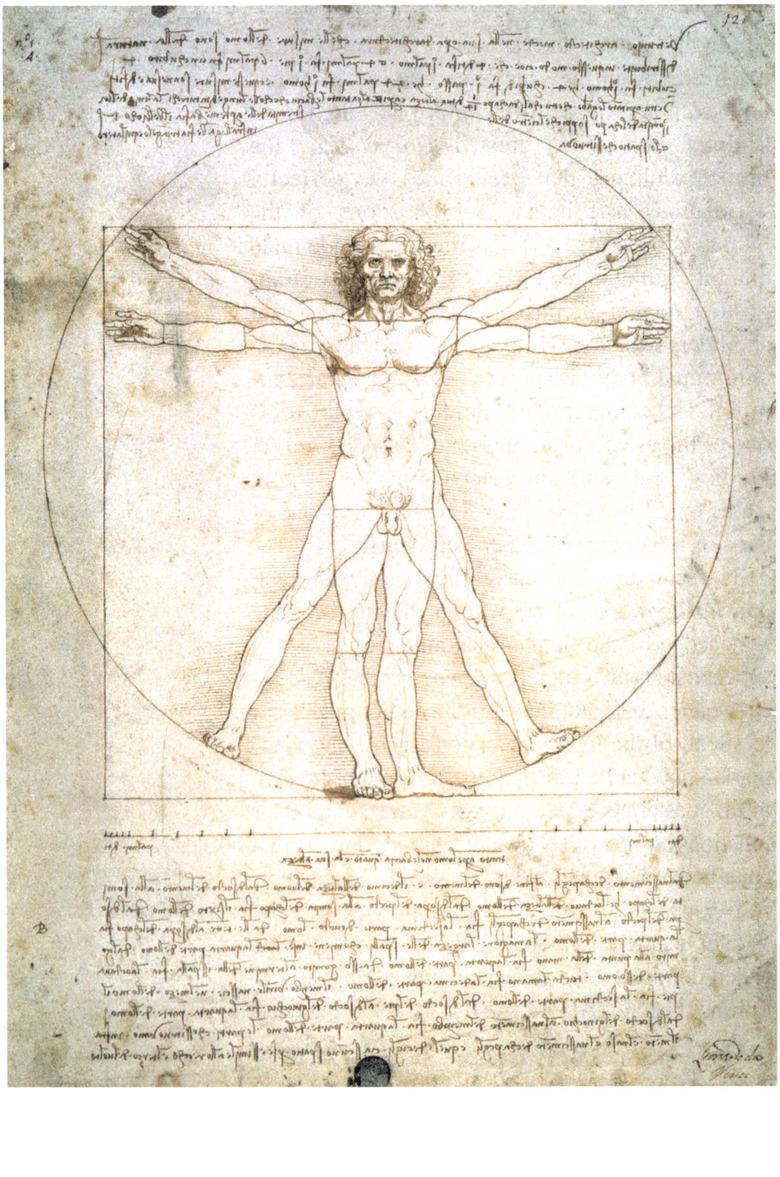

Fig. 1.2 An example of Leonardo da Vinci's manuscript showing human anatomy and proportions (Courtesy of Bridgeman Art)

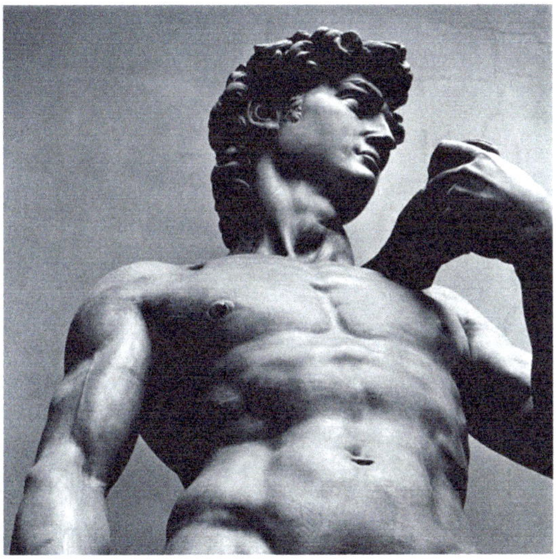

Fig. 1.3 Michelangelo's *David*

external obliques is clearly visible in Michelangelo's *David*.

In 1747, the intimate relationship between art and anatomy was again exemplified by the collaborative efforts of artist Jan Wandelaar and anatomist Bernhard Siegfried Albinus [1]. Their atlas, *Tabulae Sceleti et Musculorum Corporis Humani*, showcases the musculoskeletal system in a series of exquisitely detailed engravings (Fig. 1.4). Further evidence of the importance and prominence of anatomical art in the eighteenth century lies in the works of French artist Jacques Fabien Gautier d'Agoty [1]. D'Agoty's *The Flayed Angel* demonstrates the layered architecture of the back musculature by splaying open the superficial layers (Fig. 1.5). We look on in wonder and awe. Our fascination with uncluttered human anatomy continues today and is nurtured by our access to museums and exhibitions that celebrate the human form. These include the Museo Zoologico La Specola at the University of Florence, where hundreds of life-size wax models were sculpted from cadaver dissections between 1771 and 1814. More recently, the exhibition *Körperwelten* showcases real human specimens that have been preserved by plastination, a technique pioneered by the anatomist Gunther von Hagens. Von Hagens' work reveals anatomy in motion—running, lifting, stretching, and dancing—and has captivated the public at exhibitions all around the world since 1995.

The celebration of our physicality in the natural world is expressed through our study of anatomy, art, and aesthetics. Since art may be considered the endeavor toward perfection, we may consider artistic body sculpting as an attempt to achieve perfect human form. Although "perfect" human form hardly exists and is in any case subjective, there are several determinants of physical attractiveness as well as aesthetic ideals that we can consider to strive toward our goal of achieving beautiful physical form. These include symmetry, proportions, curves, ratios, and indices.

Greek sculptors and artists strove to reduce what they observed as perfect human form to order, by measuring features and proportions, thus quantifying aesthetic ideals. Phidias used a special ratio, approximating 1.618, for many of his creations. This golden ratio, or phi (ϕ), after Phidias, appears to hold special importance in aesthetics in the natural world.

A beautiful body can be considered to be one that attracts our attention and elicits a positive emotional response. Beauty and function are also intimately related, so that a beautiful body is one that functions well. As humans, we have evolved with finely honed mating strategies, complete with the evolved desire to seek mates who exhibit signs of youth and health. Both sexes have the innate desire to reproduce and to seek mates that exhibit physical signs of reproductive health [2]. These cues to health, strength, and fertility include muscular definition and athleticism in males and curvaceousness in females. The surgeon performing advanced body sculpting aims to improve attractiveness by enhancing muscular definition and curvaceousness.

We inherit many physical attributes, including body type and shape. In the 1940s, American psychologist William Sheldon proposed a classification of body types that is still widely used today [3]. This system of somatotypology describes three main body types: ectomorph, mesomorph, and endomorph (Fig. 1.6). An ectomorph is typically tall and thin with low fat content, narrow shoulders, and high metabolism. Ectomorphs find it difficult to gain weight.

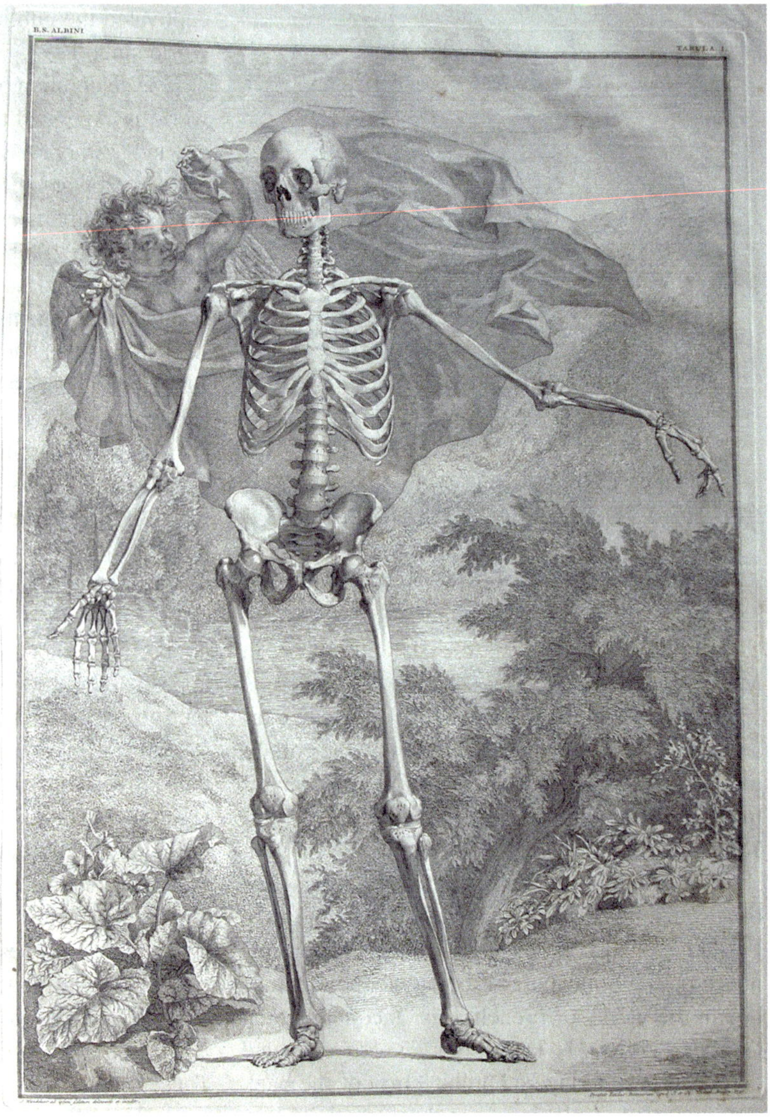

Fig. 1.4 Engraving of an animated skeleton from *Tabulae Sceleti et Musculorum* (Courtesy of Bridgeman Art)

Mesomorphs are muscular and lean, with medium bones and a solid torso. They may gain some fat if calorific intake is too high or exercise is deficient. Endomorphs have big bones, a wide waist, and a tendency toward fatness. Endomorphs gain weight easily and require high-intensity exercise and dieting to become lean. Through diet and exercise, all body types have the ability to increase muscle tone and mass, reduce body fat, improve posture, and acquire other physical manifestations of health and beauty.

Liposuction Technology and Body Art

For exercise and diet-resistant fatty deposits, liposuction has been utilized as a surgical solution for unwanted convex adiposities for decades. The introduction of the tumescent technique by Klein in the 1990s transformed the safety of suction-assisted lipoplasty [4]. However, traditional liposuction has inherent limitations based on instrumentation and technique, relegating it to

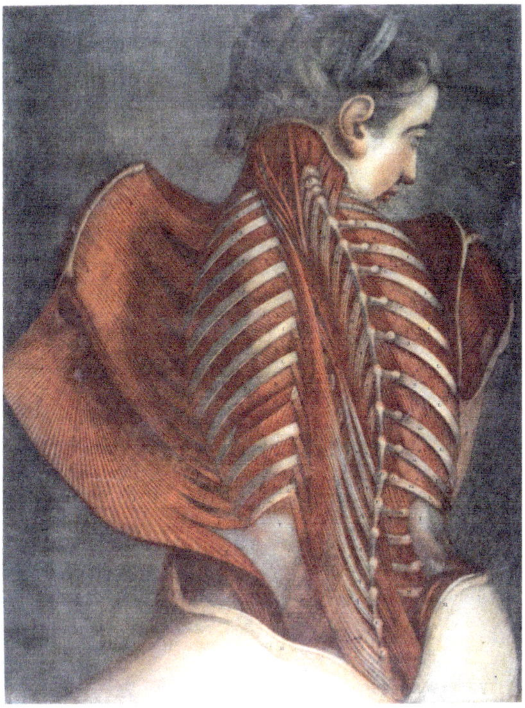

Fig. 1.5 D'Agoty's *The Flayed Angel* revealing the muscular and bony anatomy of the back (Courtesy of Bridgeman Art)

a procedure indicated primarily for debulking and unrefined body contouring.

In 2000, Sound Surgical Technologies introduced an efficient third-generation ultrasound-assisted lipoplasty technology called VASER, an acronym for vibration amplification of sound energy at resonance [5]. The introduction of VASER allowed efficient and safe emulsification of fat in deep and superficial planes through cavitation while preserving vascular and neural structures. It also represented the sculptor's chisel in a new technique that would change the concept of surgical body contouring. Pioneered by Hoyos in 2002, VASER-assisted high-definition lipoplasty (VAHDL) radically altered the tenets of lipoplasty in aesthetic surgery [6]. The human body can be sculpted like a work of art, working in all subcutaneous planes, by adding and subtracting fat with delicate instruments and refined techniques. The subdermal plane is no longer a no-go area, controlled deformities are desirable, and muscular definition is attainable through lipoplasty by revealing the underlying anatomy.

High-definition body sculpting requires experience in basic lipoplasty as an initial step. Equally important are an appreciation of the human form, aesthetic ideals, and an understanding of anatomy, technique, and safety. The latter three are described later in this book. Let us first mention form, considered to be the outward visible shape of an object.

Human Form

Human form, shape, and size have several determinants. These include the underlying skeletal framework, muscle mass and tone, and distribution and volume of subcutaneous fat. Many anatomical features are named after the geometric form they resemble, including deltoid, rhomboideus, trapezius, and scalenus muscles. Poor posture, related to lack of exercise or infirmity, also affects the shape of the body (Fig. 1.7). An understanding of human aesthetics requires an appreciation of various shapes and lines that delineate the human body in repose and in dynamic states. These forms include "C" curves, "S" curves, and "R" curves (Fig. 1.8). Curves are essential cues to human reproductive health, endocrine status, athleticism and strength, and longevity. In women, physical features that produce attractive curves include lumbar lordosis, convexities of the chest and buttocks, and muscular definition in the calves (Fig. 1.9). In men, well-developed muscle mass also produces curves, although the form tends to be more angular rather than curvaceous (Fig. 1.10). Undesirable curves appear when there is muscle atrophy, obesity, or advancing age when posture deteriorates and hormonal changes occur. With poorly developed abdominal wall muscles, for example, the intra-abdominal organs are displaced and the abdomen protrudes (Fig. 1.11). Since lipoplasty affects only subcutaneous abdominal fat, it is not a solution for abdominal protrusion secondary to muscle wall weakness or intra-abdominal fat. This requires a specific exercise program to improve core body strength and flatten the

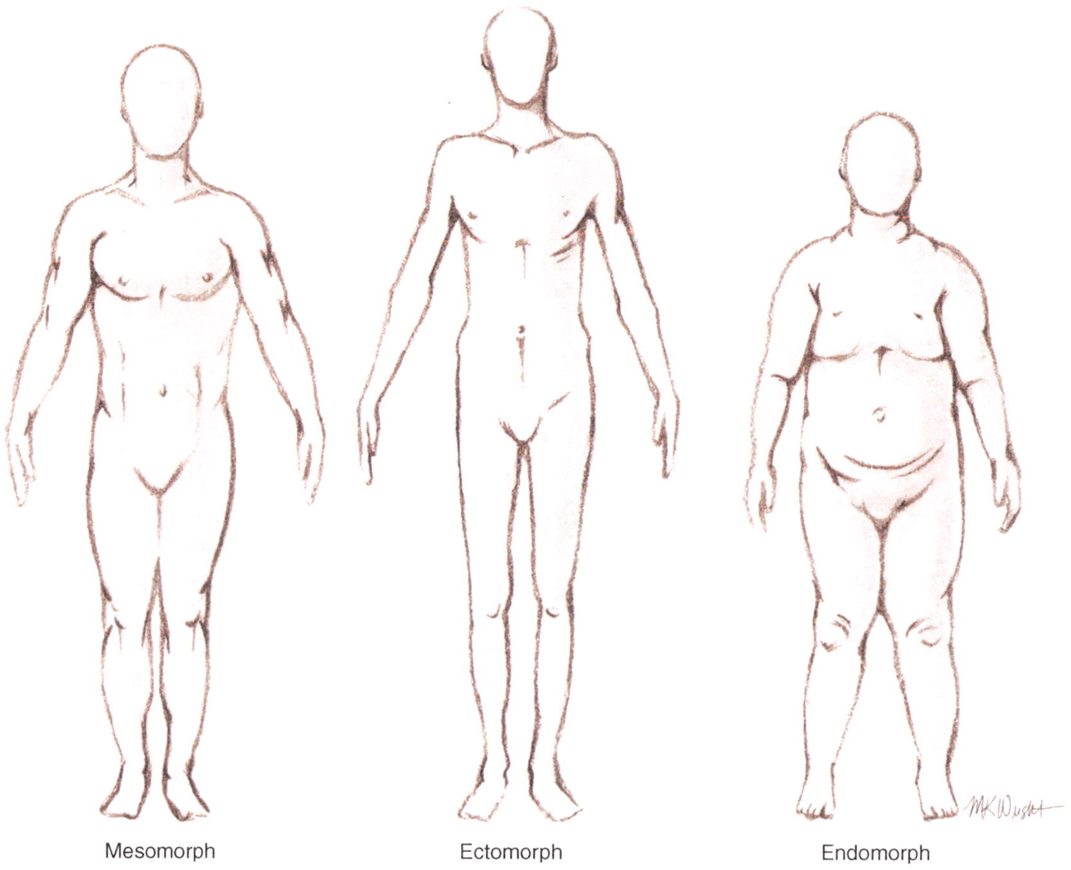

Fig. 1.6 Sheldon's three main body types

abdomen, often in combination with lipoplasty to reduce stubborn subcutaneous fat.

Physical attractiveness, especially female beauty, has been the subject of extensive research over a number of decades by experts in the fields of biology, psychology, and anthropology. Unsurprisingly, there is no unifying or undisputed answer to the question, "what determines physical attractiveness?" In other words, beauty is still somewhat in the eye of the beholder. That which is considered beautiful human form changes temporally and geographically. From the available literature, however, we can propose aesthetic ideals based on ranges and constants that describe measurements such as body mass index, waist-hip ratio, and curvaceousness. Throughout nature, symmetry and ideal proportions are also intimately related to health, vitality, and beauty.

Symmetry and Proportions

Students of art, anatomy, and aesthetic surgery will be captivated by the unique arrangement and design of the human body. Cells are arranged as units to form tissues, tissues work synchronously to form organs, and organs work harmoniously to function within the body. Proportions have always played a central role in art. Leonardo da Vinci's *On the Proportions and on the Movements of the Human Figure* and Albrecht Dürer's *Four Books on Human Proportions* detail human proportions and highlight the importance that harmony and proportions play in aesthetics and in art.

Probably the most significant measurement in human proportions and aesthetics is the golden ratio mentioned before in this chapter, approximating 1.618 (ϕ). This ratio, measureable throughout nature, explains dynamic symmetry in human

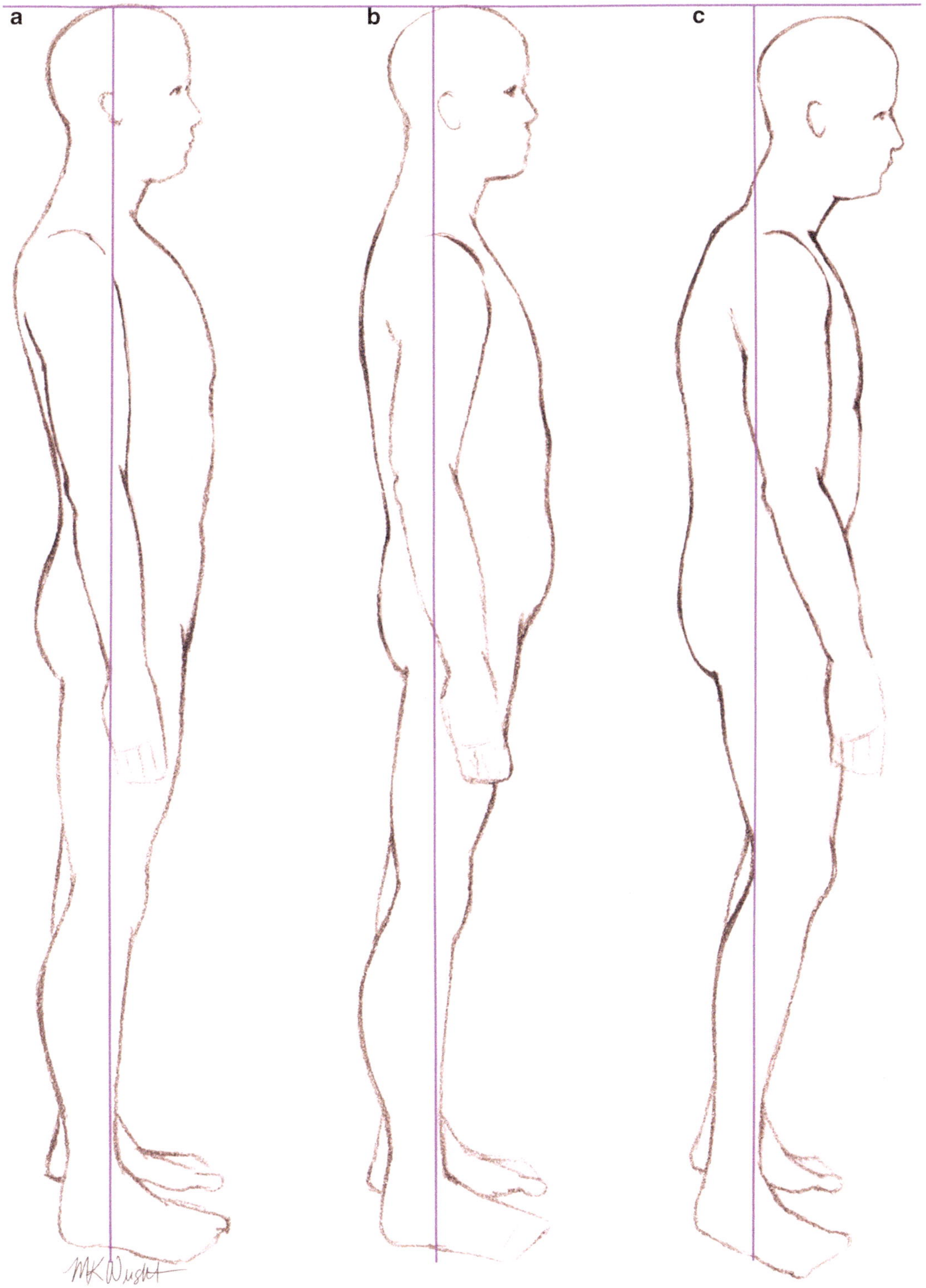

Fig. 1.7 How posture affects form. (**a**) Normal upright posture produces good form. (**b**) Shoulders forward and abdomen protruding. (**c**) Shoulders slouched forward, back curved, and neck hanging forward, producing poor form

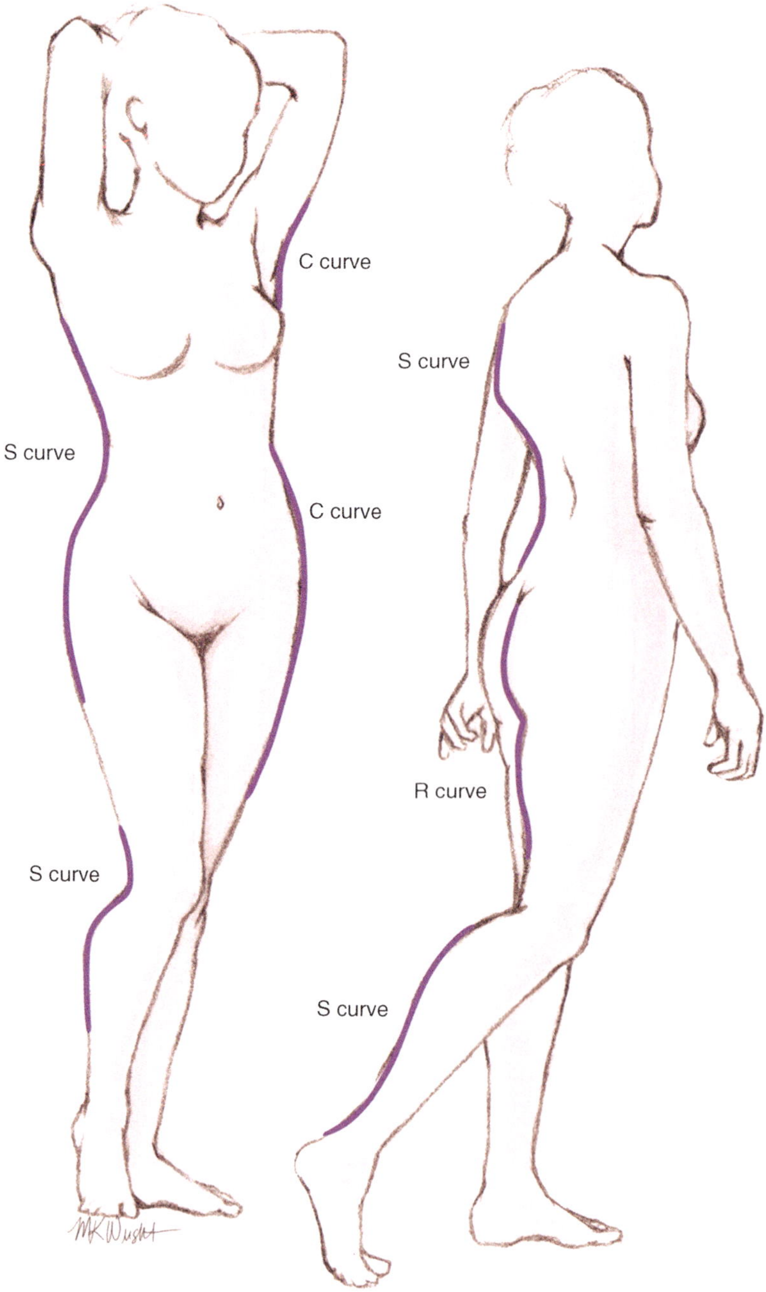

Fig. 1.8 Aesthetic curves in the human form

proportions. Mathematically, dynamic symmetry is expressed in the Fibonacci series, a series of numbers where any number in the series is the sum of the previous two numbers: 1; 1+1=2; 1+2=3; 2+3=5; 3+5=8.... Each number within a sum divided by the previous number approximates 1.62 (ϕ). When there is dynamic symmetry, numerous human proportions and aesthetically pleasing ratios approximate ϕ (Fig. 1.12).

The proportions of vertical body height are fairly consistent. The body length from the suprasternal notch to the sole of the feet can be divided into thirds. One-third forms the torso from the sternal notch to the symphysis pubis, one-third

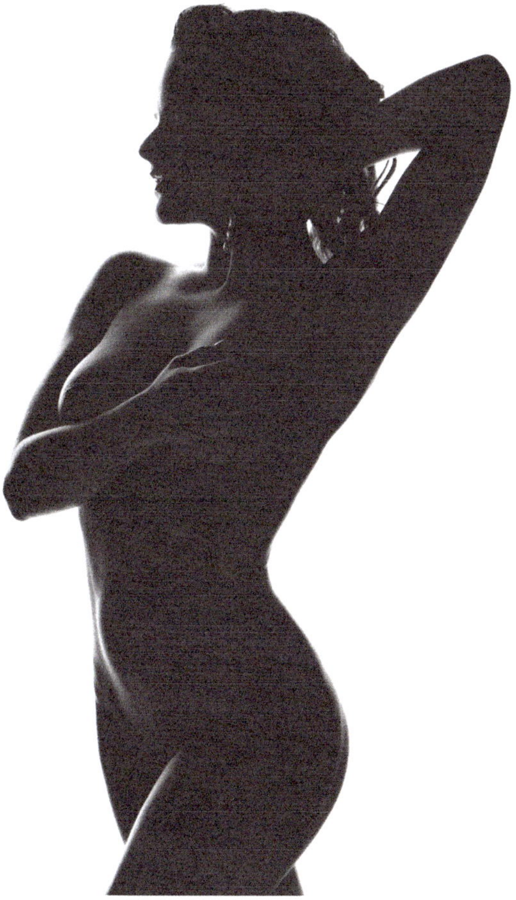

Fig. 1.9 Beautiful female form is evident in the natural curves of lumbar lordosis, the gluteal convexity, the breasts, and the subtle convexity created by the periumbilical fat

comprises the thigh length from the anterior superior iliac spine to the patella, and the lower leg length from the patella to the sole is also one-third of the body height. The head height is one-eighth of the total height, and the neck is half of the head height (Fig. 1.13). Further proportions relative to total height are provided by George Hebert in his work, *Muscle et Beauté Plastique Féminine* published in 1919 (Fig. 1.14).

Aesthetic Ideals and the Science of Beauty

Standards of female beauty vary over time and across cultures [7]. In nineteenth-century America, two opposite images of female beauty

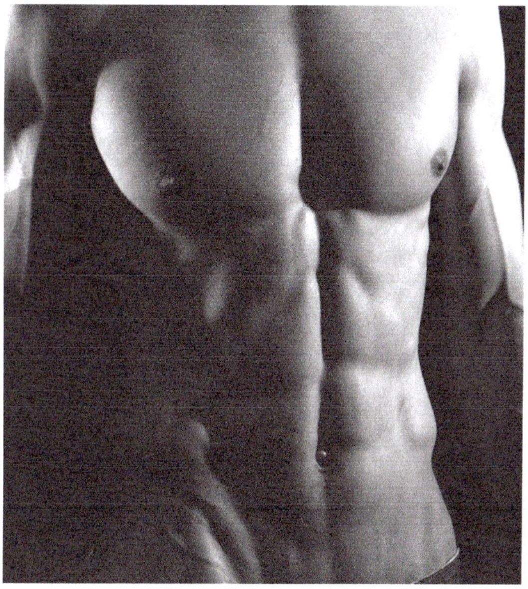

Fig. 1.10 Straight lines and angles predominate in aesthetically ideal male form

were presented: the slight and frail "steel-engraving lady" and the plump and curvaceous "voluptuous woman" [8]. This disparate image of feminine beauty continued into the early twentieth century. However, a trend toward slenderization occurred in the 1920s, as the body seemed to lose its curves and the focus on image was on the legs and face. In the 1930s, the *Esquire* magazine illustrator George Petty provided a new aesthetic ideal: a toned, athletic yet curvaceous girl with long, muscular legs (Fig. 1.15). Petty's successor at *Esquire*, Alberto Vargas, provided yet another aesthetic ideal in the 1940s and 1950s. He preserved the muscular athletic look of the Petty girl but added large breasts (Fig. 1.16). The trend toward larger breasts as an aesthetic ideal continued into the 1960s as "bosom mania" and probably still exists today to some extent, given the rising number of breast augmentations performed annually [9]. Since men place a great deal of importance on physical appearance in a mate, women go to greater lengths than men to conform to an aesthetic ideal. This involves cosmetics, fashion, and sometimes surgery. High-definition lipoplasty has become popular recently due to advances in technique, coupled with the demand for a toned athletic appearance, even in women.

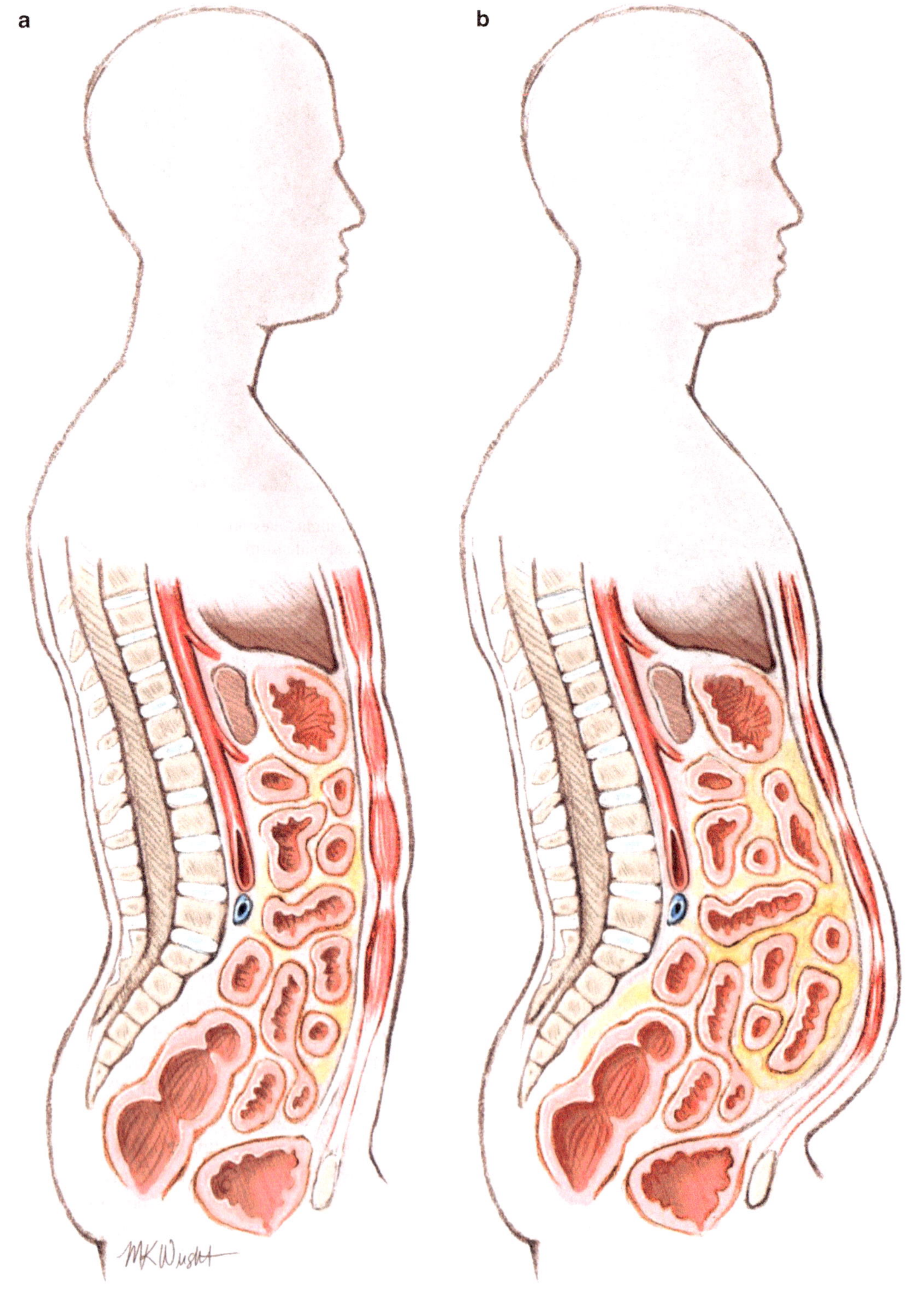

Fig. 1.11 (**a**) Flat abdomen with toned anterior abdominal wall muscles. (**b**) The abdomen protrudes when the muscles are weak. Excess intra-abdominal fat worsens abdominal wall protrusion

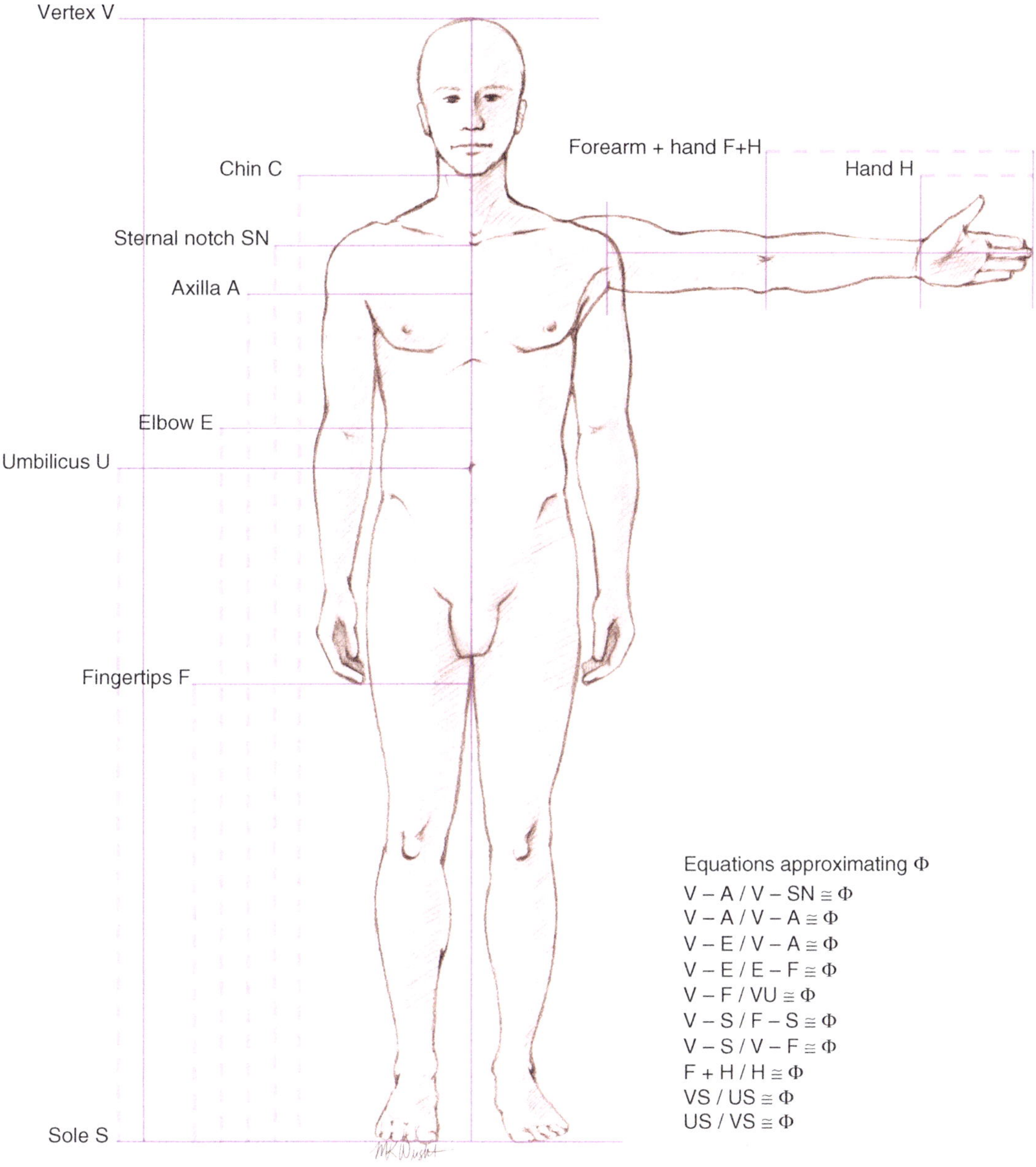

Fig. 1.12 Dynamic symmetry in human form

Three proposed and well-researched determinants of beauty are waist-to-hip ratio (WHR), body mass index (BMI), and curvaceousness [10]. Several studies conclude that the most attractive WHR, measured by dividing the circumference of the waist by that of the hips, is 0.7 [10–12]. Interestingly, the measurements of Miss America pageant winners for many years have consistently approximated this optimum ratio. Since estrogen has the effect of depositing fat in the hip area and preventing deposition in the abdomen, it follows that premenopausal women

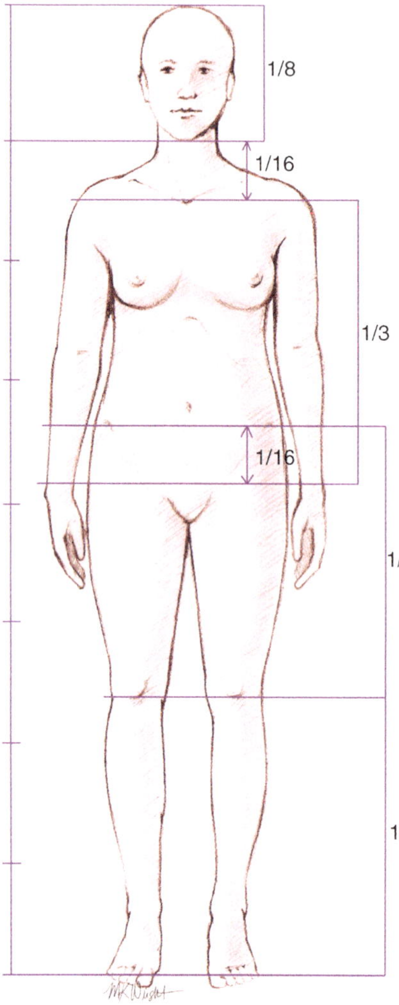

Fig. 1.13 Human proportions related to vertical body and head height

with normal estrogen levels will have lower WHR than women who have reached menopause. Lipoplasty procedures that remove fat from the waist and transfer it to the hips aim to lower the WHR and improve attractiveness (Fig. 1.17). Body mass index (BMI), calculated by dividing the body weight in kilograms by the height in meters squared, can be considered to be an index of overall fat percentage. Although a BMI in females of 20–25 is normal, studies reveal that a BMI of 20 is considered optimally attractive [13]. Curvaceousness is the degree of "hourglass shape" of a woman, such that the breasts and hips are relatively large and the waist relatively slender. A more curvaceous body is a cue to reproductive health and is considered more attractive to a male [2]. Lipoplasty, breast augmentation, and fat grafting to buttocks improve curvaceousness by amplifying these indices. The relative importance of WHR and BMI as models of physical attractiveness is debated. Since there is a positive correlation between the two, when BMI increases, so too does WHR. Cornelissen et al. proposes an explanation for this positive relationship between WHR and BMI based on a biologically intuitive additive model of fat deposition [14]. This model suggests a method for separating WHR associated with BMI (WHR_{BMI}) and that not related to BMI (WHR_{NONBMI}) but due to underlying musculoskeletal frame and endocrine-related and genetically determined body fat distribution. The analysis of Cornelissen and others conclude that it is primarily BMI, and not WHR, that determines measurements of physical attractiveness [14, 15]. In cross-cultural studies, BMI was found to account for over 75 % of the variance in attractiveness ratings, whereas WHR failed to emerge as a strong predictor [16]. There is still a role for WHR in attractiveness judgments, and improved WHR has been shown on fMRI studies to activate in observers regions of the brain associated with neural reward mechanisms, such as the anterior cingulate cortex and nucleus accumbens [17].

For men, attractiveness ratings propose that a low waist-to-chest ratio is desirable [18]. This "V"-shaped body form results from increased muscular mass in the chest and upper back, combined with minimal fat and good muscular tone in the abdominal wall. The tendinous intersections of rectus abdominis can be seen and appreciated in individuals with minimal fat overlying the anterior abdominal wall.

Men place a higher value on women's appearance than women do on men's. Nonetheless, body image plays an important role in the psyche of both sexes. A healthy, curvaceous, and toned appearance in women represents a cue to vitality

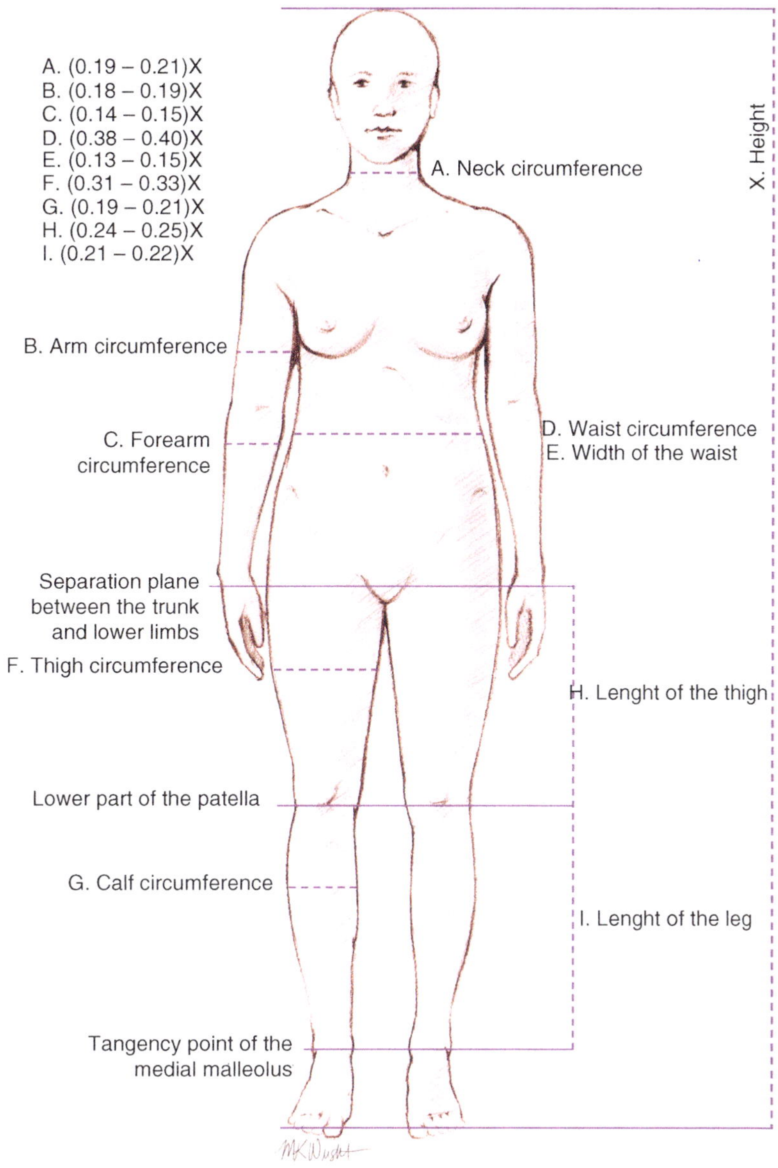

Fig. 1.14 Proportions relative to total height after George Hebert's *Muscle et Beauté Plastique Féminine*

and reproductive health and plays a major role in physical attraction. Similarly, a powerful, muscular, and athletic appearance in men also signifies reproductive health and strength, both desirable to mates in evolutionary terms. Cardiovascular and resistance exercises, together with a healthy lifestyle and eating habits, contribute significantly to the BMI and appearance of the human body. Advanced lipoplasty techniques can also be employed to remove stubborn fat and reveal the underlying muscular anatomy, contributing further to physical attractiveness and desirability.

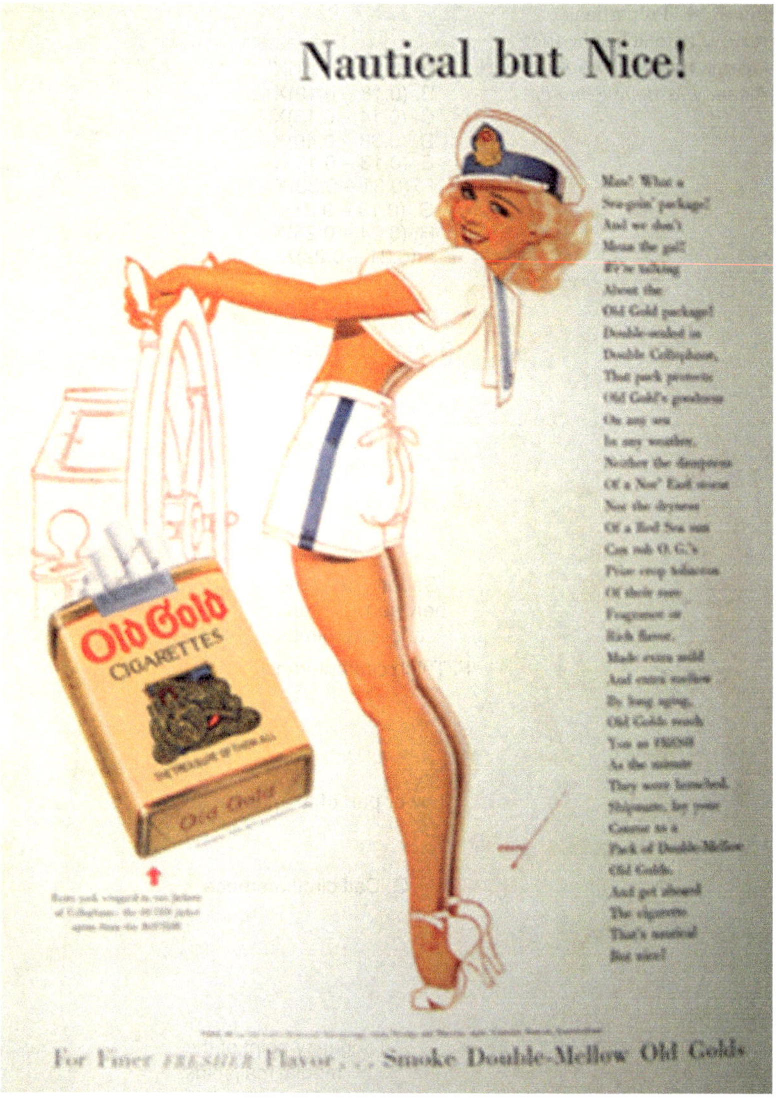

Fig. 1.15 The Petty girl (c.1938). George Petty's illustrations portrayed attractive women as athletic and toned with long muscular legs (From *Alberto Vargas* by Reid Stewart Austin; foreword by Hugh Hefner. Introduction and text copyright © 2006 by Reid Stewart Austin; images copyright © by The Estate of Max Vargas. By permission of Bullfinch. All rights reserved)

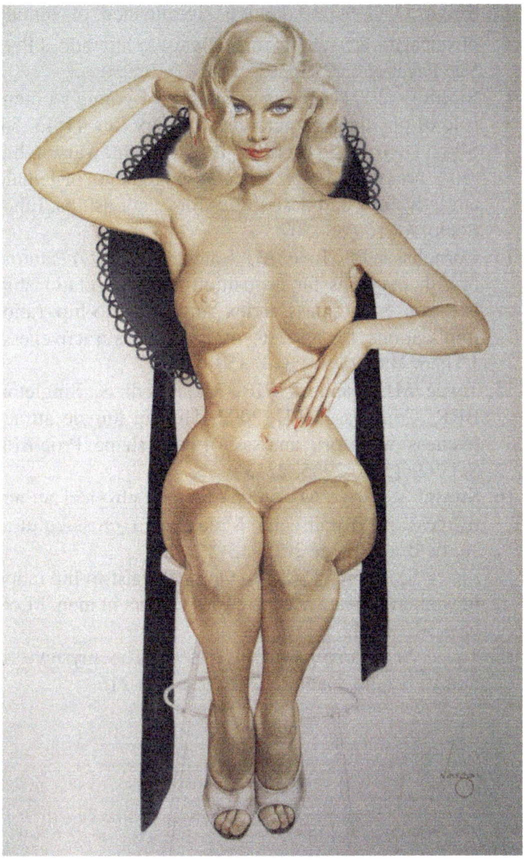

Fig. 1.16 *Ivory and Black* by Alberto Vargas (c.1955) (From *Alberto Vargas* by Reid Stewart Austin; foreword by Hugh Hefner. Introduction and text copyright © 2006 by Reid Stewart Austin; images copyright © by The Estate of Max Vargas. By permission of Bullfinch. All rights reserved)

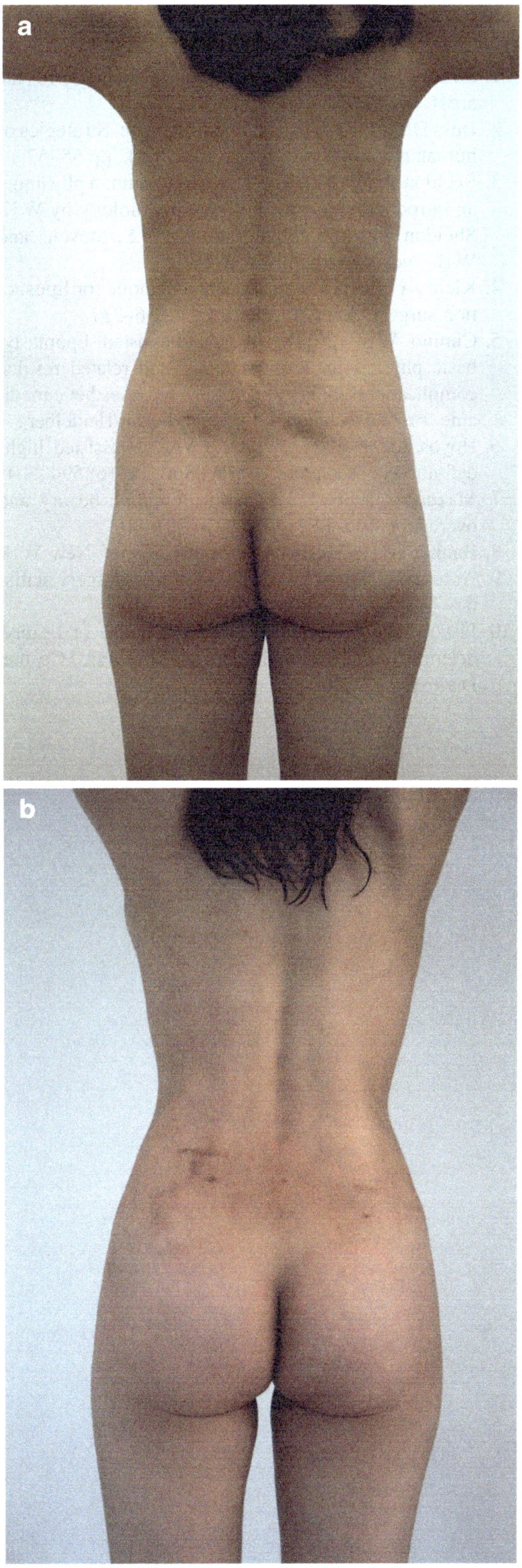

Fig. 1.17 Before (**a**) and after (**b**) lipoplasty and fat grafting to improve contours and waist-hip ratio

References

1. Simblet S (2001) Anatomy of art. In: Anatomy for the artist. DK Publishing, New York
2. Buss DM (2003) The evolution of desire. Strategies of human mating. Basic Books, New York, pp 55–57
3. Sheldon WH (1940) The varieties of human physique: an introduction to constitutional psychology by W.H. Sheldon with the collaboration of S.S. Stevens and W.B. Tucker. Harper, New York
4. Klein JA (1987) The tumescent technique for liposuction surgery. Am J Cosmet Surg 4:236–237
5. Cimino WW (2011) Ultrasound-assisted lipoplasty: basic physics, tissue interactions, and related results/complications. In: Prendergast PM (ed) Aesthetic medicine. Art and techniques. Springer, Berlin/Heidelberg
6. Hoyos AE, Millard JA (2007) VASER-assisted high-definition liposculpture. Aesthet Surg J 27(6):594–604
7. Mazur A (1986) US trends in feminine beauty and overadaptation. J Sex Res 22(3):281–303
8. Banner L (1983) American beauty. Knopf, New York
9. American Society for Aesthetic Plastic Surgery statistics. Website: www.cosmeticsurgery.org
10. Fisher ML, Voracek M (2006) The shape of beauty: determinants of female physical attractiveness. J Cosmet Dermatol 5(2):190–194
11. Singh D (1993) Adaptive significance of female physical attractiveness: role of waist to hip ratio. J Pers Soc Psychol 65:293–307
12. Singh D (2004) Mating strategies of young women: role of physical attractiveness. J Sex Res 41:43–54
13. Singh D, Young RK (1995) Body weight, waist to hip ratio, breast, and hips: roles in judgements of female attractiveness and desirability for relationships. Ethol Sociobiol 16:483–507
14. Cornelissen PL, Toveé MJ, Bateson M (2009) Patterns of subcutaneous fat deposition and the relationship between body mass index and waist-to-hip ratio: implications for models of physical attractiveness. J Theor Biol 256(3):343–350
15. Toveé MJ, Hancock PJB, Mahmoodi S, Singleton BRR, Cornelissen PL (2002) Human female attractiveness: waveform analysis of body shape. Proc Biol Sci 269(1506):2205–2213
16. Swami V, Toveé MJ (2005) Female physical attractiveness in Britain and Malaysia: a cross-cultural study. Body Image 2(2):115–128
17. Platek SM, Singh D (2010) Optimal waist-to-hip ratios in women activate neural reward centers in men. PLoS One 5(2):e9042
18. Toveé MJ, Cornelissen PL (1999) The mystery of human beauty. Nature 399(6733):215–216

2 Muscular and Surface Anatomy

Introduction

Sculpting the human body in order to improve definition is impossible without a thorough knowledge of muscular anatomy. The surgeon must also develop an artist's eye so that the form ideally created by the superficial musculature can be "visualized" and then revealed through selective lipoplasty techniques [1, 2]. In most individuals with a normal body mass index, an athletic and toned appearance can be created through high-definition body sculpting by removing fat and highlighting major muscle groups [2]. The anatomy and form of the most important muscles and muscle groups for high-definition lipoplasty are detailed in this chapter. These include muscles of the trunk, shoulder, upper arm, hip, thigh, and leg. The salient features of the muscular anatomy relevant to body contouring are outlined, such as the origin, insertion, orientation, form created, and relationship to adjacent muscle groups.

Trunk Muscles

The trunk muscles consist of large and small groups arranged anteriorly and posteriorly over the abdomen and back, respectively. They also include the chest wall muscles. They form the muscular body wall, where they connect the rib cage to the bony pelvis. The trunk muscles have various actions on the torso, including flexion, extension, lateral bending, and rotation. The definition of the trunk muscles provides an appearance of athleticism, strength, and health. In men, the posterior trunk muscles create a V-shaped form, or triangular wedge; the broad latissimus dorsi tapers inferiorly to a narrow waist (Fig. 2.1). Anteriorly, the fleshy bellies of the rectus abdominis bulge between tendinous intersections, and the pectoralis major provides a convex muscular mass over the chest (Fig. 2.2). In women, the anterior and posterior trunk muscles between the rib cage and pelvis narrow the waist. Posteriorly, the broad V shape is lacking, but the smaller erector spinae provide attractive definition on either side of the midline (Fig. 2.3). Anteriorly, a subtle shadow over linea alba and at the lateral borders of the rectus abdominis creates beautiful definition of the female abdomen (Fig. 2.4) [2].

Rectus Abdominis

This vertically oriented paired strap muscle occupies most of the central part of the anterior abdominal wall (Fig. 2.5). It is narrow and thick inferiorly and broader and flatter in the upper abdomen. The rectus abdominis arises from the symphysis, crest, and pecten of the pubis and runs upward to insert into the xiphoid process and costal cartilages of the fifth to seventh ribs. Its main action is to flex the trunk. The inferior part of the rectus abdominis is covered only on its anterior surface by the rectus sheath, and above the costal margin, the muscle lies directly

A.E. Hoyos, P.M. Prendergast, *High Definition Body Sculpting*,
DOI 10.1007/978-3-642-54891-8_2,

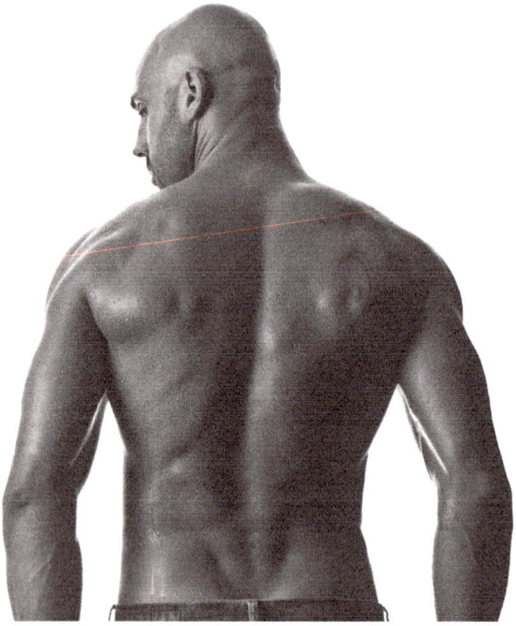

Fig. 2.1 The posterior male trunk. A "V" shape is produced by the back muscles tapering inferiorly to a narrow waist

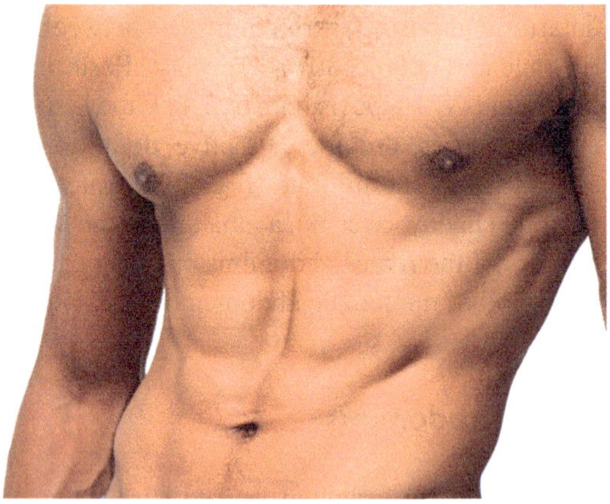

Fig. 2.2 Anterior male abdomen. The major muscle groups and their tendinous intersections create a highly defined appearance

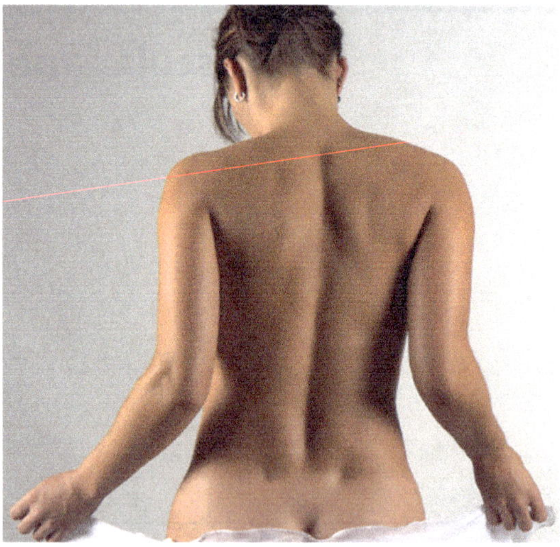

Fig. 2.3 Definition and form of the female back. Note the midline groove between the spinous muscles and the dimples in the lower back marking the location of the posterior superior iliac spines

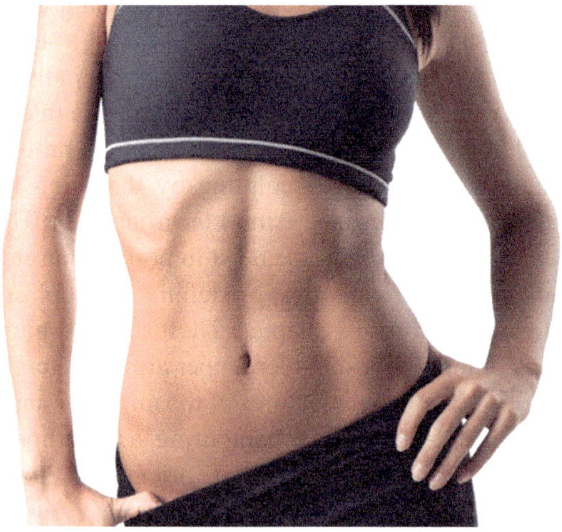

Fig. 2.4 Anterior female abdomen. The most defining features in the athletic female abdomen are the linea alba and linea semilunaris

on the costal cartilages. The paired rectus abdominis is separated in the midline by the linea alba and by three horizontal tendinous intersections. These fibrous bands are usually located at the level of the xiphoid process, at or just above the umbilicus, and halfway between these two. A fourth tendinous intersection may be visible below the umbilicus and marks the location of the arcuate line. The tendinous intersections on one side may be in line with the contralateral side or may be at different levels, giving an asymmetrical appearance to the anterior abdominal musculature. The intersections closest to the umbilicus tend to run horizontally,

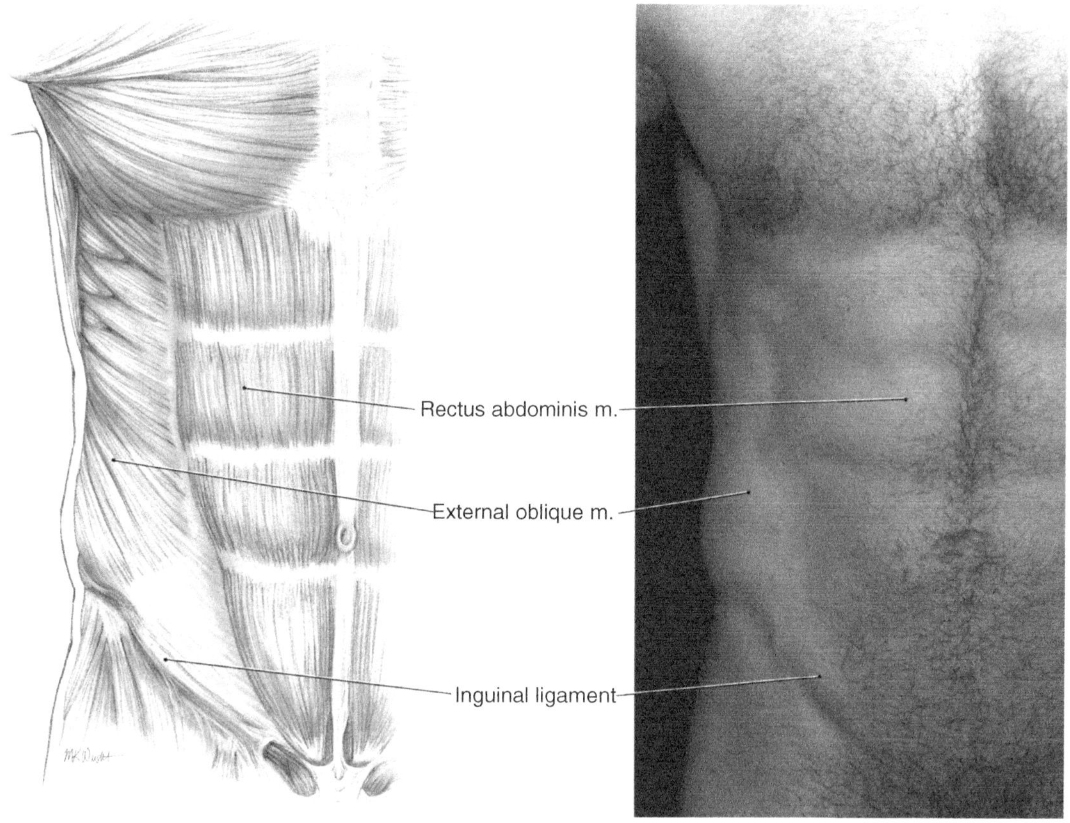

Fig. 2.5 Rectus abdominis. This represents the most important muscle in high-definition body sculpting of the anterior abdominal wall

whereas the uppermost tendinous intersections often run more diagonally. The orientation of tendinous intersections is highly variable, and all may be horizontal. Careful palpation of the anterior abdominal wall in slim individuals confirms the surface anatomy. The intersections divide the muscle into segments of fleshy protruding bellies that create the quintessential muscular male abdomen commonly referred to as the six-pack [2]. The superior borders of the upper segments usually coincide with the inferior margin of the pectoralis major, but variations exist. The muscle may continue superiorly under the pectoralis major or may end lower down, exposing the costal cartilages and creating a depression between the lower border of the pectoralis major and the superior border of the rectus abdominis. The borders of the segments created by the intersections are rounded. The lateral border of the rectus abdominis is often visible as a vertical groove in the anterior abdominal wall between the ninth costal cartilage and the pubic tubercle. This semilunar line typically runs along a line drawn from the midpoint of the clavicle to the middle of the thigh. It starts superiorly as a depression just below and medial to the nipple in men, runs inferiorly between the anterior limits of the muscular part of the external oblique and the lateral border of the rectus abdominis, and expands into a triangular area over the aponeurosis of the external oblique above the inguinal ligament. In the midline, diastasis or separation of the recti muscles with widening of the linea alba occurs following pregnancy or as a congenital deformity and may result in an abnormally convex abdominal contour. Plication of the anterior or posterior rectus sheath, sometimes combined with plication of

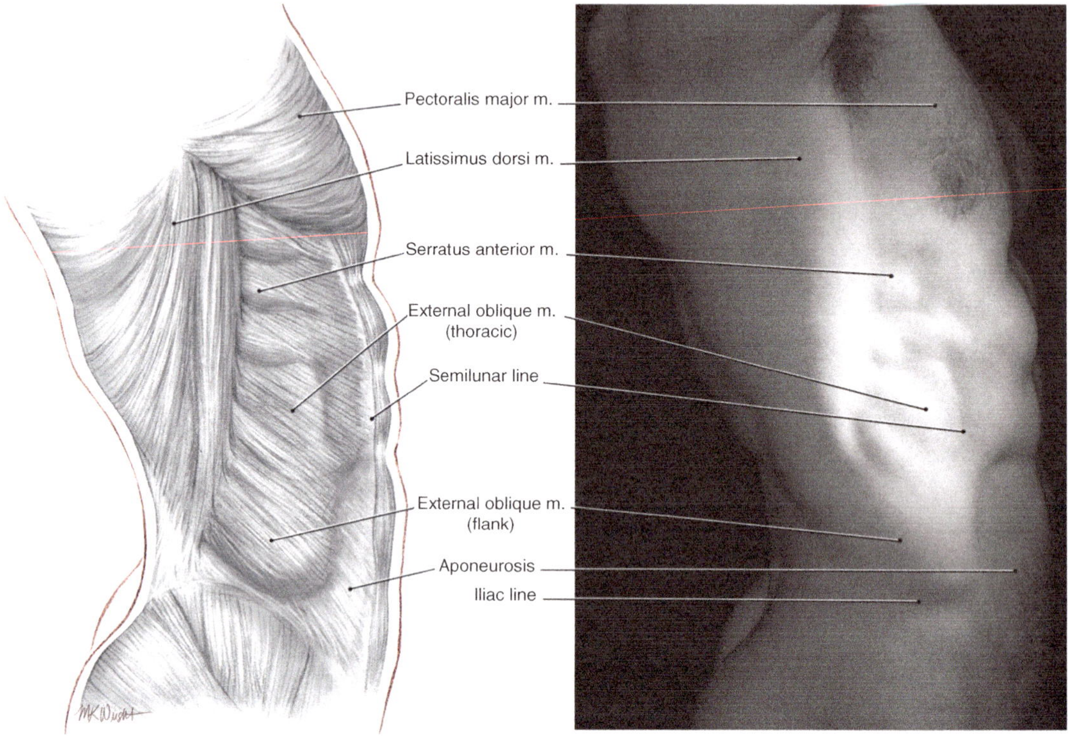

Fig. 2.6 The lateral abdominal wall. The external oblique muscle predominates, superiorly as the thoracic portion and inferiorly as the less well-defined flank portion

the external oblique aponeurosis, improves this myoaponeurotic deformity [3]. When the body is hyperextended, stretching the skin and muscle over the rib cage, a thoracic arch is easily seen where the costal cartilages meet the sternum in the midline. Even at rest, this may be seen in females and in thin individuals. The arch forms an angle of approximately 90° in males and 60° in females. In males, a more rounded arch is created by the costal margin laterally and the highest tendinous intersection of the rectus abdominis medially. The umbilicus or navel lies within a defect in the linea alba, opposite the fourth lumbar vertebra, and about midway between the xiphoid process and symphysis pubis. In athletic males, a sharp rim is usually present at the upper border of the umbilicus, whereas the lower border is less well defined. In females, a periumbilical fat pad deepens the navel and obscures its borders.

External Oblique

This muscle forms the fleshy part of the lateral abdominal wall as its fibers pass inferiorly and inferomedially superficial to the other flat muscles (Fig. 2.6). It originates from the external and inferior surfaces of the lower 7–8 ribs. The external oblique has two parts: an upper thoracic portion and a lower flank portion. The thoracic portion consists of separate elongated bundles of muscle that run parallel to one another and in a straight line from the external surfaces of the ribs to their aponeurosis at the semilunar line. The lower fibers of the thoracic portion form a transitional zone above the flank portion that coincides with the waist. The anterior edge of the thoracic portion of the external oblique is jagged or irregular where it inserts into its own aponeurosis as separate bundles. The flank portion of the muscle runs from the external surfaces of the inferior ribs to the anterior half of the lip of the iliac crest posteriorly and the external oblique aponeurosis and linea alba anteriorly. The flank pad represents a fleshy trapezoid between the ribs and pelvis that wraps around the waist. This comprises the flank portion of the external oblique anteriorly and a flank fat pad posteriorly. Even with good muscular development, external oblique muscle fibers are not visible in the smooth, convex flank pad. The inferior margin of the flank pad is the iliac line. Since the muscle fibers of the external oblique insert into the iliac crest, an iliac line lower than this is created by ptotic fat, and not muscle. The most posterior fibers of the flank portion of the external oblique pass vertically from the lower two ribs to insert into the iliac crest, creating a posterior free border. These fibers do not insert into the thoracolumbar fascia and constitute the anterior border of the inferior lumbar triangle of Petit, with posterior and inferior borders formed by the latissimus dorsi and iliac crest, respectively. Unusual cases of herniation through Petit's triangle have been reported [4]. This triangle is usually covered with the fat pad. The external oblique becomes aponeurotic medially at the midclavicular line and inferiorly at the spinoumbilical line (between anterior superior iliac spine and umbilicus). The aponeurosis passes anterior to the rectus abdominis as part of the rectus sheath and decussates with aponeurotic fibers of the contralateral external oblique, internal oblique, and transversus abdominis at the midline. The external oblique aponeurosis passes the midline to be continuous with the aponeurosis of the contralateral internal oblique. Functionally, the external oblique and the contralateral internal oblique can be considered as a digastric muscle, since their simultaneous action flexes and rotates the abdomen, as occurs when the shoulder is turned toward the contralateral hip. The inferolateral fibers of the external oblique, below the spinoumbilical line, turn backward and upward between the anterior superior iliac spine and the pubic tubercle to form the inguinal ligament. A triangular tendinous expansion occurs just below the spinoumbilical line and lateral to the rectus abdominis. There may be a slight groove above and parallel to the inguinal ligament in this area created by the internal oblique muscle lying beneath. The tip of the tenth rib marks the base of the rib cage and the superior limit of the abdominal portion of the external oblique [5]. A small triangular depression along the semilunar line occurs here in athletic people. Subdermal lipoplasty is used to create a controlled depression in this area to enhance definition of the anterolateral abdominal wall.

Serratus Anterior

This quadrilateral muscle originates anteriorly as fingerlike bundles from the external surfaces of the upper 8–9 ribs and wraps around the rib cage to insert into the vertical, medial edge of the scapula. It acts to draw the scapula laterally and around the rib cage, as in punching. The inferior part of the muscle rotates the tip of the scapula laterally, raising the arm. In muscular individuals, the anterior parts of the lowest 3–4 digitations of the serratus anterior can be seen on the lateral chest wall as they mingle with fibers of the external oblique (Fig. 2.7). The superior bundle is usually seen immediately below or at the inferior margin of the pectoralis major. The digitations of the serratus anterior are easily distinguished from the external oblique as thicker, more pronounced bundles of muscle that are oriented more horizontally relative to the fibers of the external oblique. A line drawn from the male nipple to the posterior superior iliac spine approximates the anterior extent of the visible portion of the serratus anterior over the torso as seen in profile view [5]. The rest of the serratus anterior is hidden from view by the pectoralis major superiorly and the latissimus dorsi posteriorly or is present between the two where it forms the medial wall of the axilla. Posteriorly, the mass of the serratus anterior can be appreciated where it bulges underneath the flat latissimus dorsi muscle that covers it. Its posterior limit sometimes extends more medial to the scapula where its fibers insert into part of the rhomboid major. Defining the serratus anterior plays an important role in high-definition body sculpting in male patients.

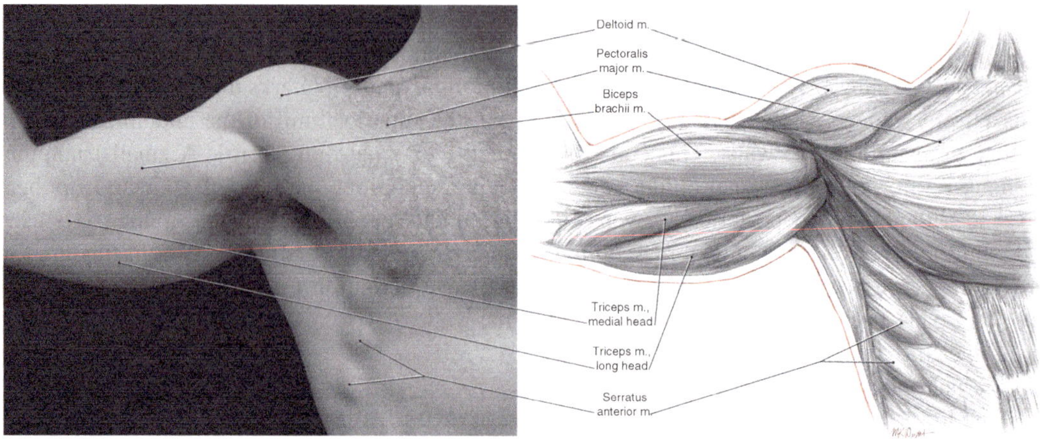

Fig. 2.7 The superolateral abdominal wall. The serratus anterior is clearly visible as three bulging slips of muscle below the lateral aspect of pectoralis major

Pectoralis Major

The pectoralis major forms most of the muscle bulk of the chest and gives the chest a smooth, convex form, particularly when the muscle is well developed (Fig. 2.8). It originates from the medial half of the clavicle, anterior surface of the sternum, costal cartilages of the first 6–7 ribs, and inferiorly the superior part of the external oblique aponeurosis of the abdomen. Based on its origin, the pectoralis major can be divided into clavicular, sternocostal, and abdominal portions. All portions of the pectoralis major insert into the lateral lip of the intertubercular groove on the anterior surface of the humerus. The clavicular portion arises from the clavicle and its fibers pass laterally and downward until they are adjacent to and parallel with fibers of the deltoid. Here the muscle bundle of the clavicular portion passes over other portions of the pectoralis major. The sternocostal portion passes almost horizontally, and the abdominal portion passes upward and laterally, deep to the other portions. Depending on the position of the arm, the pectoralis major adducts, rotates forward, flexes, and extends the humerus. Superiorly, the muscle tends to be flatter against the rib cage, whereas the inferior part of the muscle has more mass and provides a smooth convexity. The inferior margin of the pectoralis major is straight and horizontal or slightly downward sloping from medial to lateral. There is a rounded sweeping form laterally as the muscle passes upward toward the axilla. This may be interrupted by a separate curvature created by the abdominal portion of the muscle as it arises from the abdominal aponeurosis and passes toward and then beneath the sternocostal portion of the pectoralis major. A pectoral fat pad near the nipple contributes to the volume and anterior convexity of the chest. Laterally, the muscle forms the anterior wall of the axilla. Between the clavicular portion and deltoid, there is a triangular fossa, the deltopectoral fossa. A groove continues from this inferolaterally between the two muscles as the deltopectoral groove, in which lies the cephalic vein. In the midline, there is a medial depression or groove over the sternum between the insertions of both pectoralis major muscles. This is more pronounced in muscular individuals. As the origin of the muscle moves away from the midline inferiorly, the space between the left and right pectoralis muscles forms a triangular depression above the xiphoid process. Techniques used to contour the chest in males include adding volume to the clavicular portion with fat grafting and defining the borders of the sternocostal portion by removing fat in the upper abdomen and toward the axilla.

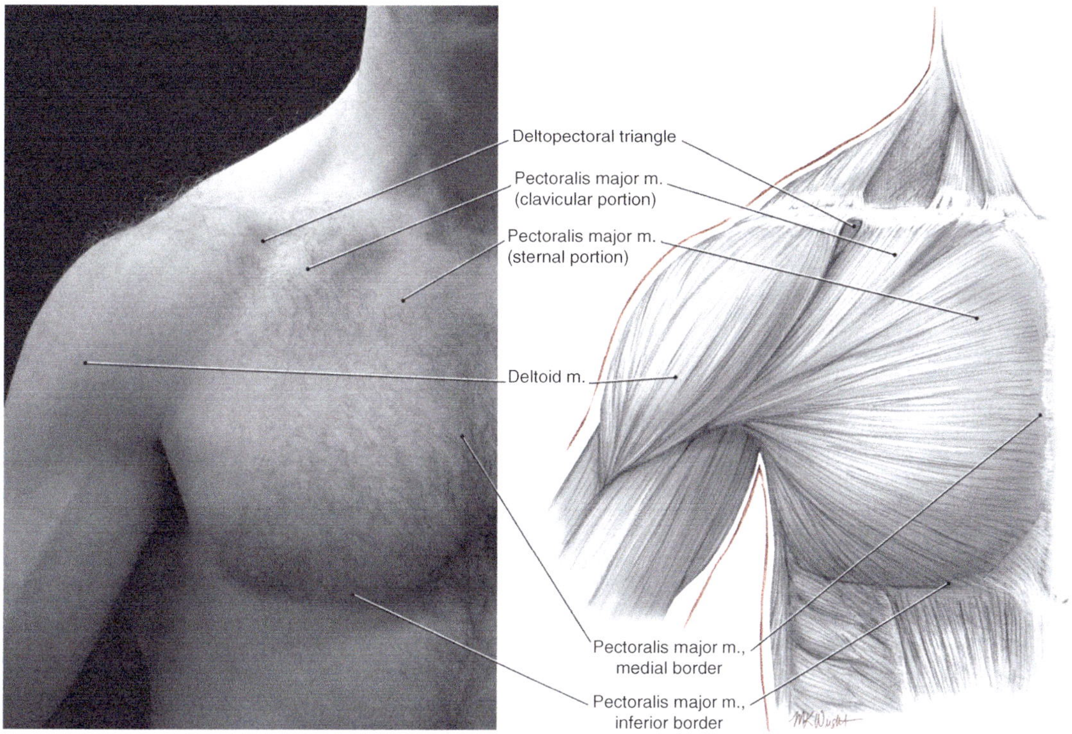

Fig. 2.8 Pectoralis major. This muscle forms the mass of the male chest

Latissimus Dorsi

The latissimus dorsi is a triangular sheetlike muscle that passes from the midline to the arm like a cape, covering the deeper muscles of the mid and lower back (Fig. 2.9). It originates from the spinous processes of the seventh to twelfth thoracic vertebrae, those of all of the lumbar and sacral vertebrae, the posterior one-third of the iliac crest, and the external surfaces of the lower three ribs. The muscle bundles converge toward the axilla and insert via a tough, square tendon into the proximal humerus proximal to the insertion of the pectoralis major. As they converge, they wrap around the teres major, forming a sling that forms the posterior wall of the axilla. The teres major forms part of that wall but appears superior and lateral to the latissimus dorsi on frontal view. The form created by both latissimus dorsi muscles is that of an inverted triangle or "V." The upper fibers of the latissimus dorsi pass horizontally from the midline and form the superior free edge of the muscle as they pass laterally at about the same level as the inferior margin of the pectoralis major anteriorly. They cover the tip of the scapula, teres major, and serratus anterior. The tendon of origin of the latissimus dorsi creates a line or curve from the midline over the thoracic vertebrae to the crest of the ilium. The latissimus dorsi and its tendon are draped over the deeper muscles, including the erector spinae, teres major, and serratus anterior. When these muscles contract or when the latissimus dorsi is stretched over them, their form is seen as bulges and shadows beneath. The lateral border of the latissimus dorsi extends upward and laterally from the waist. Although the form of the muscle is normally evident in its middle and superior portion, inferiorly, the dorsal fat pad obscures both it and the inferior flank portion of the external oblique.

Erector Spinae

The erector spinae comprises a group of muscles that fill the gutter on either side of the vertebral

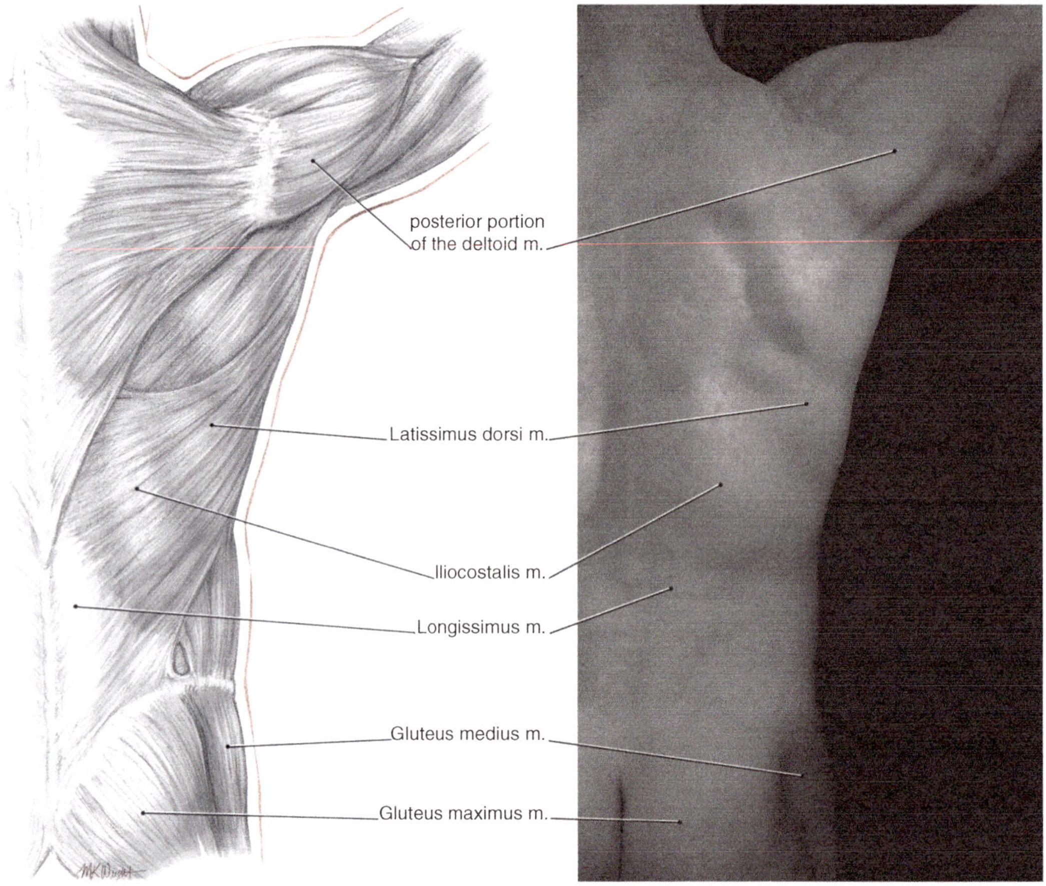

Fig. 2.9 Muscles of the back. In men, the latissimus dorsi contributes to the "V"-shaped form

column. The erector spinae group is mostly tendinous at its origin, becomes thick and fleshy in the lower back, and then tapers to form several thin slips of muscle before they end at their insertion points along the ribs and vertebrae. From lateral to medial, the erector spinae consists of the iliocostalis, longissimus, and spinalis (Fig. 2.9).

The iliocostalis forms a lateral muscle mass in the lower back. It originates from the posterior third of the iliac crest, from the lateral and median crests of the sacrum, and—through the erector spinae aponeurosis—from the spinous processes of the lumbar vertebrae. The iliocostalis has three portions, according to insertions. The iliocostalis lumborum inserts into the posterior aspects of the inferior six ribs. The iliocostalis thoracis contains muscle slips that run from the inferior six ribs to the first six ribs, and the iliocostalis cervicis runs from the first six ribs to the transverse processes of C6–C4 [6]. The form of the iliocostalis lumborum can often be appreciated through the thin anterior layer of thoracolumbar fascia that covers it.

The longissimus lies medial to the iliocostalis and also contains three portions: thoracis, cervicis, and capitis. The longissimus thoracis runs from the medial part of the posterior iliac crest and from the spinous processes of L3 to the sacrum and inserts into the base of transverse processes L1 to L5 and to the tips of transverse processes T1 to T12 as well as to the adjacent ribs. Slips from the longissimus cervicis and longissimus capitis pass to the cervical processes and mastoid process, respectively. Like the iliocostalis and longissimus, the spinalis comprises three parts, although this muscle is thinner and less consistent. The spinalis runs close to the midline with its lowest extent reaching L3. As such, it does not contribute significantly to the surface anatomy and form of the lower back.

Multifidus

The multifidus is a fleshy muscle that fills the space on either side of the midline between the spinous and transverse processes. It stabilizes the vertebral column and assists in extension, lateral flexion, and rotation of the back. The multifidus contributes to the elongated mass in the lower back on either side of the midline where it lies deep to the longissimus and spinalis.

Shoulder and Arm

The main prominence of the shoulder is attributed to the muscular mass of the deltoid that cups the shoulder joint. There is a seamless progression from the definition of the chest to the shoulder as the clavicular portion of the pectoralis major lies alongside and almost blends with the anterior portion of the deltoid. In turn, the middle portion of the deltoid points downward toward the upper arm muscles that lie on either side of its insertion. The major muscles of the shoulder and arm should not be ignored when sculpting the chest and torso.

Deltoid

This triangular muscle has three parts: anterior, middle, and posterior. The anterior portion originates from the lateral third of the clavicle, the middle portion from the acromion, and the posterior part from the inferior surface of the spine of the scapula. All portions insert into the deltoid tuberosity on the midportion of the humerus. The deltoid raises the arm anteriorly, laterally, and posteriorly. The anterior portion is usually well defined as a distinct teardrop-shaped muscle, separated from the pectoralis major by the deltopectoral triangle and groove (Fig. 2.8). There is a less well distinct groove between the anterior and middle portions of the deltoid. The middle portion gives the shoulder a rounded appearance on front view and inserts lower than the anterior and posterior parts. The posterior portion is visible as a mass that separates the deltoid from the long and lateral heads of the triceps (Fig. 2.10). The tendon of the clavicular portion of the pectoralis major passes under the tendon of the anterior portion of the deltoid. The latter inserts into the deltoid tubercle on the anterior surface of the humerus. The other two parts of the deltoid insert into the lateral aspect of the humerus. When the arm is rotated medially or laterally, the shape and

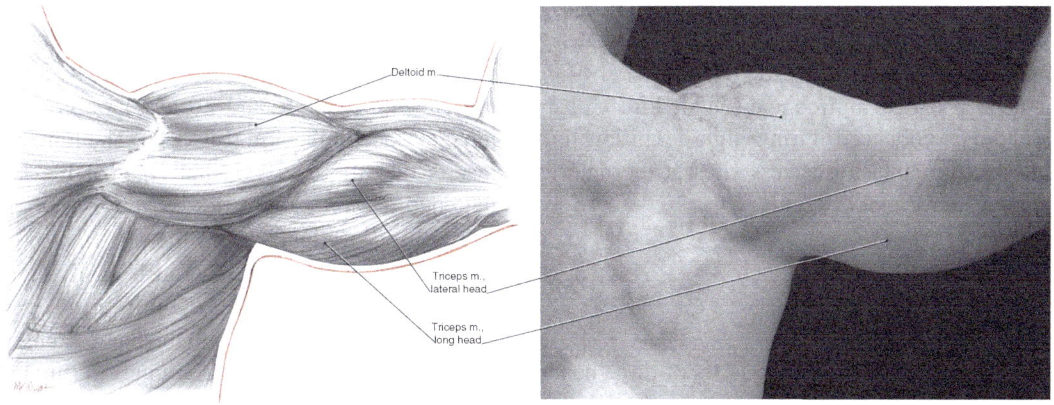

Fig. 2.10 Posterior view of the shoulder muscles. The deltoid is a prominent mass and separated from the arm extensors by a distinct groove

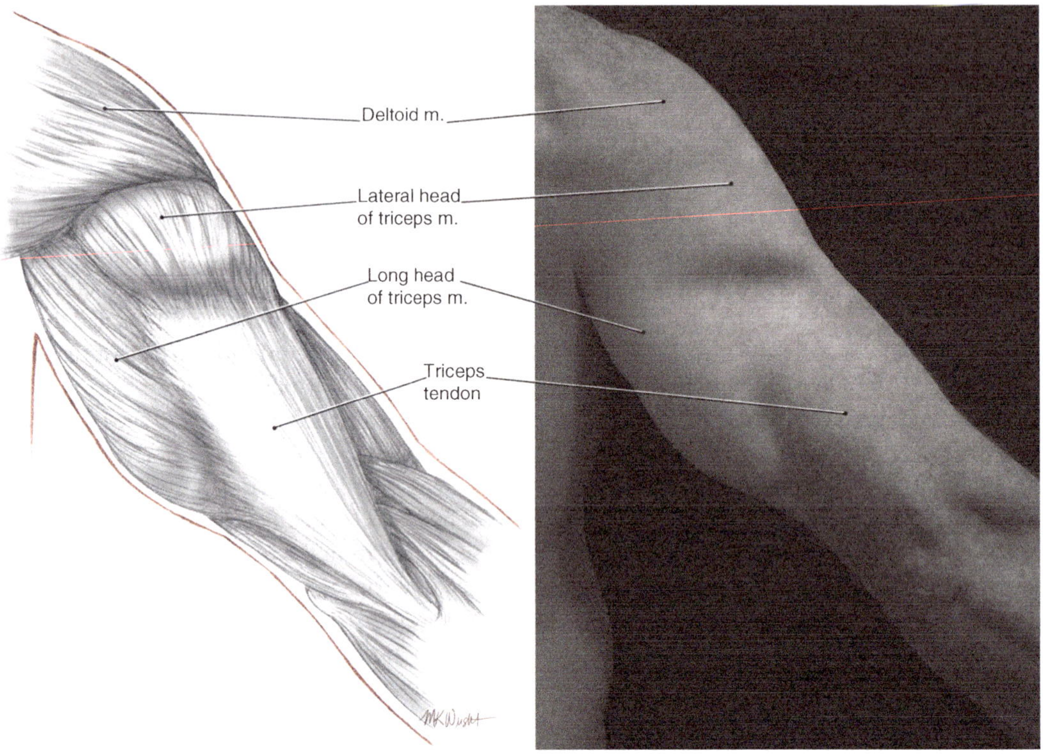

Fig. 2.11 Muscles of the posterior aspect of the upper arm. Note the grooves between the deltoid and the triceps and between the long and lateral heads of the triceps and their tendon

form of the deltoid changes slightly as the insertion points twist and the muscle moves accordingly. Unlike the anterior and posterior portions, the middle portion of the deltoid is multipennate. Tendon branches within the muscle and muscle fascicles attach obliquely to the tendons. In slim, muscular individuals, the muscle bundles can be seen to interdigitate diagonally, producing a segmented appearance over the lateral aspect of the shoulder. The definition and rounded form of the deltoid is enhanced during high-definition lipoplasty from incision access sites at the anterior and posterior axillary folds.

Triceps

The large triceps muscle consists of three heads: long, lateral, and medial. The long and lateral heads provide most of the surface form of the posterior upper arm and form a prominent bulge just distal to the rounded contour of the deltoid (Fig. 2.11). The medial head lies deeply and contributes to the volume and thickness of the arm. The long head of the triceps arises from its tendon between the teres major and teres minor, below the glenoid fossa of the scapula. It crosses the shoulder joint and forms the main mass of the posterior upper arm. Proximally, tendinous fibers from the scapula compress the long head when it is contracted, visibly dividing the belly of the muscle into anterior and posterior parts on the inner surface of the arm (Fig. 2.7). The long head inserts into the upper medial edge of the large flattened tendon of insertion of the triceps. The lateral head originates from the proximal posterior surface of the humerus and is easily visible as a mass on the lateral aspect of the arm near the deltoid. It inserts high up into the flat, rectangular triceps tendon. A thin part continues to run down along adjacent to the lateral part of the triceps tendon, creating a taillike form when the arm is tensed. All of the triceps heads insert via their tendons into the posterior aspect of the proximal

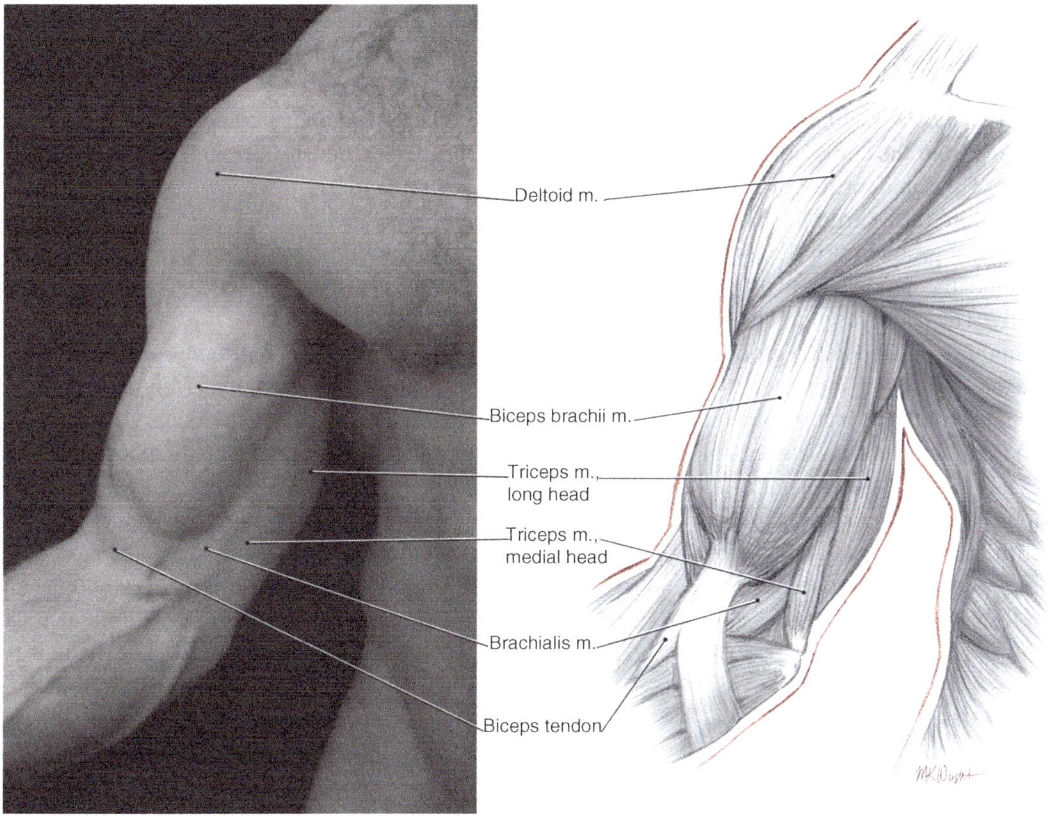

Fig. 2.12 Arm flexors. The biceps brachii forms the most defined mass on the anterior arm. The brachialis provides mass from beneath

olecranon. A cylindrical form that comprises part of the medial head of the triceps can be appreciated on the inner surface of the arm where it emerges from between the biceps brachii and the long head of the triceps about halfway down the arm (Fig. 2.7). It is possible to enhance the groove between the medial head and the biceps anteriorly and the medial head and the long head of the triceps posteriorly using very superficial and delicate ultrasound-assisted lipoplasty in this area.

Biceps

The prominent convex form over the anterior aspect of the upper arm is provided mostly by the mass of the biceps brachii (Fig. 2.12). When well developed, the biceps brachii typifies strength, athleticism, and aesthetically ideal upper arm form. The long head of the biceps originates from the supraglenoid tubercle of the scapula. The short head originates from the coracoid process of the scapula. The biceps brachii emerges from beneath the pectoralis major and creates a groove between the two muscles, particularly when the arm is abducted and externally rotated. This groove is often accentuated by high-definition sculpting to highlight the separation between the muscles. The long and short heads of the muscle travel over the humerus but do not attach to it. Instead, they insert into the tuberosity of the radius via the biceps tendon deep between the flexors and extensors of the forearm. The two heads of the biceps brachii usually appear as one bulging form over the upper arm, although sometimes the separation between the two heads can be seen running longitudinally over the muscle just medial to the cephalic vein. In the inner part of the arm, the belly of the short head of the biceps creates a convex prominence that is directed toward the axilla. As the short head emerges from underneath the pectoralis major, it is joined by the coracobrachialis on its medial side. The coracobrachialis is a cylindrical muscle that runs from the coracoid process to the medial aspect of the midportion of the humerus. In the middle third of the arm, the biceps brachii is separated by a groove from the long head of the triceps and the medial head of the triceps more distally. The neurovascular bundle lies within the brachial fascia deep to the groove. When the arm is flexed to 90° and supinated, the rounded inferior margin on the biceps brachii is prominent. With flexion against resistance, the bicipital aponeurosis becomes prominent as a thin sharp tendinous sheet that crosses from the biceps brachii over the medial aspect of the elbow. This aponeurosis passes medially and wraps around the forearm flexors.

Brachialis

The brachialis provides width to the flexor half of the upper arm. It is a broad flat muscle that lies on the humerus behind the biceps brachii. The brachialis originates from the anterior lower part of the humerus and crosses the elbow joint to insert into the coronoid process of the ulna. On anterior view, the brachialis is seen to protrude laterally from behind the biceps brachii (Fig. 2.12). A depression or groove at the superolateral origin of the brachialis on the humerus marks the junction of the brachialis and the deltoid. Closer to the elbow, its medial fibers form the floor of a concave space bordered anteriorly by the bicipital aponeurosis and posteriorly by the medial head of the triceps. The brachial vessels occupy this space.

Thighs and Hips

In properly selected patients, superficial lipoplasty to create controlled depressions between major muscle groups enhances definition and improves the aesthetics of the lower limb. Autologous fat grafting into and around the hip muscles plays an important role in gluteal sculpting and in improving the silhouette and waist-hip ratio in female patients. The major muscles that should be considered in contouring and sculpting the hip region and lower limb are described in this section.

Gluteus Maximus

The gluteus maximus contributes to the convexity of the posterior buttocks and forms most of the buttock volume in slim individuals (Fig. 2.13). It originates from the posterior gluteal line of the inner upper ilium (from the iliac crest), the posterior lateral surface of the sacrum, the coccyx, and the sacrotuberous and sacroiliac ligaments. Most of the muscle fibers run inferolaterally, curving around the hip to insert into the iliotibial tract. Deep fibers from the lower portion of the muscle insert into the gluteal tuberosity on the posterior proximal surface of the shaft of the femur. The muscle bulk creates a convex form posteriorly that contributes to the desirable "S" curve formed by the gluteus maximus and the lumbar lordotic curve superiorly (Fig. 2.14). A depression is formed over the posterior superior iliac spine since the medial fibers of the gluteus maximus originate from, but do not cover, the spine. A triangle is formed between the two depressions or dimples on either side of the midline and the gluteal cleft. Thorough lipoplasty in this sacral triangle helps define the superior borders of the buttocks. A gluteal fat pad covers the inferior medial border of the gluteus maximus and forms the medial part of the infragluteal fold. Laterally, the gluteus maximus tapers between the long head of the biceps femoris and vastus lateralis. The inferiorly pointing form of the muscle here may be visible in male patients, but in female patients the overlying gluteal fat usually obscures the form of the muscle. Additionally, a band of fascia across the inferior part of the gluteus maximus creates a deep infragluteal crease when the hip is extended. This crease extends from the gluteal cleft in the midline for a variable distance laterally depending on the volume of the buttock and tone of the skin. Gluteal augmentation using autolo-

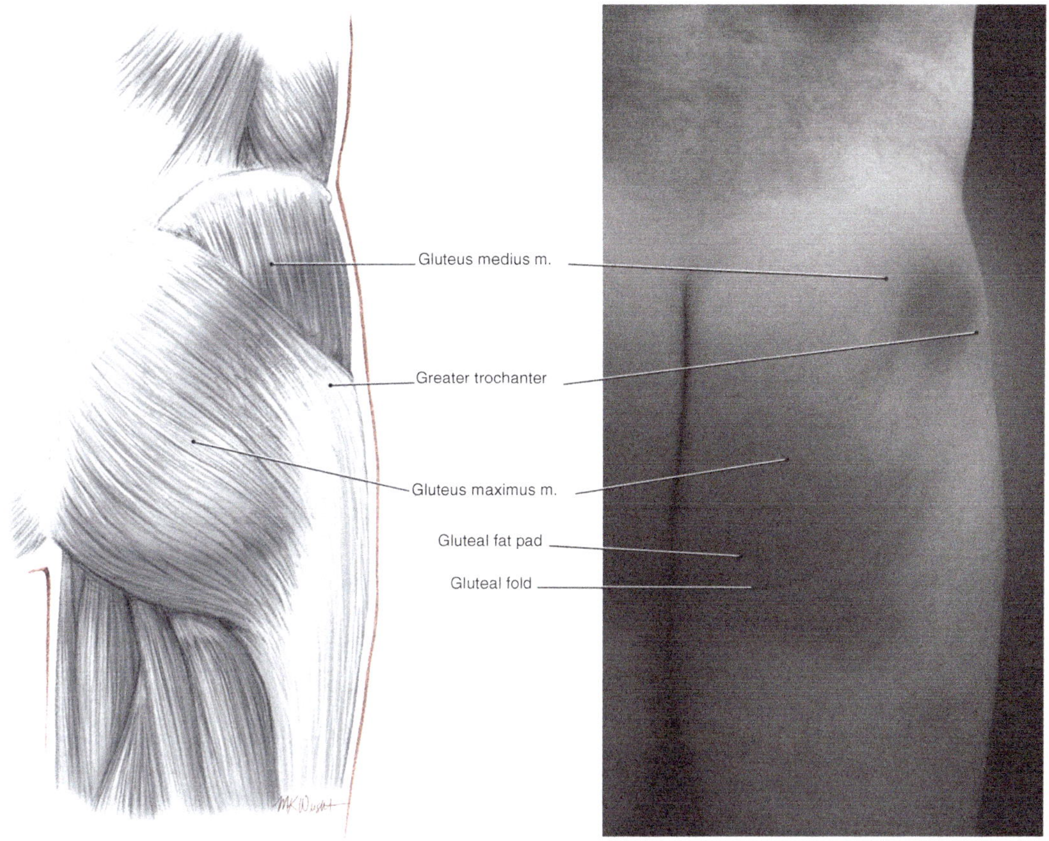

Fig. 2.13 Gluteus maximus. This muscle provides mass, shape, and projection to the buttocks

gous fat can be performed from an access site in the infragluteal crease with the patient in the prone position. On profile view, a concavity occurs between the greater trochanter and muscle fibers of the gluteus maximus where the muscle inserts into the iliotibial tract. The iliotibial tract covers the vastus lateralis and passes inferiorly to insert into the lateral condyle of the tibia. The muscle bulk of the gluteus maximus posteriorly and the gluteus medius superiorly creates a "C"-shaped form with the greater trochanter lying centrally (Fig. 2.14).

Gluteus Medius

Anterior to the gluteus maximus lies the gluteus medius, a strong fan-shaped muscle that runs from the anterior part of the lateral aspect of the ilium to the lateral surface of the greater trochanter (Fig. 2.14). The posterior part of the gluteus medius is hidden deep into the anterior fibers of the gluteus maximus. Anteriorly, the gluteus medius is bounded by the thin teardrop-shaped tensor fascia lata that passes from the iliac crest just posterior to the anterior superior iliac spine and inserts on the iliotibial tract just above the level of the infragluteal fold.

Iliopsoas

Although the form of the iliopsoas cannot usually be appreciated on the surface, it forms the floor of a triangular space bounded superiorly by the inguinal ligament and laterally by the sartorius. The iliopsoas comprises two muscles: iliacus and psoas major. The iliacus originates from the iliac

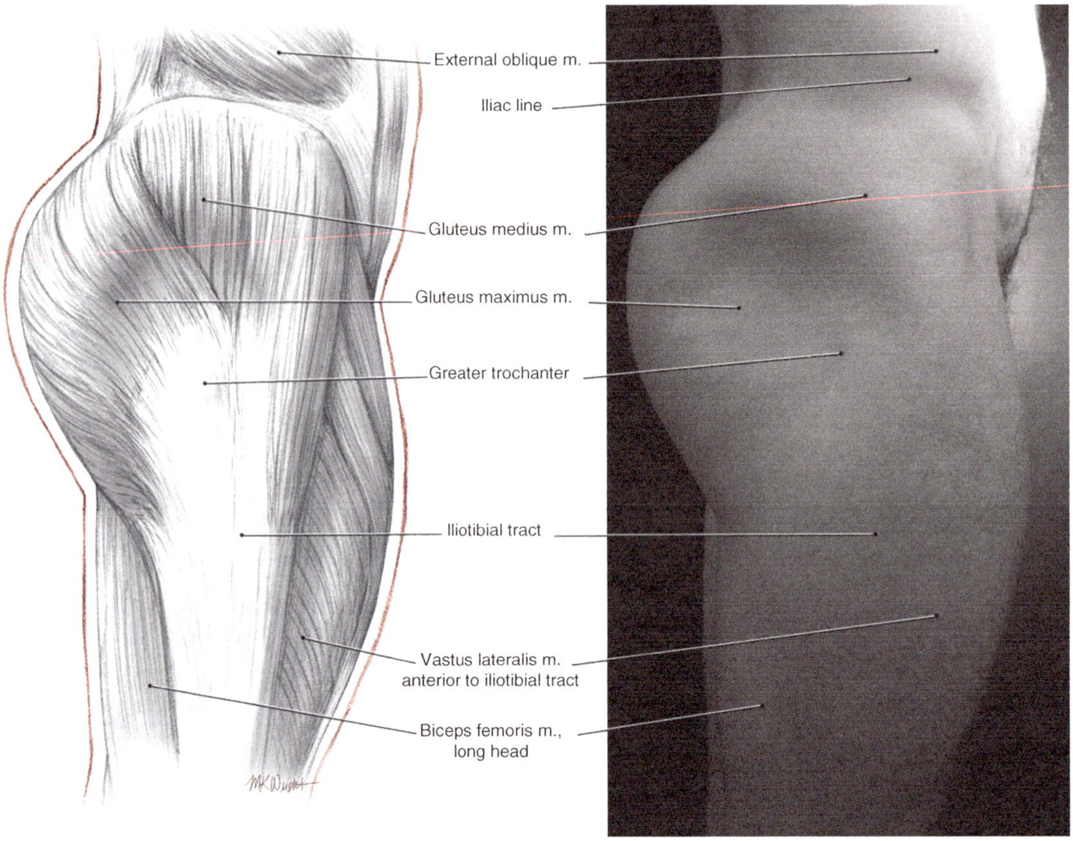

Fig. 2.14 Lateral aspect of the thigh and hip. The gluteus maximus projects posteriorly and continues anteriorly with the gluteus medius. Note the shadow between the biceps femoris and the iliotibial tract of the lateral thigh

fossa and sacrum and inserts into the shaft of the femur just below the lesser trochanter. The psoas major originates from the transverse processes and bodies of the lumbar vertebrae and inserts into the lesser trochanter of the femur. Lipoplasty over the iliopsoas just inferior to the inguinal ligament makes the ligament appear more prominent and defines the inferior extent of the abdomen.

Quadriceps

This large muscle group forms a large bulky mass over the anterior thigh. The quadriceps femoris consists of four muscles: vastus lateralis, vastus intermedius, vastus medialis, and rectus femoris. The form of the muscles, except the vastus intermedius, can be appreciated on the surface, particularly when the knee is forcefully extended (Fig. 2.15). The muscle bellies taper inferiorly toward their strong quadriceps tendon. The vastus lateralis originates from the anterior surface of the greater trochanter and along the linea aspera on the posterior surface of the shaft of the femur. The muscle sweeps over the anterolateral aspect of the thigh creating a convex form. The more bulky inferior portion ends abruptly at the quadriceps tendon below the insertion of the adjacent rectus femoris insertion into the tendon. Laterally, the iliotibial tract passes from the greater trochanter, along the lateral thigh over the vastus lateralis, and inserts into the lateral condyle of the tibia. A concave space is formed above the knee laterally that is bordered by the iliotibial tract posteriorly, the distal limit of the vastus lateralis belly superiorly, and the patella

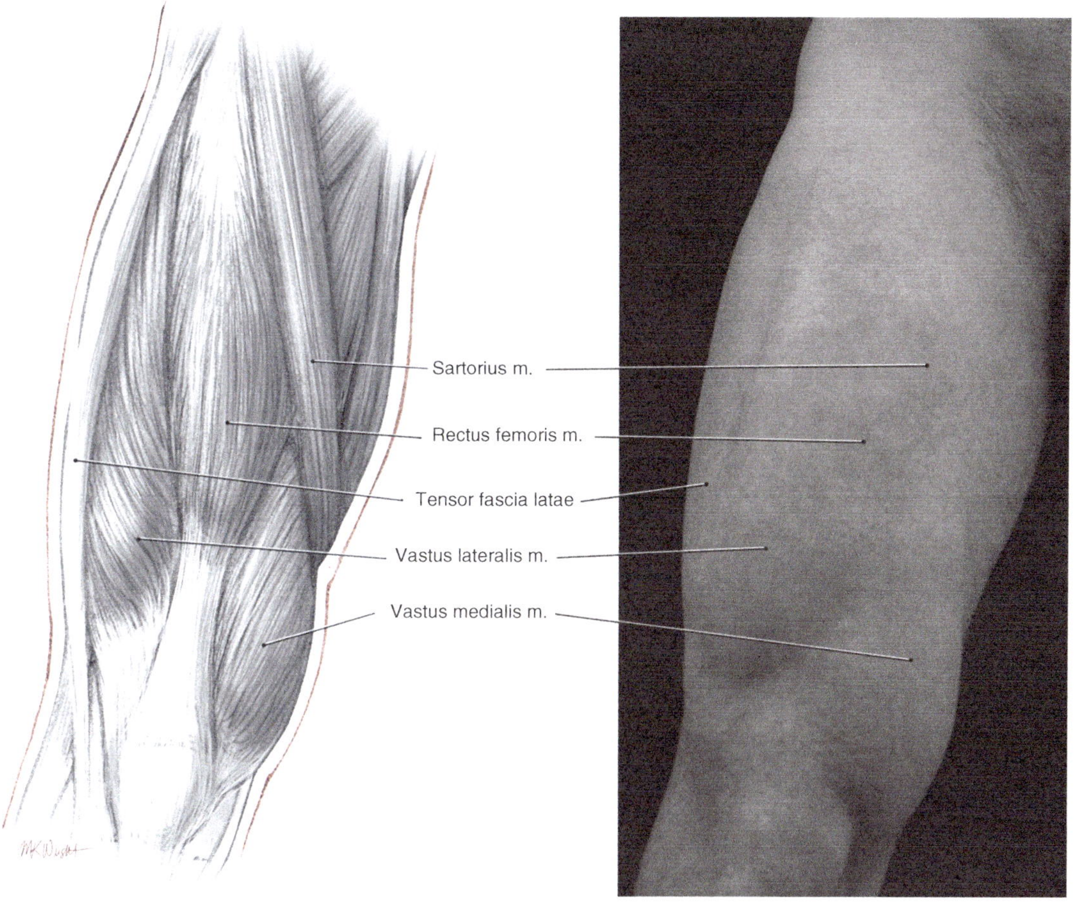

Fig. 2.15 Muscles of the anterior thigh. Except for the vastus medialis, there is little muscle mass immediately adjacent to the patella. The fat pads around the knee are contoured to define the knee and taper the thigh

anteriorly. An obvious groove is usually present along the lateral thigh that separates the quadriceps anteriorly from the hamstrings posteriorly (Fig. 2.16). This extends from the gluteus maximus to the posterior aspect of the iliotibial tract before the latter inserts into the tibia and represents an area of focused sculpting to enhance the definition of the thigh muscles.

Unlike the vastus, the rectus femoris crosses both the hip joint and the knee joint. It acts to flex the hip and extend the knee. Rectus femoris arises from the anterior inferior iliac spine and inserts into the patella first and then the tibial tuberosity via the patellar tendon. Near its origin superiorly, the form of the muscle belly is not easily appreciated as it is hidden between the tensor fascia lata laterally and the sartorius medially. The fusiform muscle belly occupies the upper two-thirds of the anterior thigh and tapers inferiorly before joining its tendon between the muscle bellies of the vastus lateralis and vastus medialis. The vastus medialis gives rise to the medial teardrop-shaped form on the lower medial thigh. It originates from the linea aspera and medial supracondylar line of the femur and inserts into the quadriceps tendon and upper outer part of the patella. The form of the vastus medialis is lower than the convexities of the rectus femoris and vastus lateralis, extending down medially to the level of the patella or below this level. The fat below the inferior margin of the vastus medialis can be removed to define the knee and improve the tapered appearance of the thigh.

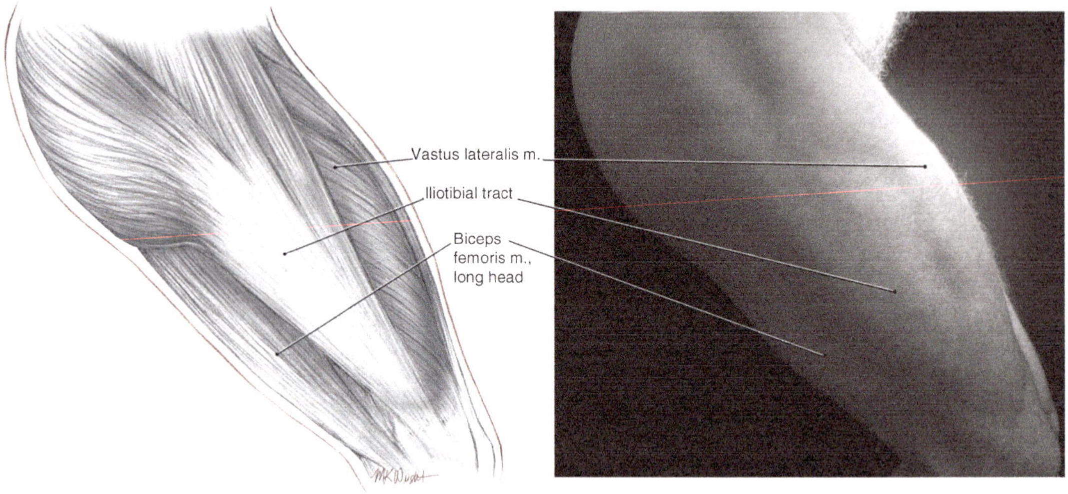

Fig. 2.16 The lateral thigh. The groove between the flexors and extensors becomes more visible upon hip and knee flexion, as in squatting

Hamstrings

This muscle group forms the posterior thigh compartment and consists of the long and short heads of the biceps femoris laterally and the semimembranosus and semitendinosus medially. The individual muscle forms are not very pronounced on the surface, except for the tendons that border the popliteal fossa when the leg is flexed. Hip and knee flexion usually produces a groove or ridge between the long and short heads of the biceps femoris and vastus lateralis.

The short head of the biceps femoris originates from the linea aspera of the femur. The long head, semimembranosus, and semitendinosus originate from the ischial tuberosity of the pelvis. Both heads of the biceps femoris insert into the head of the fibula. The semimembranosus inserts into the posterior part of the medial condyle of the tibia, whereas the semitendinosus inserts lower down on the medial aspect of the proximal shaft of the tibia. It is difficult to distinguish the long head from the short head of the biceps femoris when the knee is extended. However, with knee flexion, the two forms separate. The short head joins the common biceps tendon from posteriorly, forming a tough flat sheetlike structure that becomes very prominent with knee flexion. This thin ridge forms the lateral margin of the popliteal fossa. When the knee is flexed, a triangular fossa forms between the biceps tendon and vastus lateralis.

Sartorius

The sartorius is a long thick ropelike muscle that creates a cylindrical form on the anterior and inner thigh between the forms of rectus femoris and the adductor muscles (Fig. 2.17). It originates from a point just below the tip of the anterior superior iliac spine and spirals down the inner thigh and around the vastus medialis, to cross the knee joint and insert into the upper medial shaft of tibia below the medial condyle. Removing fat over the adductor compartment in the medial thigh can improve definition of the medial border of the sartorius. Medial to the

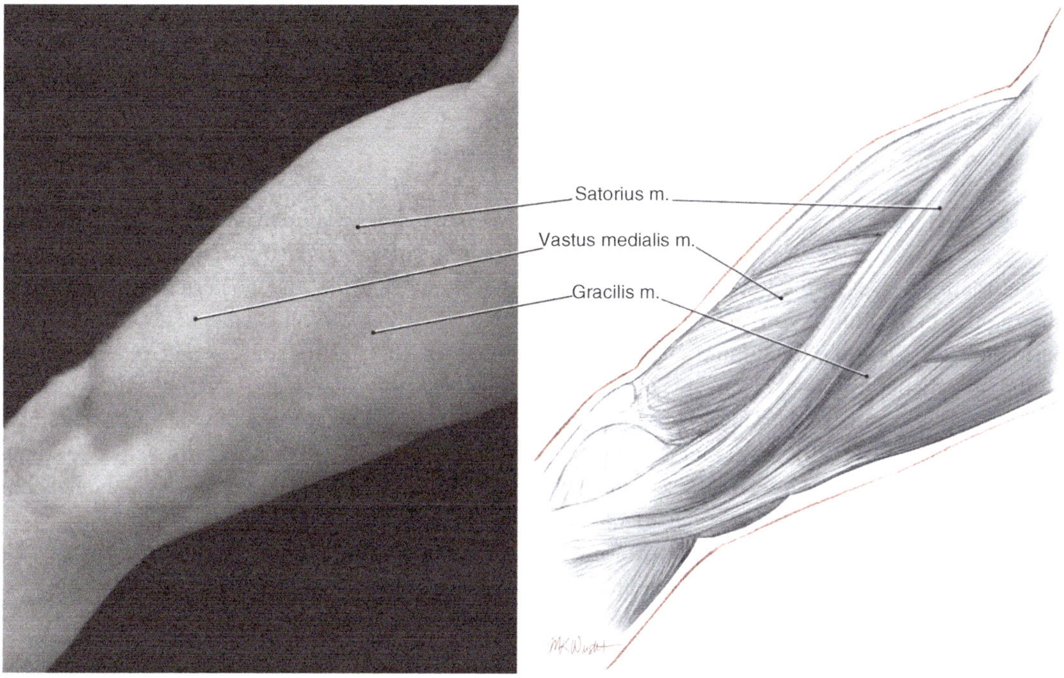

Fig. 2.17 The medial thigh muscles. The sartorius is a landmark between the quadriceps and adductors. Fat is removed medial to the sartorius along its length and over the adductors to improve the contours of the inner thigh

knee, the sartorius forms a thick band that is sometimes obscured by overlying medial knee fat pads.

Adductor Group

The adductor longus, adductor magnus, and gracilis lie in the upper inner thigh and contribute to the mass in this part of the upper leg. The adductor magnus is the largest of the three muscles and forms the mass of the medial part of the posterior thigh, blending with the semimembranosus and semitendinosus that lie laterally. The adductor longus arises just below the pubic tubercle and expands into a flat belly toward the femur. It inserts into the middle third of the posterior surface of the femur. It lies in front of the other adductors, but its form is hardly visible on the surface. The gracilis arises from the pubic arch, passes down along the inner thigh, and inserts into the superior medial aspect of the tibial shaft below the medial condyle. The tendon of origin of the gracilis may be visible when the legs are abducted; both the muscle bellies themselves are rarely seen as a distinct entity. During high-definition sculpting, thorough fat removal over the adductor compartment medial to the sartorius defines this area, but the forms of the individual muscles are not usually separated.

Increased muscular definition of the thigh is achieved by accentuating the groove between the vastus lateralis and biceps femoris. A shadow is created by thorough superficial fat removal along the vertical ridge between the extensor and flexor compartments. The muscle masses around the knee are defined by removing the knee fat pads superiorly and medially to define the vastus medialis and vastus lateralis above and the sartorius medially.

Lower Leg

The attractive curves of the lower leg are attributable to the main muscles in the posterior compartment of the leg: the lateral and medial heads of the gastrocnemius and soleus [1, 2]. These provide smooth convex prominences in the superior part of the lower leg that taper and narrow inferiorly toward the ankle. They insert through the tough Achilles tendon into the calcaneus. The delicacy of the ankle relies on a prominent Achilles tendon with very little fat medial and lateral to it. Sculpting the lower leg is performed with fine instruments to remove superficial subcutaneous fat around the forms of the gastrocnemius and soleus and on either side of the Achilles tendon.

Gastrocnemius

The medial and lateral heads of the gastrocnemius form the main muscle bulk of the calf. The medial head arises from the medial condyle of the femur and the lateral head from the lateral condyle. The medial head is larger than the lateral head and forms a convex bulge that is slightly lower than the lateral head (Fig. 2.18). The medial head occupies the superior medial quadrant of the posterior aspect of the lower leg and wraps around to cover part of the medial aspect of the leg. The lateral head wraps around to the lateral aspect of the leg to a lesser degree. Both heads are teardrop-shaped forms that end inferiorly where the muscle inserts into the broad flat gastrocnemius tendon. This tendon covers the posterior lower aspect of the leg and fuses with the tendon of the soleus beneath it to form the Achilles tendon. The key to successful contouring of the leg is to reveal the convex forms of the gastrocnemius and taper the leg inferiorly toward the sharply defined Achilles tendon.

Soleus

The soleus originates from the posterior surface of the head and superior shaft of the fibula and the soleus line on the posterior surface of the tibia. The belly of the soleus lies deep to the heads of the gastrocnemius and gives the calf thickness. Its lateral and medial edges may be seen to bulge from beneath the gastrocnemius tendon when the foot is plantar flexed. The soleus inserts into the posterior surface of the calcaneus via the Achilles tendon.

Fat Distribution

Subcutaneous fat is present in nearly every region of the body in varying quantities. The fat lies predominantly in the superficial fascia between the skin and muscles and is more plentiful on the trunk compared to the limbs. In general, females have a greater percentage of body fat compared to males, particularly over the pelvic region: hips (iliac crest), gluteal muscles, and upper thigh [7]. Regional fat anatomy and volume play an important part in the aesthetics of human form, particularly in females where breast fat and hip fat improve curvaceousness. Although fat is present throughout the body, certain areas have a propensity to accumulate relatively more fat in men and women. In females, fat tends to accumulate around the hips and buttocks (Fig. 2.19). In men, the most prominent fad pads are usually in the chest, abdomen, and flanks (Fig. 2.20). Lipoplasty performed to improve muscular definition typically involves removing the majority of the subcutaneous fat that obscures the appearance of the muscular form beneath, leaving only a thin subdermal layer. Augmentation of muscles is achieved by autologous fat transfer intramuscularly, for example, in the pectoralis major or gluteus maximus.

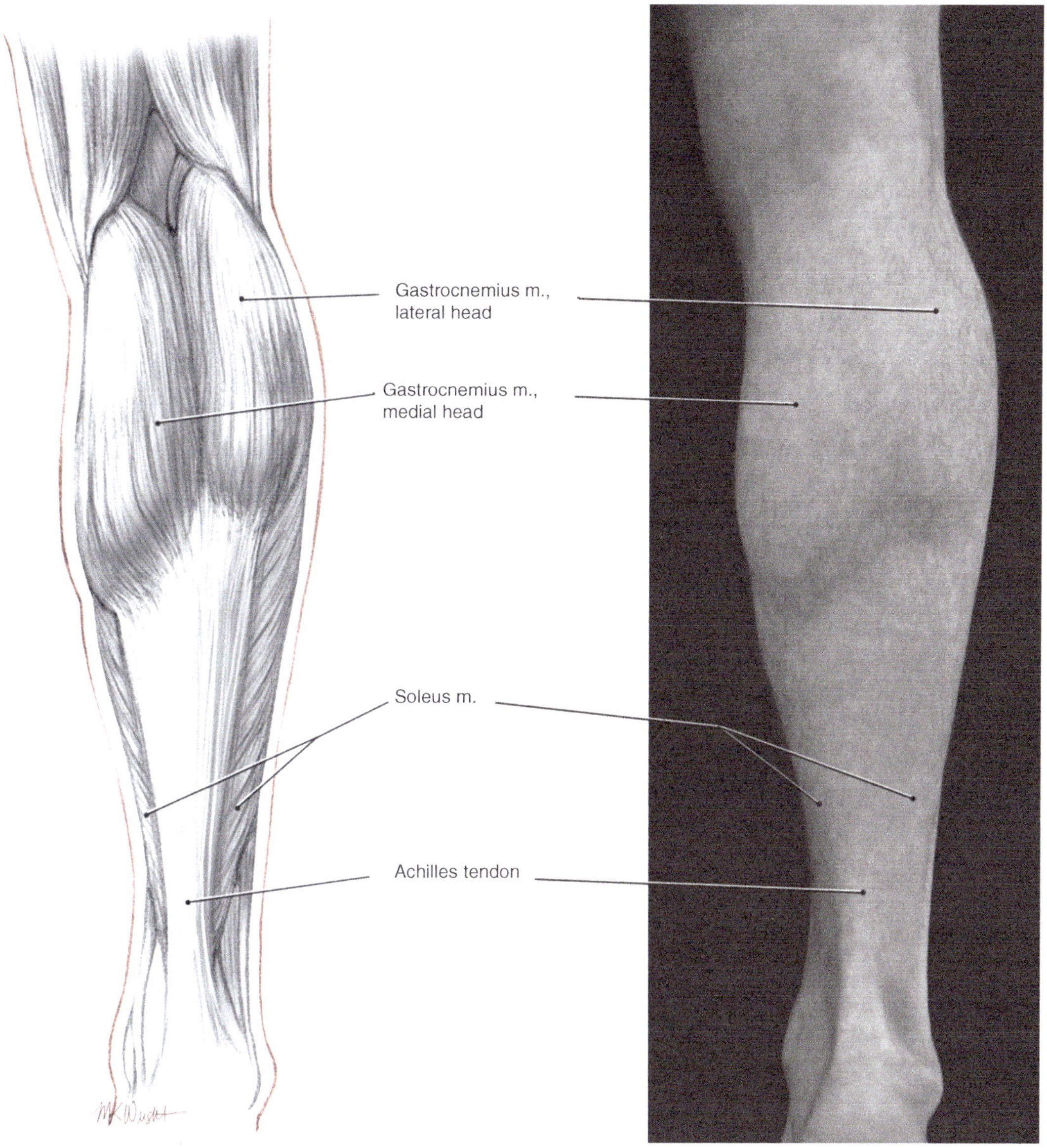

Fig. 2.18 Muscles of the leg. The medial and lateral heads of the gastrocnemius form convex masses that give the leg its contours

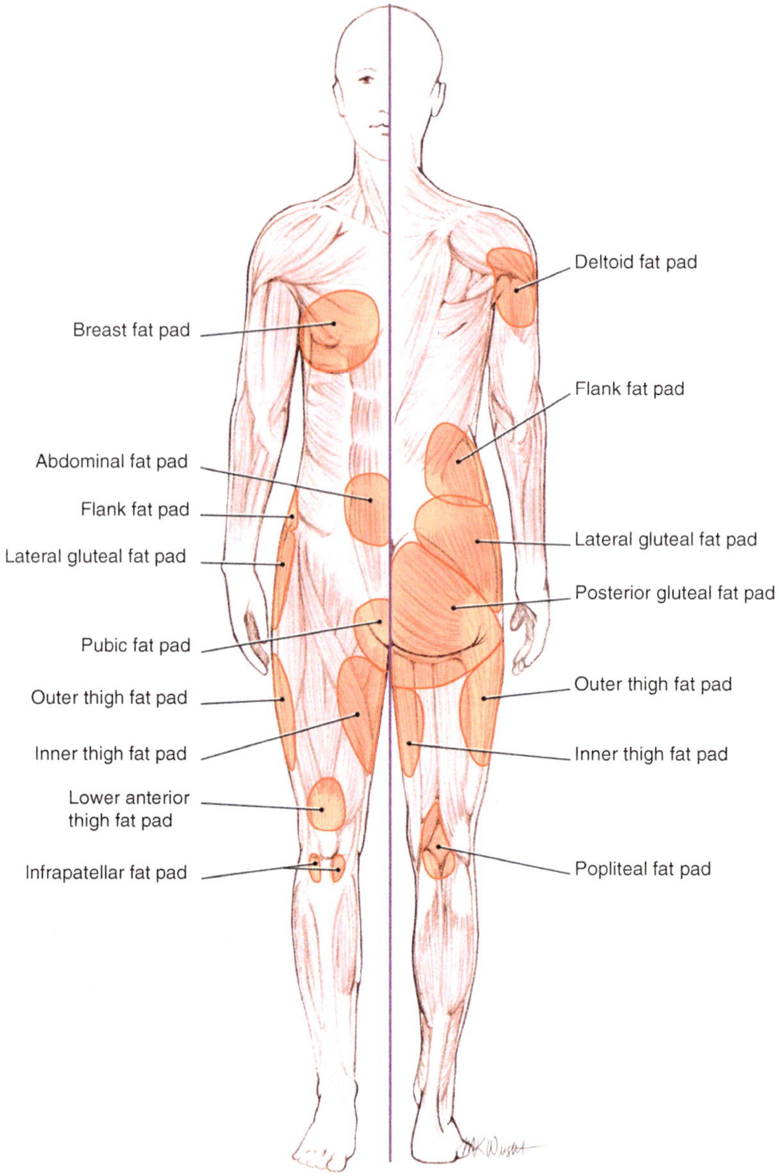

Fig. 2.19 Fat pads in the female

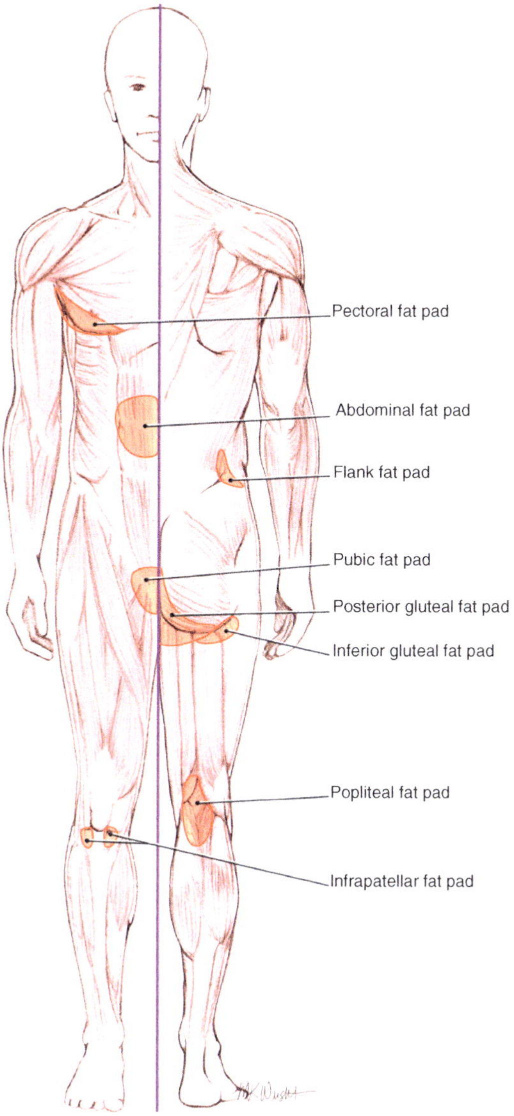

Fig. 2.20 Fat pads in the male

References

1. Rubins DK (1976) The human figure: an anatomy for artists. Penguin Books, New York
2. Simblet S, Davis J (2001) Anatomy for the artist. DK Publishing, New York
3. Nahas FX (2001) An aesthetic classification of the abdomen based on the myoaponeurotic layer. Plast Reconstr Surg 108(6):1787–1795
4. Florer RE, Kiriluk L (1971) Petit's triangle hernia: incarcerated: two case reports. Am Surg 37(8): 527–530
5. Hale RB, Coyle T (1977) The rib cage. In: Anatomy lessons from the great masters. Watson-Guptill, New York, p 24
6. Williams PL (1995) Gray's anatomy: the anatomical basis of medicine and surgery, 38th edn. Churchill Livingstone, Edinburgh, p 811
7. Goldfinger E (1991) Human anatomy for artists. The elements of form. Oxford University Press, Oxford, p 289

The Concept of Human Sculpting: Light, Shadow, and Form

3

Introduction

Sculpting the human body in order to improve definition involves a careful process of selective lipoplasty to reveal underlying structures: muscles, tendons, and bony landmarks. A sound knowledge of osteology and myology is a prerequisite for high-definition sculpting; you have to know *what* you are defining before you can learn *how* to define it. The muscles and soft and hard tissue structures that lie beneath the subcutaneous fat contribute to the beautiful and organized irregularity that comprises the human form. No part of the human body is flat, nor is it completely convex or uniformly curved. Subtle irregularities, contrasts, and angles contribute to physical attractiveness in slim and athletic individuals, provided they are harmonious. Various convex forms, elegantly linked through transition zones and spaces, with myriad planes, curves, and contrasts unite to create the whole.

High-definition body sculpting is a form of free-standing sculpture or sculpture "in the round." The completed masterpiece is meant to be viewed from all sides and is surrounded entirely by space. The beauty of the final work is manifest through the interplay between light and shadow. The palette, therefore, of the lipoplasty surgeon is black and white. Forms that fall away from the light source appear darker than those rising toward it. By developing artistic skills and an appreciation for the interaction between light and form, the surgeon can begin to define the anatomy and traits that represent cues for physical attractiveness. Instead of traditional materials, such as wood, bronze, or marble, the lipoplasty surgeon's sculpting substrate is fat [1–3].

Lipoplasty as Sculpting

Techniques in lipoplasty have evolved considerably over the last century. In 1921, Dujarrier used a crude curetting technique to remove fat from the lower limb of a ballerina dancer. This led to gangrene that necessitated an amputation [4]. Schrudde, a German surgeon, described his method of "lipexheresis" using a special uterine curette through small incisions [5]. Unsightly scars, bleeding, infection, and irregularities plagued early fat removal procedures and hindered progression in the field. The curette method by Kesselring and Meyer was noted to be only beneficial for the greater trochanteric regions, and attempts by Goodstein and Hoefflin to use a cannula with a sharp trailing edge acting as a curette in the subdermal tissues resulted in lymphorrhea and skin necrosis [6]. In 1975, Giorgio and Arpad Fischer published their work using cannulae with rotating blades, or planatomes, to suction fatty deposits [7]. Ilouz and Fournier followed with their formidable work on the development of liposuction and were instrumental in popularizing the technique among physicians of several specialties throughout the world. Although office-based surgery was performed over a

A.E. Hoyos, P.M. Prendergast, *High Definition Body Sculpting*,
DOI 10.1007/978-3-642-54891-8_3, © Springer-Verlag Berlin Heidelberg 2014

100 years ago, initially, liposuction was only practiced under general anesthesia in a hospital setting [8]. It was not feasible to remove large volumes of fat using blunt or sharp instruments under standard infiltrative local anesthesia, since the doses required for body contouring would have almost certainly resulted in lidocaine toxicity. The practice of liposuction was revolutionized in 1987 when Jeffrey Klein published his ingenious technique of anesthetizing large areas of subcutaneous fat using a mixture of diluted local anesthetic and epinephrine [9].

The advent of the tumescent technique, refinements in the procedure, improved instrumentation and the development of new technologies have lead to an increase of popularity of body conturing surgery [10]. In 2011, lipoplasty was the most common aesthetic surgical procedure in the USA with over 325,000 procedures completed [11]. Modern lipoplasty has evolved from a basic, debulking, fat removal to a form of artistic body sculpting. Smaller multi-holed cannulae have replaced larger single-holed ones to provide smoother, more precise results. Power-assisted lipoplasty (PAL) instruments efficiently and evenly remove fat through gyration, rotation, or nutation. Third-generation ultrasound-assisted lipoplasty (UAL) technology and instrumentation allow very gentle lipo-emulsification even in superficial subcutaneous planes. While some improved definition may be possible with traditional suction-assisted methods, high-definition lipoplasty cannot be realized safely without these modern technological tools.

Removal vs. Revealing

In order to achieve a postoperative result that is aesthetically appealing, harmonious, and balanced, we must approach the human form with the eye of a sculptor. Although fat removal is part of high-definition body sculpting, it is not the chief aim. Traditional liposuction in overweight patients focuses on *removal*, whereas high-definition lipoplasty in patients of normal weight focuses on *revealing*. In essence, the advanced lipoplasty surgeon is a sculptor revealing the elegant underlying muscular and bony anatomy. The sculptor starts with the armature and adds clay to sculpt the human form; the surgeon starts with a form and modifies it by removing excess, adding in deficient areas, and creating controlled deformities that represent clues to suggest the underlying anatomy [3].

Chief Lines

As a sculptor, the surgeon considers the chief lines in the form. Anteriorly this runs from the suprasternal notch, through the midline of the sternum, and along the depressed linea alba. The posterior chief line runs along the midline of the back as a gulley between the erector spinae group. On profile, the posterior chief line depends on posture, spinal anatomy, and gluteal soft tissue volume. The latter can be augmented during lipoplasty to enhance the beautiful "S" curve that continues from the lumbar lordotic curve above. Anteriorly, breast projection in females and upper pectoral fullness in males dominate the chief line. The actual appearance of the chief lines, lines of contrast, and surface definition are produced as a result of the interaction of light and shadow. Gradations of light and shadow determine our perception of surface form and, ultimately, our perception of beauty [1–3].

Light and Shadows

The patterns of light reflection and absorption from surfaces determine what we see. In general, the skin is semi-matte, and light reflects from skin in a uniform way referred to as form light [12]. Convex forms are perceived as smooth, three-dimensional structures because they display gradations of light and shadow. The aspect of the form that directly faces the light source appears lighter; the part that rolls away from the light appears darker or shaded. From the light part of the form to the darker part, there is a tonal progression. By using tonal progression, an appearance of fullness or depth is created where shadow becomes more pronounced moving away from the light. If this artistic concept is ignored, isolated shadows with sharp borders may produce

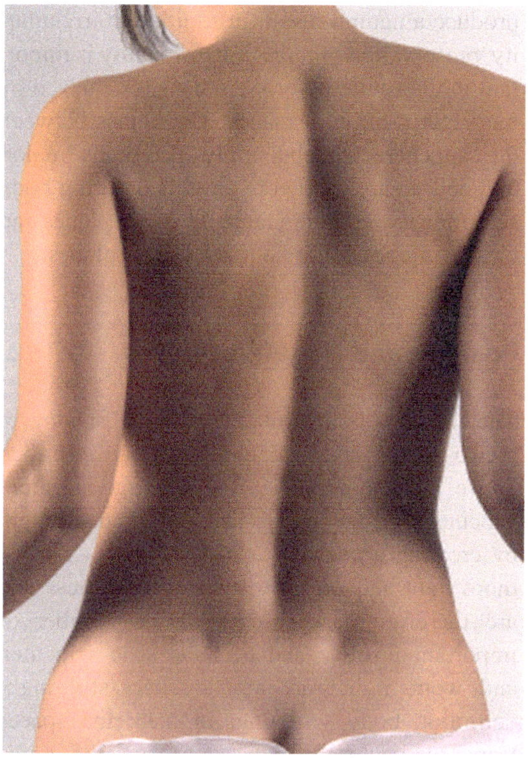

Fig. 3.1 Light and shadow revealing definition over the female back. The posterior chief line lies as a shadow between the paravertebral muscles. Two shadows are present over posterior superior iliac spines, creating the sacral triangle with the intergluteal cleft

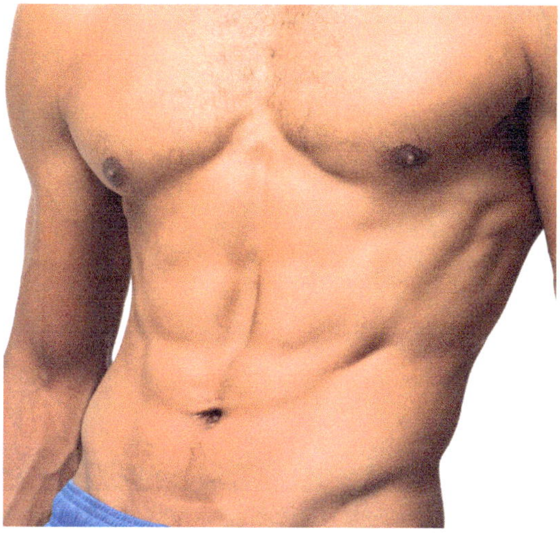

Fig. 3.2 Shadows in the male abdomen that create definition. The shadows below the nipple, below the tip of the tenth rib, and below the flank portion of external oblique are created during high-definition lipoplasty

an unnatural appearance. In abdominal lipoplasty, for example, this can lead to an undesirable wood-like appearance. In art, this is referred to as over-modeling. Allowing contours to project convexly ensures relatively more light reflection. Depressions between or adjacent to convex forms are created to hide these spaces from light so that they bathe in shadow and appear darker. In addition, by removing fat selectively in these spaces, the convexities appear relatively augmented. In this way, contouring over the chest wall around the female breast enhances the appearance and perceived size of the breasts. Similarly, creating darker shadows around the bellies of rectus abdominis makes the muscle segments appear to project. Even small or subtle shadows play an important role in the improvement of definition and creation of a natural appearance: the shadows over the posterior superior iliac spines that form the sacral triangle (Fig. 3.1), the shadow below the tip of the tenth rib, and the shadow between the linea semilunaris and the inferior border of the pectoralis major (Fig. 3.2).

Contours and Form

It is important to have an appreciation for appropriate form to plan and perform successful body sculpting. In this regard, considerations in human form include volume, contrast, continuity and discreteness, and organization [9]. The body consists of major and lesser forms, and each should have appropriate volume or fullness. In men, fullness is desirable in the upper pectoral region, deltoids, and biceps. High-definition lipoplasty may utilize autologous fat grafting to augment the pectorals and deltoids. In women, the buttocks and breasts frequently require augmentation to improve fullness and curvaceousness [13]. Lesser forms are smaller, but not less important, forms that often rest on major forms and contribute to the appearance of athleticism. These so-called packed forms include the convexities of the rectus abdominis between tendinous intersections and slips of the serratus anterior over the lateral aspect of the torso. These forms are enhanced by sculpting shadows around them rather than by directly augmenting them with fat [2, 3].

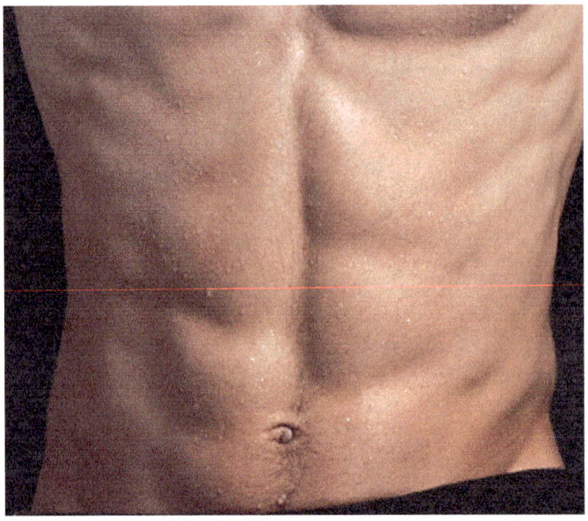

Fig. 3.3 The regularly irregular human form. Note that the tendinous intersections are at different levels on each side

The undulating major and lesser forms that comprise the human body are continuous with one another to the extent that there is harmony, but they do not blend so seamlessly that there is uniform smoothness. Each discrete form is separated subtly from surrounding ones by small transition zones, little ramps that lead from one form to the next. Small cannulae are used to shape these transition zones, which usually receive less light than the forms they define. The slightly shaded transition zones improve muscular definition. Contrast is a notable feature in the aesthetics of form. The large form of the pectoralis major contrasts with the serratus anterior inferiorly. The converging muscle fibers of the pectoralis major and deltoid contrast with the vertically oriented fibers of the rectus abdominis. Contrasts catch our eye and interrupt the homogeneity that might otherwise relegate the human form to an uninteresting mass of uniformity and sameness.

The contrasting forms, shadows, and spaces that comprise the human form are arranged in an organized way. There is an attractive irregularity about the surface anatomical features, but they are regularly irregular. For example, horizontal tendinous intersections in the rectus abdominis occur in pairs, but left and right pairs are not always at the same level (Fig. 3.3). Other examples of irregularity include tendon insertion morphology and asymmetry within the umbilicus. These features must be preserved in order to produce a natural result. In addition to irregularity, preservation of three dimensionality is important in the sculpting process. This is achieved by the superposition of planes. The planes between the upper rectus abdominis, pectoralis major, and deltoid are created or amplified during body sculpting by removing fat in the lower planes and preserving or adding fat to the higher planes.

Positive and Negative Spaces

The concept of manipulating light and shadow to create forms and define features is described above. We can add a shadow by removing more subcutaneous fat in a localized area and add light by creating a convexity. Positive spaces receive more light and negative spaces receive less and are therefore darker. There are a number of important positive and negative spaces in men and women that are key to successful high-definition body sculpting. In men, the spaces frame the pectoralis major and rectus abdominis anteriorly and define the lower back muscles posteriorly (Fig. 3.4). Similarly, in women the negative spaces enhance the appearance of the breasts and rectus abdominis, but horizontal tendinous intersections are untouched to avoid masculinizing the female abdomen (Fig. 3.5). The techniques required to create negative spaces are discussed in subsequent chapters. Negative spaces are carefully marked preoperatively and require more thorough and superficial liposuction. The techniques used to achieve shade, tonal progression, and the superpositions of planes are a significant departure from traditional methods of liposuction.

Advanced Lipoplasty Techniques

The specific techniques required to define each anatomical area are described in subsequent chapters. The principles are outlined here.

Intraoperatively, there are three main steps in high-definition body sculpting: infiltration, emulsification, and aspiration. Autologous fat grafting follows to complete the contouring procedure.

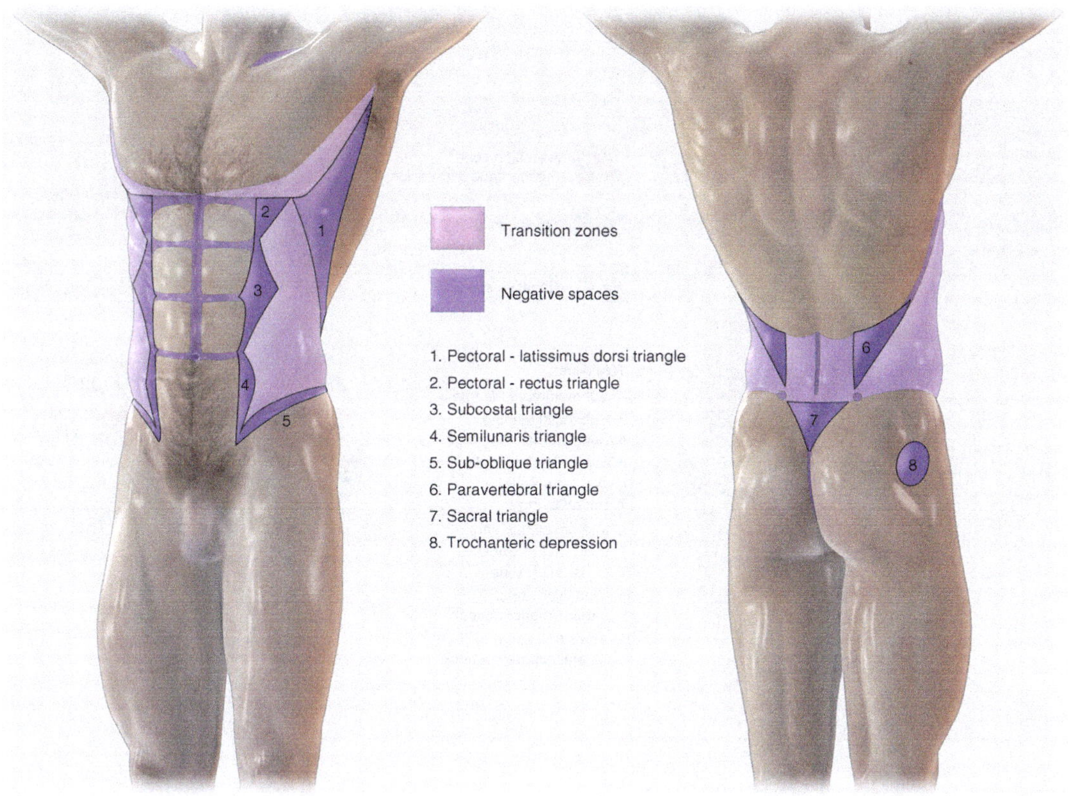

Fig. 3.4 Negative spaces and shadows in the male torso

Infiltration

The infiltration of tumescent fluid into the subcutaneous fat compartments is the first step in body sculpting. The tumescent technique is described in Chap. 5. Typically, a large volume of saline, admixed with epinephrine, sodium bicarbonate, and varying quantities of lidocaine, is infiltrated into the subcutaneous treatment planes until the tissues are firm. Tumescent anesthesia may obviate the need for sedation or general anesthesia. When general anesthesia is used, the tumescent infiltrate is usually prepared with a much smaller quantity of local anesthetic. This initial step produces a relatively bloodless field due to the profound vasoconstrictive properties of epinephrine. The fluid environment is essential for the safety and efficacy of ultrasound-assisted lipoplasty. For high-definition lipoplasty, fluid must be infiltrated very superficially in the subdermal layer as well as deeper layers to protect the tissues during the delivery of ultrasound. A peau d'orange or dimpled appearance in the skin is normal when the fluid is infiltrated very close to the dermis.

Emulsification

The second step in high-definition body sculpting is the delivery of ultrasound to the entire treatment area to emulsify fat. Third-generation ultrasound-assisted lipoplasty (UAL) using the VASER® system (Valeant Pharmaceuticals North America LLC, Bridgewater NJ) is employed to optimize safety and efficacy. The VASER® system is described in more detail in Chap. 6. Thorough emulsification in the superficial subdermal plane is performed first to re-drape the skin and enhance the skin tightening effect. This is followed by a deeper emulsification to reduce vol-

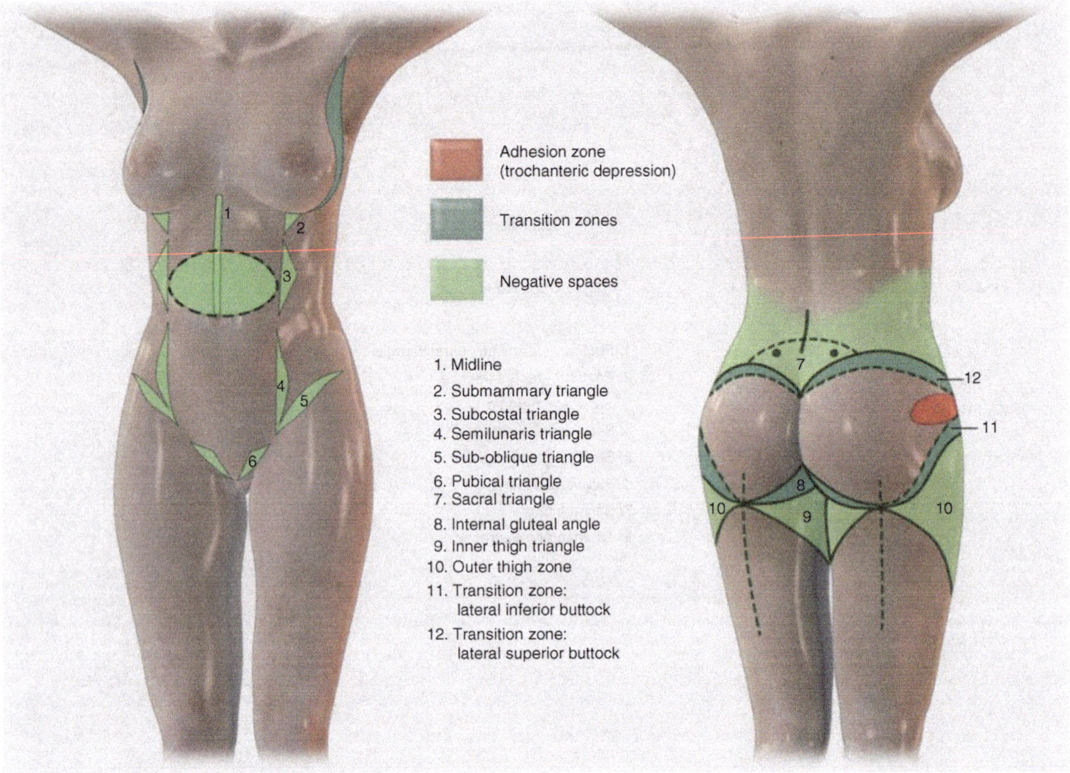

Fig. 3.5 Negative spaces and shadow in the female torso

ume. Slow, gentle but deliberate strokes are used to pass the titanium probes through the fatty tissue until little or no resistance is felt. The probes should not be passed forcefully or held tightly; an appropriately chosen probe at the correct setting glides effortlessly through the pearls and lobules of fat without harming blood vessels or nerves.

Aspiration

The first step in aspiration is to remove the emulsified fat in the deeper planes using either 4.6, 3.7, or 3.0 mm cannulae. Power-assisted technologies can be used to accelerate this phase. The author uses the PowerX (Valeant Pharmaceuticals North America LLC, Bridgewater, NJ) device for debulking. The extent and areas of debulking are dictated by the preoperative markings. Where convexities are desired, less fat is removed; where negative spaces are desired, fat is removed more thoroughly. After debulking, the 3.0 mm cannula is used to treat the superficial plane. In order to define muscle groups and create shadows, it is necessary to create controlled deformities. These are deliberate irregularities, created by removing almost all of the fat in the subdermal layer.

Controlled Deformities

The creation of controlled deformities occurs in the last phase of high-definition body sculpting and is the most challenging and least forgiving

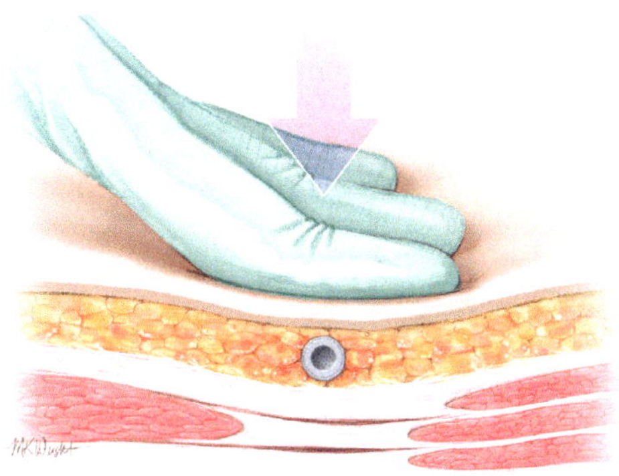

Fig. 3.6 Compression. Controlled localized pressure is exerted over the aspiration cannula to sculpt negative spaces and controlled irregularities. Note: compression is never used over ultrasonic probes

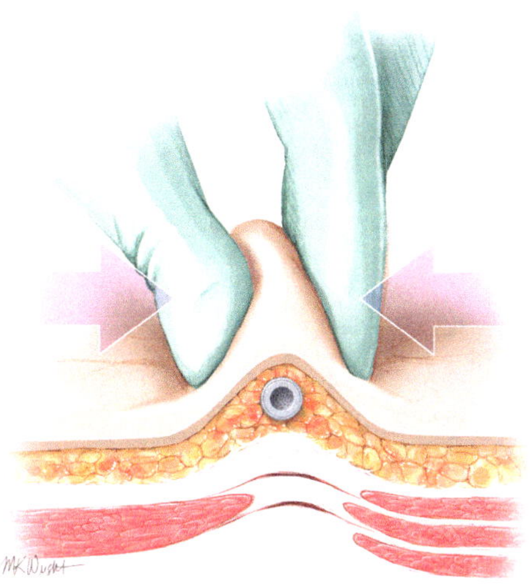

Fig. 3.7 Pinching. Subcutaneous fat is grasped and compressed around the cannula. This technique is particularly useful to enhance the shadow over linea semilunaris

step in the procedure. These negative spaces and controlled deformities are formed using compression and pinching techniques. During compression, the tissue is pressed down over the tip of the cannula with the guiding hand (Fig. 3.6). A concavity is gradually formed by repeated passage of the fine cannula through the compressed tissue. Pinching facilitates the removal of subdermal fat by grasping the skin and squeezing it around the cannula tip (Fig. 3.7). This technique is particularly useful for creating shadows along the linea semilunaris. As the sculpting procedure progresses, the shadows begin to show and the three-dimensional forms are created. The deepest groove contains the darkest shadow and represents the area that received the most thorough liposuction. These grooves are blended with surrounding forms by removing progressively less fat as the negative space rolls toward a positive space. This tonal progression is achieved by reducing the compression over the cannula and by reducing the number of strokes in each subcutaneous track. The endpoint for high-definition body sculpting is the visual result. The surgeon should be able to appreciate the definition at the end of the procedure (Fig. 3.8).

Fat Grafting

Once the required degree of definition has been achieved, harvested fat is used to augment convex forms, particularly the buttocks, breasts, deltoids, male chest, and calves. Large 60 and 20 ml syringes and 3–4 mm Toomey cannulae are used using a retrograde linear threading technique. The subcutaneous and intramuscular planes receive the fat in multiple fine strokes to ensure small parcels are left rather than large boluses. These techniques are described in Chap. 7.

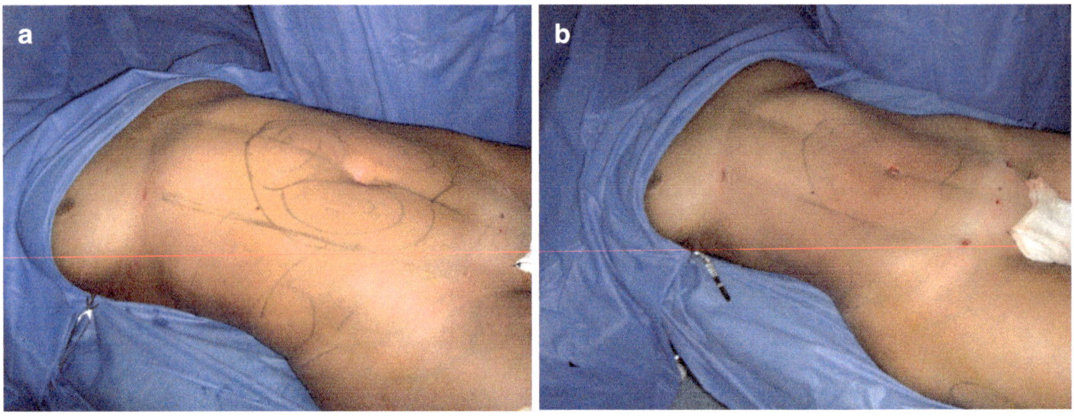

Fig. 3.8 The definition should be appreciated at the end of the procedure: (**a**) before; and (**b**) after the fat extraction in both superficial and deep layers

References

1. Schider F (1957) An atlas of anatomy for artists. Dover Publications, New York
2. Rubins DK (1976) The human figure: an anatomy for artists. Penguin Books, New York
3. Simblet S, Davis J (2001) Anatomy for the artist. DK Publishing, New York
4. Flynn TC, Coleman WP III, Field LM, Klein JA, Hanke CW (2000) History of liposuction. Dermatol Surg 26(6):515–520
5. Schrudde J (1984) Lipexheresis (liposuction) for body contouring. Clin Plast Surg 11(3):445–456
6. Shiffman MA (1997) The liposhaver in facial plastic surgery. Arch Otolaryngol Head Neck Surg 123(10):1144
7. Fischer A, Fischer G (1976) First surgical treatment for molding body's cellulite with three 5 mm incisions. Bull Int Acad Cosmet Surg 3:35
8. Current issues in dermatologic office-based surgery. Joint American Academy of Dermatology/American Society of Dermatologic Surgery Liaison Committee (1999) J Am Acad Dermatol 41(4):624–634
9. Klein JA (1987) The tumescent technique for liposuction surgery. Am J Cosmet Surg 4:236–267
10. Prendergast PM (2011) Liposculpture of the abdomen in an office-based practice. In: Body contouring. Art, science, and clinical practice. Springer, Berlin
11. The American Society for Aesthetic Plastic Surgery: cosmetic surgery national databank statistics 2011; ASAPS website: www.surgery.org
12. Ryder A (2000) The artist's complete guide to figure drawing. A contemporary perspective in the classical tradition. Watson-Guptill Publications, New York, p 84
13. Fisher ML, Voracek M (2006) The shape of beauty: determinants of female physical attractiveness. J Cosmet Dermatol 5(2):190–194

Preoperative Assessment and Preparation for High-Definition Body Sculpting

4

Introduction

More than any other form of body contouring surgery, high-definition lipoplasty requires a special collaboration between the surgeon and the patient. The unique nature of the advanced lipoplasty techniques, including the extent of contouring, superficial fat removal, and creation of sculpted irregularities, requires that the patient understands every aspect of the procedure so that informed decisions can be made. From the initial consultation, the patient-doctor relationship develops and is central to success in high-definition body sculpting. The patient learns what the procedure entails, suitability, preoperative and postoperative care, and all of the potential side effects and complications associated with the procedure. One of the keys to success is for the surgeon to determine expectations and then set realistic ones based on the patient's physical condition. Since body dysmorphic disorder occurs in 7–15 % of patients seeking cosmetic surgery, some patients will not be satisfied regardless of how successful the surgeon believes the procedure to be [1]. These patients must be identified and excluded from treatment. On the other hand, patients who may previously have been refused traditional liposuction based on a paucity of fatty tissue may benefit greatly from high-definition ultrasound-assisted lipoplasty. These patients typically desire an athletic, toned, or muscular appearance and already exercise regularly and are extremely motivated. Patient wishes are determined during an initial consultation.

Consultation

Patients present to a practice offering high-definition lipoplasty (VASER hi-def™ or VASER 4D Sculpt™) often following media coverage of the procedure or having reviewed the procedure on the Internet or on a website. Invariably, they will already have formed some expectations as to what they might look like following the procedure: athletic arms, sexy curves, and six-pack abs. The patient's enthusiasm and excitement must be tempered somewhat with a detailed medical discussion of the procedure and steps involved in high-definition lipoplasty. To this end, it is crucially important that the person conducting the initial consultation is the surgeon who proposes to perform the procedure, not a patient adviser, nurse, or other staff member. The consultation should be conducted in a comfortable environment and should not be rushed. A cursory discussion lasting less than 15 min is insufficient and is not in the best interests of both the patient and the surgeon. With a relaxed, pragmatic, and honest discussion, the patient and the surgeon develop a positive rapport. A patient who does not trust the surgeon fully may be dissatisfied with the outcome regardless of the surgical result.

A.E. Hoyos, P.M. Prendergast, *High Definition Body Sculpting*,
DOI 10.1007/978-3-642-54891-8_4,

Rather than leading the patient by asking, for example, "what is the problem?", allow the patient tell their own story. Opening the consultation with "what are you interested in?" is usually sufficient and does not imply that there is *any* problem. An obese patient who requests to remove "all fat" is clearly unrealistic and should raise a red flag. Patients of normal body weight who wish to reduce bulges and define features in exercise and diet-resistant areas are realistic. Common requests in female patients include toned arms, flat abdomen, reduced bulges in inner thighs, improved curves, and an overall athletic appearance. In men, "six-pack" abdominal wall definition, sculpted pectorals, muscular arms, and removal of superfluous fat in the flanks are the requests most commonly received during a consultation for high-definition lipoplasty. All of these requests can be addressed during VASER-assisted high-definition lipoplasty, either as one extensive procedure or in staged procedures either under general anesthesia or tumescent local anesthesia, with or without sedation.

The procedure must be explained to the patient in detail in terms that are easy to understand, avoiding unnecessary medical jargon. This discussion includes a step-by-step description of the procedure itself, the technology used, and the expected benefits. The postoperative course should be described, and the importance of intensive postoperative care specific to high-definition lipoplasty should be impressed upon the patient. This includes the patient's role in strict continuous application of compression garments, nutritional support, and attendance at massage and external ultrasound or radiofrequency appointments in the early postoperative course. It is useful to explain the purpose of each facet of postoperative care and remind the patient that suboptimal results, or even complications, may arise if the patient does not adhere to postoperative instructions. The expected benefits are discussed with the patient, and the timeline for visible improvement is given. Although results in terms of improved definition are visible immediately following the procedure, the patient should expect near-complete results as soon as 1 month postoperatively, provided that postoperative care is optimized.

The fees associated with the procedure should be discussed with the patient, as well as any additional fees for touch-up procedures should they be required. Before and after photos of the surgeon's own work can be reviewed with the patient, but it is important to emphasize that every patient is different, and various factors affect results, including age, body type, skin condition, muscular anatomy and mass, comorbid conditions, and postoperative care.

During the initial consultation, it is important to enquire about the patient's history of weight loss or weight gain, exercise regime, and dietary habits. If patients have a history of significant weight fluctuations, they are likely to have reduced skin elasticity. This may affect postoperative skin retraction. Patients who do not exercise or exercise infrequently may have poor posture, abdominal protrusion secondary to reduced muscle tone, and fatty areas that may respond to exercise before surgery. It is important to stress to the patient that high-definition lipoplasty cannot be performed in isolation. It is an adjunct to a program of healthy eating and exercise.

History

A detailed past medical history should be obtained, including previous cosmetic surgery. Enquire whether the patient was satisfied with previous cosmetic procedures or not. Prior surgical procedures on the abdomen, including laparoscopic procedures, have implications for preoperative planning, particularly where surgical scars are adherent to the anterior abdominal wall or incisional hernias are suspected. Previous liposuction on the proposed treatment areas should be documented and may require specific ultrasonic probes in order to emulsify fat in fibrous areas. Cardiac and pulmonary conditions that may preclude extensive high-definition body contouring should be identified in the medical

Table 4.1 American Society of Anesthesiologists (ASA) physical status classification system

Category	Preoperative health status
ASA I	Normal healthy patient, excluding very young and very old
ASA II	Patients with mild systemic disease but no functional limitations
ASA III	Patients with severe systemic disease
ASA IV	Patients with severe systemic disease that is a constant threat to life
ASA V	Moribund patients expected to die within 24 h

history and review of systems. These include arrhythmias, cardiac failure, pulmonary edema, and chronic obstructive pulmonary disease.

It is helpful to classify the patient according to the American Society of Anesthesiologists patient-physical-status classification (Table 4.1). However, this is only a gross predictor of outcome and not a predictor of anesthetic risk [2]. A history of systemic or endocrine disorders, including hypertension, diabetes, and thyroid dysfunction, requires appropriate investigation and control prior to surgery. Ascertain whether the patient has any personal or family history of thrombosis, embolism, or coagulopathy. A complete list of medications, including herbal and nutritional supplements, should be listed. Medications that are metabolized by the liver's cytochrome P4503A4 enzymes interact with lidocaine and may increase the potential for toxicity in patients undergoing lipoplasty under tumescent local anesthesia (Table 4.2). Several supplements, herbs, foods, and spices increase bleeding risk or increase anesthetic risk and should be avoided for at least 2 weeks before and for 1 week after surgery (Table 4.3). Similarly, patients who take nonsteroidal anti-inflammatories such as aspirin and ibuprofen are at increased risk of bleeding unless they are discontinued for 10 days prior to surgery. During the history taking, all known allergies should be identified, including allergy to local anesthetics. The history should include general questions pertaining to cardiac, respiratory, endocrine, gastrointestinal, and neurological systems. A history of hypertrophic scarring, keloids, or postinflammatory hyperpigmentation may dictate placement of incisions during surgery.

Table 4.2 Drugs that interact with lidocaine

Antibiotics	*Benzodiazepines*
Ciprofloxacin	Alprazolam
Clarithromycin	Diazepam
Erythromycin	Flurazepam
Anticancer medications	Midazolam
Tamoxifen	Triazolam
Antidepressants	*Beta-blockers*
Amitriptyline	Propranolol
Clomipramine	*Calcium channel blockers*
Fluoxetine	Amiodarone
Fluvoxamine	Diltiazem
Nefazodone	Felodipine
Paroxetine	Nicardipine
Sertraline	Nifedipine
Antihistamines	Verapamil
Cimetidine	*Cholesterol-lowering medications*
Antifungals	Atorvastatin
Fluconazole	Lovastatin
Itraconazole	Simvastatin
Ketoconazole	*Immunosuppressants*
Miconazole	Cyclosporine
Antiseizure medications	*Protease inhibitors*
Carbamazepine	Indinavir
Phenytoin	Nevirapine
Valproic acid	Nelfinavir
	Ritonavir
	Saquinavir

Note: This list is not exhaustive

Table 4.3 Herbs and foods with antiplatelet or anticoagulant effects

Alfalfa	Garlic
Anise	Ginger
Arnica	Ginko
Aspen	Ginseng
Black cohosh	Horse chestnut
Borage seed oil	Licorice
Bromelain	Onion
Capsicum	Papain
Celery	Safflower
Clove	Sweet clover
Dong Quai	Turmeric
Fenugreek	Vitamin E
Fish oils (omega-3 fatty acids)	Wild lettuce

Physical Examination and Assessment

General

First, the general appearance and body type of the patient are assessed. All somatotypes—ectomorphs, mesomorphs, and endomorphs—may be considered suitable candidates for high-definition body contouring depending on their subcutaneous fat volume and distribution. The ideal candidate has stubborn areas of exercise and diet-resistant fat with a normal body weight. The body mass index is determined by dividing the weight of the patient in kilograms by the height in meters squared, BMI = weight (kg)/{height (m)}^{2}. Patients who are obese (BMI > 30) are unlikely to be suitable for high-definition lipoplasty since the removal of fat to reveal muscular definition in part of the body would highlight lack of definition elsewhere and result in disharmony. The author advises these patients to lose weight through healthy eating and exercise before high-definition body sculpting and refers to a nutritionist and a strength and fitness conditioning professional to help them achieve their goals. Patients who are overweight may benefit from traditional VASER® lipoplasty as an initial step, combined with exercise and diet, and present again at a later stage for a definitive high-definition contouring procedure.

With the patient standing, the posture and form are analyzed. Patients with good posture have a convex protrusion of the chest and concave lordotic curve of the lower back. The skeletal framework to a certain extent determines body shape. Although the bony skeleton cannot be altered through lipoplasty, body shape can be improved through selective fat resection and grafting. A subtle anterior protrusion of the left hemithorax compared to the contralateral side is common. Symmetry can be improved intraoperatively by removing more fat over the left hemithorax than the right. Attempts to create the hourglass female aesthetic ideal are made by thorough fat resection in the waist and fat grafting to the hips and gluteal area, combined with breast augmentation. In males, the inverted triangular form of the torso is achieved by resecting fat at the lower waist and preserving fat over latissimus dorsi. This is combined with pectoral fat grafting and detailed sculpting over the rectus abdominis.

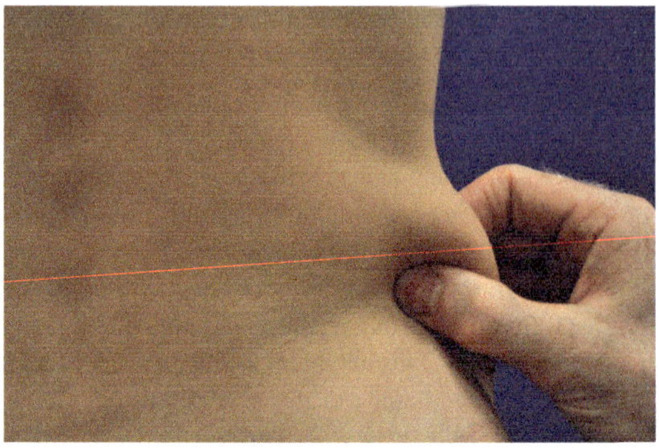

Fig. 4.1 Pinch test. The subcutaneous fat is grasped between the thumb and the forefinger to determine how much fat is amenable to resection

The general examination also includes a thorough examination of all systems, including cardiovascular, respiratory, and neurological systems. Abnormal findings should be investigated prior to surgery or general anesthesia. Examination results must be documented clearly in the medical notes.

Abdomen and Torso

The abdomen is inspected in the relaxed, standing position. Abdominal protrusion due to intra-abdominal fat, muscle wall weakness, and rectus diastasis will not improve with lipoplasty alone. To determine the degree of rectus diastasis, the patient is asked to elevate the shoulders and head from the supine position. With significant rectus diastasis, this maneuver produces central tenting and protrusion of the linea alba between the bellies of rectus. Unless myofascial plication is performed during surgery, lipoplasty alone will not flatten the abdomen completely. The skin is inspected for scars, striae, and obvious laxity. To assess the amount of fat amenable to resection, the pinch test is performed (Fig. 4.1). The fat and skin are gently grasped between the forefinger and the thumb. To reveal underlying muscular anatomy, most of this fat is

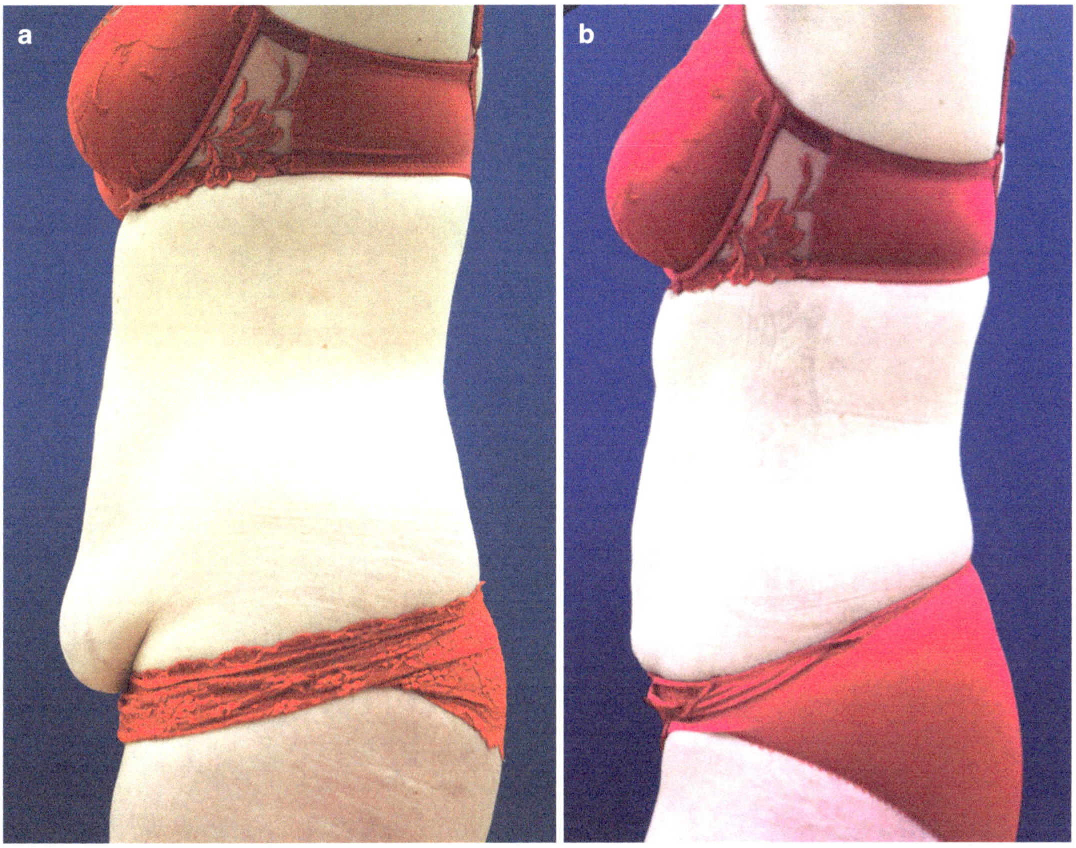

Fig. 4.2 (**a**) Before VASER®. (**b**) After VASER® lipoplasty of the lower abdomen without skin excision. Significant skin retraction has been achieved

removed through deep and superficial ultrasound-assisted liposuction. In females, a protrusion of fat or apron of fat and skin overhanging a Pfannenstiel scar is common following caesarian section. Thorough superficial ultrasound-assisted lipoplasty may occasionally be sufficient to cause skin retraction (Fig. 4.2). However, for high-definition contouring, combined lipoplasty and mini or full abdominoplasty is often necessary. The abdomen is palpated for muscle mass and tone and carefully checked for inguinal, femoral, umbilical, and incisional hernias. Patients with small to moderate amounts of subcutaneous fat and good underlying muscle tone, with no skin laxity, are the best candidates for high-definition body sculpting, even if no muscular definition is visible preoperatively.

The waist circumference and hip circumference are measured in females and the waist-hip ratio (WHR) calculated. A WHR of 0.7 is generally considered ideal [3, 4]. The contribution to body shape by the underlying bony framework is determined by palpating the costal margin and iliac crest. When aesthetic body contouring is limited by the underlying bony skeleton, a plan of fat redistribution, rather than resection alone, is often appropriate. The pinch test is performed circumferentially, over the abdomen, flanks, and back, and fat distribution is documented. For harmonious body sculpting, the abdomen and torso are treated together as one aesthetic unit, often including the upper arms.

The author routinely prints out patient photographs before the procedure and creates new contours by drawing on the photos using marker

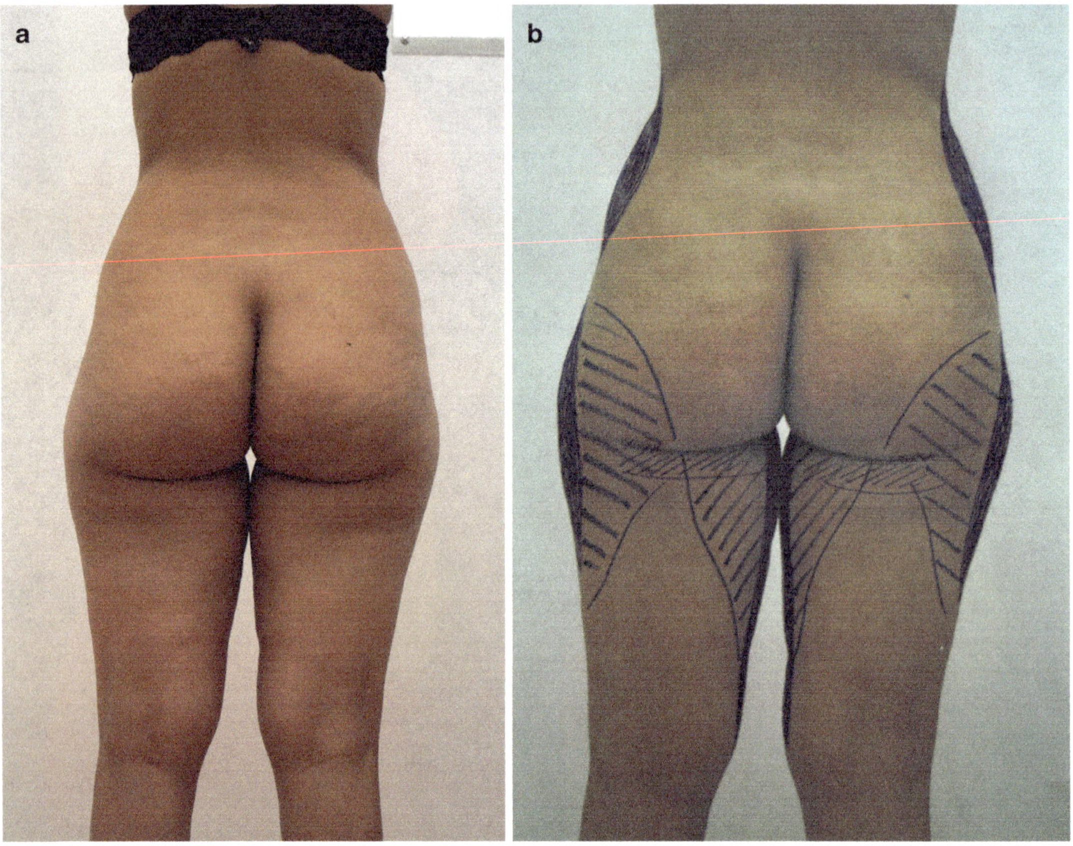

Fig. 4.3 (**a**) Preoperative photograph. (**b**) Markings made directly on printed photograph to plan procedure

pens (Fig. 4.3). This exercise helps the surgeon visualize the expected contours and decide how much fat should be taken. More importantly, it helps determine what should be left behind to achieve aesthetically pleasing contours.

Chest

In male patients high-definition body sculpting frequently involves lipoplasty of the male breasts and pectoral region. The contour of the chest is inspected from the front and profile view. The breasts may be abnormally enlarged due to excessive male breast tissue (gynecomastia), fat (pseudogynecomastia), or both fat and breast tissue. The chest may become feminized, and there may be breast ptosis. The contribution of glandular tissue to breast enlargement can usually be determined by palpation, although an ultrasound scan provides definitive information. Any abnormal masses on physical examination mandate diagnostic imaging, including mammography and ultrasonography. In order to provide an athletic, more muscular appearance in the male patient, the aim of sculpting in this area is to define and amplify the appearance of the underlying pectoral muscles. This is usually achieved by removing subcutaneous tissue from the lower chest, defining the inferior and lateral borders of pectoralis major, and grafting fat in several planes to the upper chest. Skin tone is assessed to predict postoperative skin retraction. Unless ptosis is severe, skin retraction in the male chest following ultrasound-assisted lipoplasty is excellent.

In female patients, breast size, shape, position, and symmetry are assessed in relation to overall body aesthetics. Breast augmentation, or reduction, may be considered and discussed with the patient at the time of consultation. In patients who have large breast implants, consideration must be given to access incision sites for contouring the abdomen. A breast examination should be performed before any procedure on the breast.

Arms

The arms are examined with the patient standing and relaxed to assess the general appearance, shape, and skin quality. Contouring the arms involves lipoplasty of the posterior aspect of the upper arm, although circumferential arm contouring is also possible [5–7]. With the arm abducted to 90° and flexed at the elbow, the fat on the posterior arm amenable to resection can easily be palpated. Asking the patient to extend the arm against resistance contracts triceps and helps distinguish the subcutaneous fat from the muscular compartment (Fig. 4.4). The presence or absence of definition of the deltoid, biceps, and triceps is noted and discussed with the patient. High-definition lipoplasty improves definition of the arms by revealing these muscles and highlighting the transition zones between them. During the examination, the proposed incision sites, usually at the elbow and axilla, are explained to the patient. An incision site at the posterior axillary fold provides access to treat the upper arm as well as the upper back and flank.

Buttocks, Thighs, and Calves

Mendieta describes four main buttock frame shapes: A-shaped buttocks, V-shaped buttocks, square buttocks, and round buttocks [8] (Fig. 4.5). This useful classification helps the planning process for gluteal contouring. The A-shaped frame tends toward an hourglass shape and is aesthetically more ideal than the others. While even the A-shape often requires liposuction at the waist, lower back, and point A, the other frames are best contoured with a careful combination of fat resection and fat grafting to achieve smooth contours. According to Mendieta, "volume removal must always be balanced with volume enhancement when performing body contouring surgery." High-definition body sculpting is no exception.

The size, shape, and volume of fat over the thighs and calves are assessed and documented.

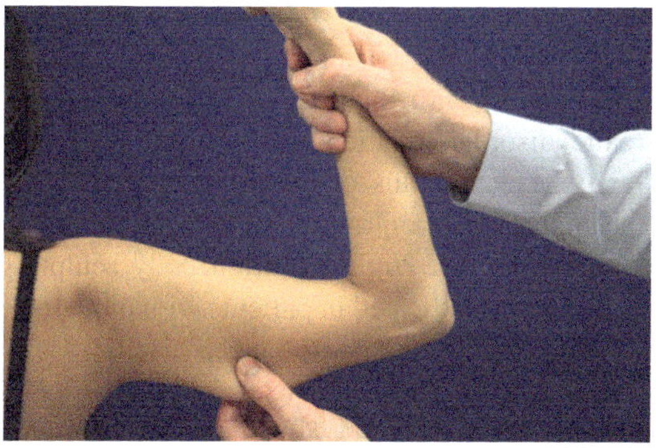

Fig. 4.4 Assessing fat over the back of the arm. The patient is asked to extend the arm against resistance to contract triceps

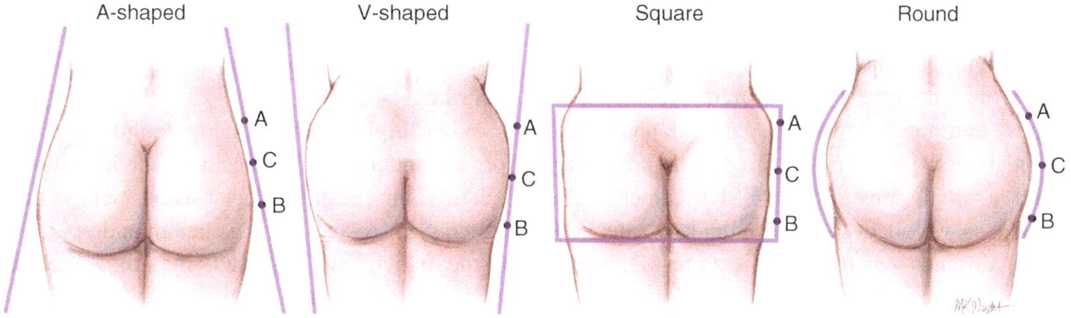

Fig. 4.5 The four main gluteal frames as described by Mendieta. The "A" frame is the closest to ideal. Each requires a different approach with varying degrees of fat resection and fat grafting

Improved shape and definition are achieved by removing excessive fat over the main muscles in the lower limbs, including the quadriceps and biceps femoris in the thighs and the gastrocnemius in the calves.

Patient Selection

The indications for standard liposuction procedures and high-definition body sculpting differ. The latter goes beyond reduction of convex adiposities to represent a true sculpting around and between muscles, combined with autologous fat grafting. Considerations for patient selection include body mass index, skin condition, condition of the abdominal wall, previous surgery, underlying medical conditions, smoking habit, and patient expectations. The ideal patient is healthy and has good underlying muscle tone with exercise and diet-resistant areas of fat. Caution must be taken when treating smokers and patients with diabetes or uncontrolled systemic disorders. Patients with significant skin laxity or panniculus of the lower abdomen are unsuitable for lipoplasty alone and often require abdominoplasty. High-definition body sculpting is also contraindicated in patients with unrealistic expectations or poor compliance.

Preparation

Following the initial consultation, once the patient has decided to proceed with the procedure, a separate visit is arranged prior to surgery. During this visit, the patient is afforded the opportunity to ask further questions or clarify concerns. The patient is measured for the postoperative compression vest and garment, and proper standardized photographs are taken, preferably with a single-lens reflex (SLR) camera. The patient is weighed again to calculate safe lidocaine dosages where the procedure is planned under tumescent local anesthesia. Blood is taken for routine preoperative investigations, including full blood count, renal and liver function, and coagulation studies. An electrocardiogram and thoracic X-rays may be obtained for patients if they are receiving general anesthesia. If there are scars tethered to the abdominal wall or suspected hernias, an ultrasound scan of the abdominal wall is essential.

The patient must understand the procedure, the risks versus benefits, and the perioperative care involved before making an informed decision as to whether to proceed or not. A consent form is required that details the procedure again and outlines potential complications (Table 4.4). The patient should be allowed to take this home and review it before it is signed. In addition, written preoperative and postoperative instructions are provided so that the patient is familiar with the perioperative requirements and commitments (Table 4.5). If the patient smokes, they must stop smoking at least 2 weeks before the surgery and refrain from smoking for at least 2 weeks postoperatively. Drugs that interact with lidocaine should be discontinued a week before surgery (Table 4.2). Medications with antiplatelet effects, including aspirin and ibuprofen, should be discontinued at least 10 days prior to surgery. Estrogens, including the oral contraceptive pill, are associated with an increased risk of thromboembolic disease and should be stopped 3 weeks prior to surgery and for 2 weeks following the procedure. Several herbal medicines and supplements have antiplatelet effects, may prolong anesthesia effects, and cause serious fluctuations in blood pressure and should be avoided for at least 2 weeks prior to surgery (Table 4.3).

The postoperative schedule, including appointments for manual lymphatic drainage massage, removal of drains, and routine checkup visits, is provided to the patient so they can prepare accordingly.

When high-definition body sculpting is performed under general anesthesia or intravenous sedation, an anesthesiologist assessment is conducted prior to surgery. The health and readiness of the patient are assessed, including medical conditions, previous anesthetic problems, airway difficulty, and likelihood of aspiration. The anesthetic plan is discussed with the patient, including interventions to reduce preoperative anxiety

Table 4.4 Consent for high-definition body sculpting

CONSENT FOR HIGH-DEFINITION BODY CONTOURING

Instructions
This is an informed-consent document that has been prepared to help inform you concerning ultrasound-asissted (VASER) high-definition lipoplasty, its risks and alternatives to treatment.

Please read this information carefully and completely. **Initial each page**, indicating that you have read the page, and **sign** the Consent for Surgery, proposed by your surgeon.

Introduction
VASERlipoplasty and high-definition body sculpting are surgical techniques that remove unwanted deposits of fat from specific areas of the body, including the face and neck, upper arms, upper and lower back, abdomen, buttocks, hips, inner and outer thighs, knees, calves and ankles. This is not a substitute for weight reduction, but a method for removing deposits of fatty tissue and improving definition. Body contouring using VASER technology may be performed as a primary procedure for body contouring or may be combined with other surgical techniques.

The best candidates for high-definition body contouring are individuals of relatively normal weight who have excess fat in particular body areas. Having firm, elastic skin will result in a better final contour after this procedure. Skin that has diminished tone due to aging, weight loss and sun damage will not reshape itself to the new contours and may require additional techniques to tighten excess skin.

The high-definition procedure is performed using advanced proprietary technology called VASER. A patented grooved solid metal probe is first inserted through small skin incisions. Ultrasonic energy emitted from sides and ends of the probe as it is passed back and forth breaks down fatty deposits. A hollow metal surgical instrument known as a cannula is then inserted and is directed through the area of emulsified fat cells. The cannula is attached to a vacuum source, which provides gentle suction to remove the emulsified fat. Because the VASER procedure is unique in that it first targets and dissolves fat cells and then draws off emulsified fat, leaving the collagen matrix intact, surgical trauma, complications and potential for post-operative pain and bruising are minimised while skin retraction is optimal.

There are a variety of different techniques used for lipoplasty (fat removal) and care following surgery. The VASER procedure can be performed under local or general anaesthesia. Tumescent local anaesthesia requires the infiltration of fluid containing dilute local anaesthetic and epinephrine into areas of fat. This reduces discomfort at the time of surgery, and reduces post-operative bruising.

Special support garments are worn after surgery to control potential swelling and promote healing, to provide comfort and support, and to help skin better fit new body contours.

Alternative Treatment
Alternatives to VASER for body contouring include no treatment at all. Diet and exercise regimens may be beneficial in the overall reduction of excess body fat.

Other forms of lipoplasty can involve traditional liposuction, laser lipolysis, radiofrequency-assisted lipoplasty, injection lipolysis and the removal of excess skin surgically. Alternative surgical treatments carry their own risks and potential complications.

HIGH-DEFINITION BODY SCULPTING INFORMED CONSENT

Risks and side-effects of high-definition body contouring
Every surgical procedure involves a certain amount of risk, and it is important that you understand the risks involved with body contouring using VASER. Although the majority of patients do not experience these complications, it is important that you understand the potential complications before treatment.

Patient selection

(continued)

Table 4.4 (continued)

Individuals with poor skin tone, medical problems, obesity, or unrealistic expectations might not be suitable candidates for LipoSelection

Allergic reactions
Rarely, local allergies to tape, suture material or topical solutions used during the procedure have been reported. More serious systemic reactions due to drugs administered during surgery or prescription medicines may require additional treatment.

Asymmetry
Due to factors such as skin tone, bony prominences, and muscle tone, which can contribute to normal asymmetry in body features, it may not be possible to achieve symmetrical body appearance through lipoplasty procedures.

Bleeding
While unusual, it is possible to have a bleeding episode during or after surgery. Should post-operative bleeding occur, it may require emergency treatment to drain accumulated blood or require a blood transfusion. Non-prescription herbs and dietary supplements can increase the risk of surgical bleeding. Do not take any aspirin or anti-inflammatory medications for 2 weeks before surgery, as this may increase the risk of bleeding. Please review our Pre-Operative Instructions and **consult your doctor before taking *anything*.**

Change in skin and skin sensation
A temporary decrease in skin sensation may occur following the body contouring procedure. This usually resolves over a period of time. Diminished or complete loss of skin sensation that does not totally resolve could potentially occur, but this is uncommon.

Chronic pain
Chronic pain and discomfort following VASER lipoplasty is unusual.

Infection
Infection is unusual following this type of surgery. Should an infection occur, treatment including antibiotics or additional surgery may be necessary. Although extremely rare, life-threatening infections such as toxic shock syndrome could occur after lipoplasty, regardless of the technology used.

Long-term effects
Subsequent alterations in body contour may occur as a result of aging, weight loss or gain, pregnancy, or other circumstances not related to the body contouring procedure. It is important to maintain lifestyle habits such as diet and exercise to maintain optimum body proportions. An increase in weight can result in disproportionate fatty deposits in areas not treated following lipoplasty.

Pulmonary complications
In extremely rare cases, fat droplets could become trapped in the lungs to create a possibly fatal complication called fat embolism. Pulmonary complications may also occur secondary to blood clots (pulmonary emboli) but this is extremely unlikely when a general anaesthetic is not used. Such complications would require hospitalisation and additional treatment.

Scarring
Although the incisions created during the LipoSelection procedure are very small and good healing is expected, abnormal scars may occur. Such scars may be enlarged or different in colour to surrounding tissue.

Seroma
This is a localised collection of fluid under the skin. Seromas are uncommon using VASER technology for lipoplasty, but should they occur, additional treatment or surgery may be required to promote drainage.

Risks and Side-Effects of VASER and high-definition body sculpting

Skin discolouration and/or swelling
Although VASER lipoplasty reduces the skin discolouration and swelling normally resulting from lipoplasty procedures, such could occur, and in rare situations, persist for extended periods of time. The incidence of permanent skin discolouration is rare.

Skin contour irregularities
As VASER lipoplasty selectively targets fat cells, leaving other essential tissues intact, skin contour irregularities and depressions in the skin are unlikley but possible. Visible and palpable wrinkling of skin

Table 4.4 (continued)

can occur, particularly when large quantities of fat cells are removed and/or skin is lacking in good elasticity. Post-operative skin contour irregularities could necessitate additional treatments including surgery.

Lignocaine toxicity
There is the possibility that large volumes of fluid containing local anaesthetic drugs and epinephrine that is injected into fat during the procedure may contribute to fluid overload or systemic reaction to these medications. Although uncommon, additional treatment including hospitalisation may be necessary.

Ultrasound technology
Risks associated with the use of ultrasound in lipoplasty treatments include the aforementioned and the following specific risks:

Burns
Ultrasonic energy may produce burns and tissue damage either at the incision site or in other areas if the probe touches the undersurface of the skin for prolonged periods of time. If burns occur, additonal treatment and surgery may be necessary.

Probe fragmentation
Ultrasonic energy produced within the probe may cause disintegration (fragmentation) of the surgical instrument. The occurrence and effect of this is unpredictable. If this should occur, additional treatment including surgery may be necessary.

Unknown risks
The long term effect on tissue and organs of exposure to short-duration, high-intensity ultrasonic energy is unknown. The possibility exists that additional risk factors resulting from the use of ultrasound with VASER could potentially be discovered.

Other
While we have attempted to assist you in building realistic expectations for your body contouring treatment, you may be disappointed with your surgical results. However infrequent, it may be necessary in your case to perform additional surgery to improve results.

It is important to read the above information carefully and have all your questions answered before signing the consent on the next page.

HIGH-DEFINITION BODY SCULPTING INFORMED CONSENT

Consent for Surgery/Procedure or Treatment

I have received and read the following information sheet: **Consent for high-definition body contouring.**

I understand that high-definition body contouring using VASER technology is an elective surgical procedure to remove body fat from specific areas of the body and improve definition.

The procedure has been explained to me in a way that I understand. I have had the opportunity to ask questions and my questions have been answered. Alternative methods of treatment have been discussed with me.

I acknowledge that no guarantee has been given by anyone as to the results I might obtain. Although a good result is expected, I understand that there are risks to the procedure or treatment proposed, as detailed in the preceeding information pages.

I consent to the administration of such anaesthetics and anxiolytics considered necessary or advisable. I understand that all forms of anaesthesia involve risk and the possibility of complications, as outlined.

For purposes of medical education, I consent to the admittance of observers to the operating room.

I consent to the disposal of any tissue which may be removed.

(continued)

Table 4.4 (continued)

Having discussed the reasonable expectations of LipoSelection with me and answered all of my questions to my satisfaction, I hereby authorise Dr __________ and such assistants as may be selected to perform high-definition body contouring and any other procedure(s) that in their judgement may be necessary or advisable should unforeseen circumstances arise during surgery.

With my signature below I hereby consent to having high-definition body contouring using VASER and to the above.

______________________________ ______________

Patient Signature Date

I, Dr ______________, certify that I or a member of staff has discussed all of the above with the patient and have answered all questions regarding the VASER-assisted high-definition body contouring procedure. I believe the patient fully understands what I have explained and answered.

HIGH-DEFINITION BODY SCULPTING INFORMED CONSENT

Photographs, Vidoetape, and/or Computer Images

Patient name (print):______________________ DOB______________

Requested by:______________________

I, the above-named patient, hereby consent that photographs, videotape, and/or computer imaging may be taken of me or of parts of my body under the following circumstances:

Pre- and post-operative photographs will be taken of my treatment for record purposes. The photographs shall be taken by my doctor or a photographer approved by my doctor. I understand that these photographs will be the property of ________________.

The aforementioned photographs and/or videotape shall be used only for medical records, research, education, or science purposes by my doctor and/or ______________. Photographs and information relating to my case may be published and republished, either seperately or in connection with eachother, in professional journals, medical books, and doctor or patient presentation materials or media, provided that in any such publication or use my name and identity is kept confidential and protected.

I have had the opportunity to discuss this consent with my surgeon and agree that all of my questions have been answered. This authorisation is granted in furtherance of medical education and other good

Table 4.5 Preoperative and postoperative instructions for high-definition lipoplasty patients

PREOPERATIVE INSTRUCTIONS

1. DO NOT SMOKE for 2 weeks prior to and 2 weeks after surgery. Smoking reduces blood circulation, slows down healing and increases complications.
2. DO NOT TAKE ASPIRIN or products containing aspirin for 2 weeks prior to or following your scheduled surgery. Aspirin affects your blood's ability to clot and could increase your tendency to bleed during surgery or during the post-operative period.
3. DO NOT TAKE DIETARY SUPPLEMENTS for 2 weeks before and after surgery. These include vitamins, ginger, ginko biloba, garlic, ginseng and fish oils. They may increase your risk of bleeding and bruising during and following surgery.
4. DISCONTINUE OESTROGENS (BIRTH CONTROL PILLS AND REPLACEMENT THERAPY 3 WEEKS PRIOR TO SURGERY AND FOR 2 WEEKS AFTER SURGERY
5. DO NOT DRINK ALCOHOL for 5 days prior to surgery. Alcohol may increase your risk of complications such as bruising.
6. IF YOU DEVELOP A COLD, COLD SORE, FEVER, OR ANY OTHER ILLNESS PRIOR TO SURGERY PLEASE NOTIFY US.
7. DAY PRIOR TO AND DAY OF SURGERY. Please shower using only antibacterial soap. Males receiving abdominal or flank treatment may prefer to shave the treatment area; females receiving abdominal or thigh treatment may prefer to shave pubic areas below the hairline
8. WEAR COMFORTABLE, DARK, LOOSE-FITTING CLOTHING on day of surgery—including a shirt that buttons all the way up the front. Wear nothing that you must put on over your head. Slip-on shoes are recommended for maximum post-operative comfort. We suggest you safeguard your car seat and bedding with a protective cover as there will be some leakage of fluid following surgery.
9. LEAVE JEWELRY AND VAULABLES AT HOME. Do not wear wigs, hairpins or hairpieces.
10. AVOID WEARING MAKEUP, FACIAL OR BODY MOISTURISERS.
11. SURGERY TIMES ARE ESTIMATES ONLY. You could be at the clinic longer than indicated.
12. ARRANGE FOR A DRIVER TO AND FROM SURGERY. We cannot discharge you to a taxi. Put a pillow and blanket in the car for the trip home.
13. IF YOU ARE RECEIVING INTRAVENOUS SEDATION OR GENERAL ANAESTHESIA, YOU MUST FAST (NO FOOD OR DRINK) FOR AT LEAST 6 HOURS PRIOR TO SURGERY

(continued)

Table 4.5 (continued)

I HAVE READ AND FULLY UNDERSTAND THE ABOVE ITEMS 1-13

____________________________________ _______________

Patient Signature Date

POST-OPERATIVE INSTRUCTIONS

IF YOU EXPERIENCE EXCESSIVE PAIN OR BLEEDING, FULLNESS OR SPREADING REDNESS IN TREATMENT AREAS, OR FEVER, PLEASE CALL US IMMEDIATELY

1. DRIVING: A family member or friend must drive you home from your surgery (it is best to have them stay and assist you for the first 24-48 hours). Please do not drive if you are taking the prescription pain medication *Tramodol*.
2. COMPRESSION GARMENTS: Following your surgery, a compression garment was placed to provide comfort and support while helping your skin conform to your new body contour. If you had treatment on your abdomen and torso, a compression foam vest may also have been applied. The day following surgery, you may remove the garment/vest once a day for laundering, sponge bathing and bandage changing (if present). Continue wearing the garment 24 hours a day for the first 2-4 weeks, followed by 12 hours a day (remove at night) for the subsequent 2-4 weeks, according to the advice of your surgeon.
3. BATHING OR SHOWERING: Sponge bathe only for the first 72 hours when removing the compression garment. After 72 hours, you may take a shower or bath when the garment has been temporarily removed. Avoid Whirl Pools and hot tubs for at least one week (until the incision sites have healed).
4. TREATMENT SITES: Please keep your dressings as clean and dry as possible, changing daily if wet to help prevent infection. Do not apply heat or ice to the surgical areas. You should expect significant drainage (oozing) of blood-tinged anaesthetic solution at the incision sites due to fluids injected during your procedure. Although the fluid may appear red, it is mostly anaesthetic solution and saline and only 1% blood. In general, the more drainage there is, the less bruising and swelling there will be. Many patients have found it helpful to use a shower curtain or other protective covering on their mattress for the first few days after their body contouring procedure. When your incisions stop draining, please clean with tap water and antibacterial soap or solutionand reapply clean, dry, sterile dressings, eg. Primapore. When the incisions have closed completely (after a few days), you may apply petroleum jelly to the incision sites. Itching, pulling, pinching, hardness, tightness and/or

Table 4.5 (continued)

numbness sensations are normal. All should subside within 24 hours to 1 week, but sometimes can last for months. This is part of the healing process and your patience is apppreciated.

5. DRAINS: Drains may have been placed in the front and/or back in order to facilitate drainage of fluid from the treated areas. These will be removed by your doctor after 24-48 hours when drainage is minimal.
6. MANUAL LYMPHATIC DRAINAGE (MLD) MASSAGE: It is recommended that you start a couse of MLD as soon as 2 days following your procedure. This specific and gentle massage shoud be performed by practitioners specifically trained in the technique. This will help to accelerate healing, reduce hardness, improve bruising and swelling and improve results. As many as 8-12 treatments can be performed, twice or 3 times per week.
7. EXTERNAL ULTRASOUND/RADIOFREQUENCY THERAPY: In addition to MLD, a postoperative treatment regimen will be given to you to improve healing and soften tissues. It is important that you remain totally compliant to this treatment schedule.
8. ACTIVITY: Rest for the first 12 hours. It is normal to experience light-headedness when rising or removing/changing your compression garments. Please have someone help you with this for the first few days after surgery. Take it easy for the first week, resuming normal activity as tolerated. Experiencing more than mild swelling and discomfort may indicate that you are overdoing it. Avoid strenuous activities, lifting over 10lbs, or aerobic exercise for 2-3 weeks. Protect incisions and any bruised areas from the sun until completely healed; use SPF30 or greater for 6 months. Avoid tanning until bruising has faded, which normally takes 10-14 days.
9. DIET: If you experience any post-operative nausea, try carbonated drinks and dry crackers to settle your stomach. Take your post-operative medications with food to minimise irritation. If your stomach feels normal, start slowly with liquids and bland foods, progressing to soups, and finally a normal diet as tolerated. Drink plenty of clear fluids.
10. ALCOHOL: As well as refraining from drinking alcohol for at least 5 days before surgery, it is especially important that you do not consume alcohol as long as you are taking over-the-counter or prescription pain medication following surgery as they may interact.
11. SMOKING: We continue to stress the importance of not smoking. Smoking reduces blood circulation to skin and tissues and delays healing. Do not smoke at all during the first 14 days following the procedure.
12. EXPECTATIONS: Remember, the goal of your treatment is not weight loss but improved contour and definition. In fact, since the body retains fluids in response to surgery, you may notice a temporary weight gain, resolving over the first week. In addition, remember that for the majority of people the goal is significant improvement, not perfection. Lower abdominal patients may experience significant swelling in the pubic area. Post-operative discomfort usually takes the form of deep muscle soreness and normally improves over the folllowing 2-7 days. Slight temperature

(continued)

Table 4.5 (continued)

elevation and flushing of the face, neck, and upper chest could last 48 hours. You may initially experience a mild depression that should begin lifting after the first week, once you see the bruising and swelling fade. Menstrual irregularities (premature or delayed monthly onset) are a common side effect to surgery. If areas on the thighs were treated, you may have swelling in your calves and ankles for up to 3 weeks.

13. POST-OPERATIVE MEDICATIONS. Please take the antibiotics and pain medications as advised or prescribed by your doctor. If you have no allergies, you may start with regular paracetamol (1000mg every 6 hours). If this does not relieve discomfort or pain, you can take the prescription pain medication in addition to the paracetamol. Do not take aspirin, Brufen or Neurofen. If antibiotics are prescribed, it is very important you complete the full course.
14. POST-OPERATIVE APPOINTMENTS. For maximum healing and optimal long-term results, you must follow the schedule of appointments that are made following your surgery.

I HAVE READ AND FULLY UNDERSTAND THE ABOVE ITEMS 1-12

________________________________ ______________

Patient Signature Date

and postoperative nausea and vomiting. Although the general health of the vast majority of patients undergoing high-definition body sculpting is good, specific conditions such as hypertension and cardiac disease are assessed and must be controlled before surgery in patients undergoing any lipoplasty procedure.

References

1. Glaser DA, Kaminer MS (2005) Body dysmorphic disorder and the liposuction patient. Dermatol Surg 31(5):559–560
2. Levin N (2007) Preanesthetic assessment of the cosmetic surgery patient. In: Friedberg BL (ed) Anesthesia in cosmetic surgery. Cambridge University Press, Cambridge, p 172
3. Singh D (1993) Adaptive significance of female physical attractiveness: role of waist to hip ratio. J Pers Soc Psychol 65:293–307
4. Singh D (2004) Mating strategies of young women: role of physical attractiveness. J Sex Res 41:43–54
5. Lyos AT (2012) Circumferential para-axillary superficial tumescent (CAST) liposuction for upper arm contouring. In: Shiffman MA, Di Giuseppe A (eds) Cosmetic surgery. Art and techniques. Springer, Berlin/Heidelberg, pp 981–992
6. Chamosa M, Murillo J, Vázquez T (2005) Lipectomy of arms and lipograft of shoulders balance the upper body contour. Aesthetic Plast Surg 29(6):567–570
7. Nguyen AT, Rohrich RJ (2010) Liposuction-assisted posterior brachioplasty: technical refinements in upper arm contouring. Plast Reconstr Surg 126(4): 1365–1369
8. Mendieta CG (2011) Evaluation based on anatomic landmarks. In: The art of gluteal sculpting. Quality Medical Publishing, St. Louis, p 10

5 Anesthesia: Tumescent, MAC, and General

Introduction

With the increase in the number and type of plastic surgical procedures that aim to improve the physical appearance and social acceptance, anesthesia can become the most feared factor by the patient, sometimes even more than the surgical procedure itself. It becomes necessary to educate the patient about the safety of the surgery and the anesthesia. Demystification of the anesthesia as a dangerous endeavor, diminishing the risk by an adequate preoperative evaluation, and performing the surgery according to the safety standards will keep high-definition lipoplasty as a safe, effective, and rewarding surgery.

We cannot forget certain issues that otherwise would disturb the desirable outcomes. These variables include lots of individual particularities, sometimes hard to figure out: from the socioeconomical level up to the particular environment for the postsurgical recovery.

It is always important to highlight and reassure all the advantages and disadvantages of the procedure and clear all the doubts, myths, and misinformation about the anesthesia. The patient is the only one who can decide about how the procedure is going to be done. For the body-contouring anesthesia, we must emphasize to the patient on how the preanesthetic drugs work and what is the appropriate pre- and postsurgical care and let them know all the possible complications of the anesthesia.

The type of anesthesia used for high-definition body sculpting depends on several factors, including the patient condition and preference, extent of procedure, staff, and facility.

This chapter describes the principles and technique for tumescent local anesthesia, monitored anesthesia care (MAC), and general anesthesia.

Preanesthesia

The first patient contact is done during the preanesthetic appointment. This must be done in a pleasant environment, with enough time and disposition to explain and clear all doubts. It is important to notice that not all the planned procedures can always be done; the possibility to perform the procedure depends in the findings of the past medical history and habits with the aim of looking for the best conditions of quality and security for the patient and the anesthesiologist.

It is always important to highlight the importance of the veracity of the information that the patient provides and letting them know that this information can be very useful to prevent complications and legal issues, and in the case of their appearance, a quick response can be provided.

Medical Record

Start the preanesthetic consultation emphasizing in establishing a good doctor-patient relationship.

A.E. Hoyos, P.M. Prendergast, *High Definition Body Sculpting*,
DOI 10.1007/978-3-642-54891-8_5, © Springer-Verlag Berlin Heidelberg 2014

The questioning must be addressed to reveal the socioeconomic status of the patient with the aim of having a conversation that the patient can plenty understand and can retrieve accurate information about past medical history. When asking about their labor performance, we can get clues about the functional class that for this type of procedures must be I/IV according to the NYHA.

Always ask about the past allergy history to the drugs used in previous anesthesia and to food, environment, and other substances used in surgery (surgical tape, iodine solutions, latex, etc.) that in one or other way can alter the anesthesia process.

Take the vital signs to keep a record of the expected hemodynamic variables of the patient according to their past medical history and the medications he/she might be in. Include heart rate, blood pressure, oximetry at ambient, height, and weight. Calculate the body mass index, which must be lower than 30 to allow the procedure and to avoid complications such as ventilatory failure, thrombosis, long bedridden periods, delay in recovery, and probable displeasure with the final outcomes.

The patient classification using the New York Heart Association (NYHA) scale gives an idea of the cardiovascular risks, functional state, and some information about the patient's habits. It is important to ask about past history of cardiovascular disease (hypertension, venous insufficiency, thromboembolic disease, myocardial ischemia or infarcts, arrhythmias), pulmonary disease (smoking, asthma, recent upper viral infections, COPD), urinary diseases (recent infections and how it was managed, chronic kidney disease), and gastrointestinal diseases (gastritis, bowel movements, irritable bowel syndrome). Remember also to note the received treatments, the efficacy of it, and the possible surgical and anesthetic issues of these treatments. All this information is valuable because the symptoms and management of any of these diseases can alter the recovery process even if the postsurgical pain is controlled and there are no surgical complications.

The past surgical history must include the number and type of procedures and surgical and anesthetic complications including dental work. Past traumatic history includes treatment, complications, sequels, and handicaps. Previous history of metabolic diseases like thyroid dysfunction or diabetes, must include: current management of the disease, last medical check-up, especific medical recommendations and latest blood tests.

The patient behavior is also important. Always ask about the use of tobacco, alcohol, and recreational drugs like cocaine, marihuana, LSD, heroin, amphetamines, etc.; check the time and frequency of use and signs of dependency. A period of at least 5 months of abstinence of tobacco, 15 days in the case of psychiatric medicines, and 3 days if there is alcohol use is recommended. We must always emphasize the importance of knowing these habits and warn the patient about the possible complications.

The physical examination must always include the vital signs record, blood pressure, heart rate, and oxygen saturation with the fraction of inspired oxygen of 21 %; weight; and height. Calculate the body mass index (BMI), which ideally must be below 30.

$$\mathrm{BMI} = \frac{\mathrm{Weight}(\mathrm{kg})}{\mathrm{Height}(\mathrm{m})^2}$$

Normal value: 18.1–24.9
Overweight: 25.0–29.9
Obesity: >30.0.

Using this index, and considering the surgical blood looses, we calculate a safe volume of fat extraction:

$$\mathrm{FH} = \mathrm{HT} \times e^{\mathrm{ivl}/\mathrm{tbv}}$$

Where FH: final hematocrit
HT: hematocrit
ivl: intra-surgical blood volume loss
tbv: total estimated blood volume
e: Euler's constant (2.71828)

This formula lets us estimate the blood losses on every stage of the surgery and not in a linear manner like what is usually done.

The lab works must include the following: complete blood count checking for platelet and white cells condition, hemoglobin, hematocrit, coagulation times (prothrombin time/PT, INR, and partial thromboplastin time/PTT), renal function (creatinine and blood urea nitrogen/BUN), pregnancy test, HIV testing, and glycemia. When there is a known pathology like thyroid disease, the specific lab work must be addressed.

It is also important to take a 12-lead electrocardiogram (EKG) and chest X-rays even though most guidelines argue that these tests should not be taken on a healthy patient, but our the experience has shown that every day, we find many "healthy" patients with EKG abnormalities like arrhythmias, electric conduction alterations, and chest X-rays with signs of obstructive disease in young people.

Having this set of tests done, we can promptly plan a presurgical management if needed or definitely contraindicate the procedure.

After getting all the medical data collected and analyzed, we proceed to assign the anesthetic risk according to the American Society of Anesthesiologist (ASA) scale and the functional class according to the New York Heart Association (NYHA). By general rule, surgery is only performed in patients with an ASA scale of II/VI or lower.

Tumescent Anesthesia

Since the introduction of tumescent local anesthesia (TLA) in 1986, this method has been widely adopted for traditional liposuction and has an unprecedented safety record [1–4]. Intravenous sedation may be performed in combination with TLA to reduce discomfort and anxiety for the patient. There is a fine line between moderate sedation, deep sedation, and general anesthesia, so it is imperative that the anesthesiologist present has the equipment and monitoring available to convert to general anesthesia if required [5]. In cases of large volume, extensive high-definition body sculpting, general anesthesia may be desirable.

During tumescent anesthesia, a mixture of physiologic saline, lidocaine, epinephrine, and sodium bicarbonate are infiltrated into fatty tissue until a state of "tumescence" is reached. Tumescence is characterized by firm, swollen tissue that is turgid and somewhat fixed (Fig. 5.1). There are several reasons for the high safety profile of liposculpture performed under tumescent local anesthesia without IV sedation or general anesthesia:

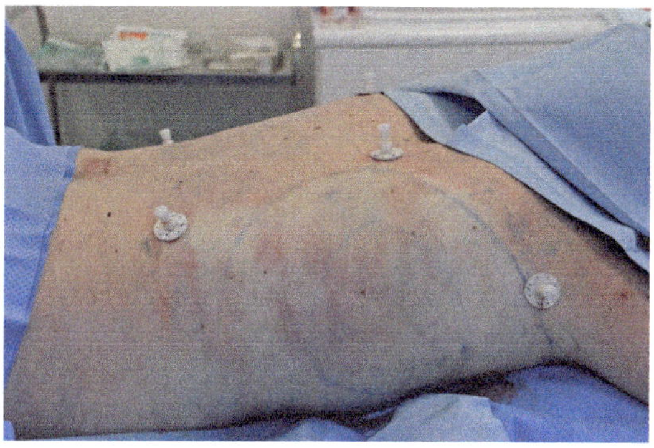

Fig. 5.1 Tumescent anesthesia. Tumescent fluid is infiltrated until the tissues become firm and rigid. Note the blanching secondary to epinephrine-induced vasoconstriction

1. The dilution of lidocaine with saline to concentrations of 0.05–0.1 % and dispersion in fatty tissue alters the pharmacokinetics entirely. The maximum safe dose of lidocaine with epinephrine increases from 7 to 55 mg/kg [6].
2. Epinephrine has a dual role. It causes vasoconstriction in the subcutaneous fat, creating an almost bloodless field, and reduces blood loss to less than 1 % of liposuction aspirate. The vasoconstriction also slows systemic absorption of lidocaine so that serum levels of lidocaine rise slowly and peak only 4–14 h after infiltration [7].
3. Tumescent local anesthesia allows liposculpture to be performed in the awake patient, eliminating the risks inherent to intravenous sedation or general anesthesia.

Proper planning prior to the procedure is required for safe and effective tumescent anesthesia. Based on experience, an estimate is made of the volume of tumescent fluid required to achieve optimum tumescence. Large abdomens with soft fat and loose or slightly lax skin require more volume to reach tumescence compared to smaller abdomens or those with no striae or laxity and good skin tone. The typical patient for high-definition sculpting has a smaller abdomen with good skin tone and requires more subcutaneous fluid to reach a state of tumescence. The concentration of lidocaine per liter of tumescent fluid is decided depending on the total volume

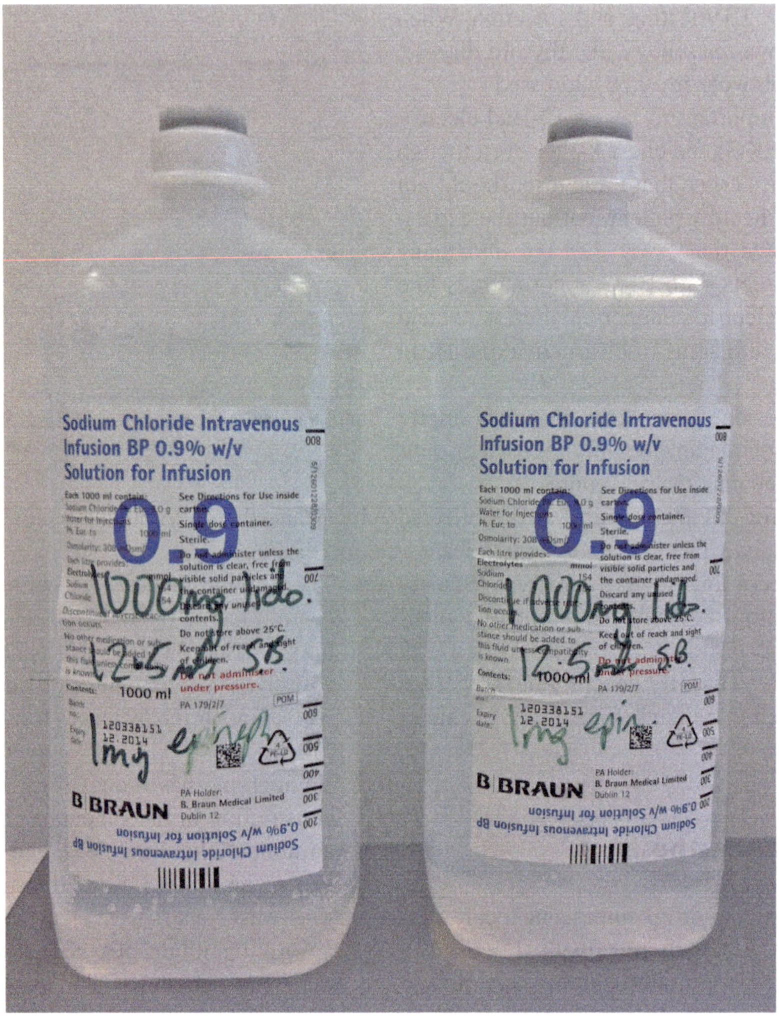

Fig. 5.2 Tumescent fluid ready for infiltration. The added components should be clearly marked on the container to avoid confusion

required for adequate tumescence during the procedure and the weight of the patient.

For lipoplasty of the abdomen, the author adds 600–800 mg lidocaine to each liter of normal saline, thus achieving an approximate lidocaine concentration in tumescent solution of 0.06–0.08 %. For superficial work and fibrous areas, up to 1,000 mg lidocaine in one liter of normal saline may be required, achieving a 0.1 % lidocaine solution. Each liter of normal saline contains lidocaine, epinephrine 1 mg, and 12.5 ml 8.4%w/v sodium bicarbonate (Fig. 5.2). The author uses no more than 45 mg/kg lidocaine. Using this limit, a 70 kg male patient receives up to 3,150 mg lidocaine. As such, if sculpting of the abdomen, flanks, thighs, and arms is required, the procedure is staged, since the volume required to anesthetize these areas with tumescent fluid would become prohibitively great. Alternatively, a more extensive procedure is performed either using intravenous sedation and a reduced concentration of lidocaine or under general anesthesia.

Tumescent anesthesia for liposculpture on the awake patient must be sufficient and properly administered in order to eliminate pain and

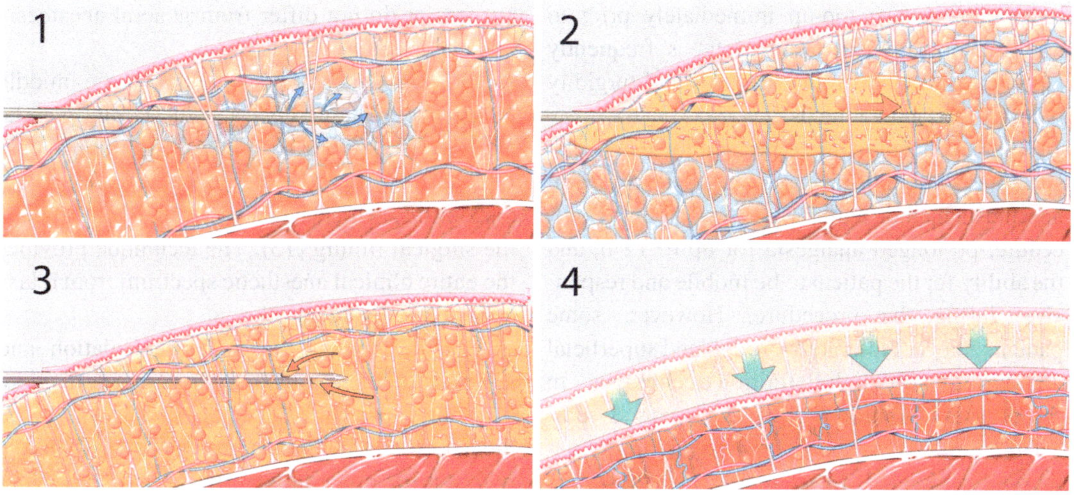

Fig. 5.3 (*1*) Infiltration of tumescent local anesthesia occurs deeply first and then superficially and subdermally. After 20 min, the fluid reaches the interlobular and intralobular spaces. Ultrasound probes should only be used in wet tissues (*2*). Then begin the extraction in the deep layers (*3*). Note the skin retraction after the superficial extraction (*4*)

discomfort, provide adequate vasoconstriction, and stabilize tissues for fat removal. A homogenous fluid-filled fat compartment is also essential for ultrasound-assisted lipoplasty to transmit sound energy and reduce complications such as burns and seromas. After the surgeon scrubs and dons full sterile surgical attire, skin preparation is performed using betadine or chlorhexidine wash and the patient is covered using disposable sterile drapes. Small volumes of 1 % lidocaine with 1:200,000 epinephrine are injected intradermally at the incision sites. Small 2–4 mm stab incisions are made using a number 11 blade. Meanwhile the 1-l bags of tumescent fluid are warmed to 37–40 °C in a warming bath to prevent hypothermia and reduce pain during infiltration [8]. The vasoconstriction properties of epinephrine in the solution are sufficient to overcome the theoretical inconvenience of vasodilatation using warmed fluid. The initial infiltration of the tumescent fluid using blunt cannula can be uncomfortable for the patient, particularly in sensitive or fibrous areas such as the epigastrium, around the umbilicus, or in the flanks. For the inexperienced liposuction surgeon, as well as the patient, this can be a source of considerable stress and may discourage the surgeon from infiltrating all fat layers completely and thoroughly. The use of sharp, large-bore spinal needles to reduce pain during infiltration should be avoided due to the risk of bleeding or perforating intra-abdominal structures. These needles can also be painful themselves. Tumescent infiltration should be slow initially (150 ml/min) and in the deep layers and increased as tolerated to 200 ml/min and continue through the more superficial layers of fat until the tissues are swollen and firm. It is important to infiltrate right up to the dermis before high-definition lipoplasty since these areas will be treated with both ultrasound delivery and suction. The operating hand should move forward and backward slowly and deliberately to fill between fat lobules at every level, while the other hand palpates the tissue from the surface, always aware of the location of the tip of the cannula. After withdrawing the cannula, a suture is placed to stem the flow of fluid from the incision site to prevent a reduction in pressure in the fat compartment.

A port is placed into the incision directly at this point to prepare for VASER-assisted lipoplasty. It is necessary to wait at least 20 min following the end of infiltration before continuing to allow complete diffusion of the tumescent fluid to all compartments within the subcutaneous tissues, including the intralobular compartments around the adipocytes (Fig. 5.3). Since tumescence is a temporary state, a top-up immediately prior to aspiration or emulsification of fat is frequently required to reestablish the firmness and turgidity required to stabilize the tissues [8].

The benefits of using tumescent local anesthesia alone without intravenous sedation or general anesthesia include a quick recovery from the procedure, prolonged analgesia for up to 12 h, and the ability for the patient to be mobile and responsive during the procedure. However, some patients may not tolerate thorough and superficial contouring with high-definition techniques. In these cases, monitored anesthesia care is indicated. Similarly, if extensive overall body contouring is planned, MAC or general anesthesia should be considered.

Monitored Anesthesia Care (MAC)

In recent years, exponential growth, complexity of cases and patients, and media attention to high-profile untoward events are accompanied with concerns for patient safety and development of safer anesthesia practices. Especially for cosmetic procedures, an exponential growth has been seen in the last decade; office-based procedures are now becoming one of the most frequent consultations.

It is well known that the basic technique of liposuction is the tumescent; however, when high-definition lipoplasty procedures involve thorough superficial liposuction and contouring of extensive body areas, it is important to consider the needs of additional intravenous sedation, hypnosis, analgesia, and anxiolysis. This can be delivered as monitored anesthesia care also known as MAC. The MAC technique is a specific anesthesia service for diagnostic or therapeutic procedures that include all aspects of anesthesia care: a pre-procedure visit, intra-procedure care, and postoperative anesthesia management [5].

By today, in the USA an increment from 3 to 11 million (1997–2007) has been reached (about 460 %), and also demands for MAC are arising as recovery time, adverse events, and surgery length are less or do not differ from general anesthesia and deep sedation [9–13].

The MAC technique stands in the middle between pure tumescent anesthesia and general anesthesia. The MAC allows infiltrating over multiples zones at higher rates with no patient discomfort, which helps to substantially reduce the surgical timing [13]. The technique provides the entire clinical anesthetic spectrum from relaxation to moderate anesthesia.

For the patient the amnesia, sedation and shorting of the surgical timing, means a more pleasant experience. The reported literature on the safety and complications of the MAC usage makes it the procedure of choice for many types of surgeries [13]; however, due to the extensive extraction work on the superficial layers, which are characteristic of the high-definition techniques, the pain is a limiting factor. The final decision of its use relies on the patient's particularities, the type of procedure, and of course the anesthesiologist considerations.

General Anesthesia

One of the goals to do the high-definition lipoplasty under general anesthesia is to do as much work as pertinent to the case to induce the maximum results. The results are more endurable when they are produced in a single procedure, because some factors can be taken out of the equation: the surgeon can concentrate in the work, not in the several distractions due to being pending of the tumescence, to a time limit, or to an infiltration limit.

The anesthesia for this purpose does not differ much to any general anesthesia [14]. However, we consider that our patients have a special right to choose a type of anesthesia that can provide a good awakening, good postoperative analgesia, and, above all, free or almost free of discomfort like nausea or hypothermia.

Thanks to the medical developments, especially in pharmacology, biochemistry, and physiology, and an improved understanding in the function and relation of the receptors with their ligands, now we have drugs available that allow achieving a better control on the autonomic functions during anesthesia [15].

Anesthetics for aesthetic plastic surgery procedures have also been improved, bringing the patient a safer and pleasant experience, starting in the presurgical management up to the postoperatory discharge [14, 15].

Premedication and Indications

Preoperative fasting must be of at least 8 h for solid food and 4 h for drinks. Explain all the surgical risks and possible surgical/anesthetic complications. Fill out the consent and make the patient and anesthesiologist sign it.

The patient prescription must include:

Gabapentin 15–20 mg/kg/day. This drug helps prevent the neuropathic postsurgical pain due to its action over the voltage dependent ionic calcium channels type N. The plasmatic levels rise very fast, letting the drug act within the first 24 h of the prescription. It should be given for 5 days including the day of the surgery.

Dimenhydrinate 1.5 mg/k single dose on the night previous to the surgery. We take advantage of the high somnolence level produced by this drug without dependence risks, and at the same time, it works in the premedication against nausea and vomit.

Always advise the patient to have a daily physical activity of at least 30 min (hiking, waking, swimming looking for pulmonary and heart conditioning) and a diet rich in fiber, proteins, and liquids to improve the bowel habits and raise the hemoglobin levels.

Due to the high altitude of the city where we have most of our patients (Bogota 2,650 m–8,612 ft), if the patient comes from the sea level, we recommend to arrive at least a week before and take an iron supplement plus folic acid once a day before lunch.

It is possible to need blood derivates during the postoperatory care; however, most of the effort is focused in avoiding this. We use normovolemic hemodilution with crystalloids in patients whose surgical blood loss will end in a hematocrit lower than 30 %.

Surgical Management

Take precautionary measures to keep a stable euthermic body temperature always avoiding hypothermia. We use a fluid heater and thermic blankets under the sterile surgical clothing. This is done to diminish the heat loss due to the use of the tumescent solution and at the same time improves the pain management and achieves a faster anesthetic recovery.

Antithrombotic therapy should include the use of anti-DVT stockings, intermittent pneumatic compression, and low molecular weight heparin at doses of 0.3–0.5 mg/kg/day for 3 days starting 4 h after the procedure.

We use a general balanced anesthetic technique (sevoflurane with a CAM 1–1.5 %, remifentanil 0.15 ug/kg, dexmedetomidine 0.15 ug/kg/min). For induction, we use midazolam 0.05–0.1 mg/kg, fentanyl 1 ug/kg/bolus, and cisatracurium 0.05–0.1 mg/kg.

Antibiotic prophylaxis is needed if the procedure lasts longer than 4 h. It is done using a first-generation cephalosporin at doses 30–50 mg/kg single dose.

Antiemetic management is done by using metoclopramide 0.1–0.3 mg/kg/day; the effect is improved by adding dexamethasone 8 mg 30 min after the intake of metoclopramide. If there is any contraindication for the use of metoclopramide, we use 4 mg of ondansetron.

For gastric protection, we use secretion inhibitors such as ranitidine and omeprazole. Analgesia is arranged by using nonsteroidal anti-inflammatory drugs (NSAIDS) like ketorolac 30 mg in bolus or diclofenac 1.5–3 mg/kg/day previously to the procedure. During the procedure, we use 1 mg/kg of meperidine IV, both to prevent pain and the tremors after surgery.

Postsurgical Anesthetic Management

The patient is taken to the postanesthetic care unit. Add supplemental wet oxygen via nasal cannula, aiming to increase the inspired fraction up to 28 %; use basic monitoring of blood pressure, pulse, and oxygen saturation; control the temperature using thermic sheets (hot air flow); control the pain using the analog visual scale; and when possible, use an elastomeric pump for ketorolac, tramadol, and ondansetron for 3 days controlled on a daily basis.

Continue the pharmacological and physical antithrombotic management but remember that early walking is the best therapy. It is done by an adequate pain control and hemodynamic stability of the patient.

The pulmonary atelectasis should be avoided and a prompt treatment must be started with respiratory therapy using bronchodilators, corticoids, and the incentive spirometer.

When the volume of fat extracted is larger than 5,000 ml, the patient must be left under medical surveillance overnight to check for the diuresis, take control of laboratory tests 12 h after the surgery looking for CBC changes, and evaluate the postoperatory blood volume. If the volume extracted is less than 5,000 ml, the patient stays for observation only 2 h.

The outpatient management must emphasize on the importance of early mild activity like walking, plenty of water intake, and a protein- and fiber-rich diet. The outpatient medication must include antibiotic therapy for 7 days and analgesia with Cox2-type NSAIDs; continue the treatment with gabapentin and iron-folate supplement.

The outpatient care is enhanced if a home nurse is included; by doing this, the postoperatory management adherence is improved and the physician can have a closer control of the recovery. The initial postsurgical evaluation must be done during the first 48 h after the procedure.

The postoperative anaesthetic management protocol described above has improved patient outcomes and reduced complications following high-definition body sculpting.

References

1. Coldiron BM, Healy C, Bene N (2008) Office surgery incidents: what seven years of Florida data show us. Dermatol Surg 34(3):285–291
2. Housman TS, Lawrence N, Mellen BG, George MN, Filippo JS, Cerveny KA, DeMarco M, Feldman SR, Fleischer AB (2002) The safety of liposuction: results of a national survey. Dermatol Surg 28(11):971–978
3. Coleman WP III, Hanke CW, Lillis P, Bernstein G, Narins R (1999) Does the location of the surgery or the specialty of the physician affect malpractice claims in liposuction? Dermatol Surg 25:343–347
4. Hanke CW, Lee MW, Bernstein G (1990) The safety of dermatologic liposuction surgery. Dermatol Clin 8:563–568
5. Urman RD, Shapiro FE (2007) Anesthesia techniques: which is the safest choice? In: Shapiro FE (ed) Manual of office-based anesthesia procedures. Lippincott Williams and Wilkins, Philadelphia, p 41
6. Ostad A, Kageyama N, Moy RL (1996) Tumescent anesthesia with a lidocaine dose of 55 mg/kg is safe for liposuction. Dermatol Surg 22(11):921–927
7. Yang CH, Hsu HC, Shen SC, Juan WH, Hong HS, Chen CH (2006) Warm and neutral tumescent anaesthetic solutions are essential factors for a less painful injection. Dermatol Surg 32(9):1119–1122
8. Sattler G, Sattler S (2007) Physiodynamic concept of tumescence. In: Hanke CW, Sattler G, Sommer B (eds) Textbook of liposuction. Informa Healthcare, Abingdon, pp 43–45
9. American Society of Anesthesiologists (2005) Position on monitored anesthesia care. ASA House of Delegates. Available at www.asahq.org/publicationsAndServices/standards/23.pdf.2004
10. Bhananker SM, Posner KL, Cheney FW, Caplan RA, Lee LA, Domino KB (2006) Injury and liability associated with monitored anesthesia care: a closed claims analysis. Anesthesiology 104(2):228–234
11. Bitar G, Mullis W, Jacobs W, Matthews D, Beasley M, Smith K, Watterson P, Getz S, Capizzi P, Eaves F 3rd (2003) Safety and efficacy of office-based surgery with monitored anesthesia care/sedation in 4778 consecutive plastic surgery procedures. Plast Reconstr Surg 111(1):150–156; discussion 157–8
12. Shapiro FE (2008) Anesthesia for outpatient cosmetic surgery. Curr Opin Anaesthesiol 21(6):704–710
13. Scarborough DA, Herron JB, Khan A, Bisaccia E (2003) Experience with more than 5,000 cases in which monitored anesthesia care was used for liposuction surgery. Aesthetic Plast Surg 27(6):474–480
14. Mustoe TA, Buck DW 2nd, Lalonde DH (2010) The safe management of anesthesia, sedation, and pain in plastic surgery. Plast Reconstr Surg 126(4):165e–176e
15. Marcus JR, Tyrone JW, Few JW, Fine NA, Mustoe TA (1999) Optimization of conscious sedation in plastic surgery. Plast Reconstr Surg 104(5):1338–1345

6 VASER Technology for Ultrasound-Assisted Lipoplasty

History

The use of ultrasound in surgical procedures is not new. Kelman introduced phacoemulsification for cataracts in 1967 after being inspired by his dentist's ultrasound device for descaling [4]. Since then, ultrasound has been used extensively in neurosurgery for selective destruction of tumors and in general surgery, particularly for cutting and coagulating during laparoscopic surgery [5]. In the late 1980s and early 1990s, Scuderi and Zocchi pioneered the application of ultrasound for selective emulsification and removal of fat for body contouring [6–8]. The first-generation ultrasound-assisted lipoplasty device was developed by SMEI Company in Italy. SMEI's sculpture consisted of large 4–6 mm solid probes that emulsified fat at a frequency of 20 kHz. In the mid-1990s, two second-generation ultrasound-assisted lipoplasty devices were introduced. Lysonix 2000 (Lysonix Inc., Carpenteria, CA) featured hollow ultrasonic cannulae of 4.0 and 5.1 mm diameter. Fat emulsification and aspiration occurred simultaneously through the golf-tee and bullet-design cannulae at a frequency of 22.5 kHz. During the same period, Mentor Corporation introduced their Mentor Contour Genesis device. This employed 3.0 and 5.1 mm hollow cannula at a frequency of 27 kHz. Excessive ultrasound delivery to the tissues with these devices compounded with the elimination of protective wetting solution due to simultaneous aspiration during ultrasound delivery resulted in significant complications [9–11]. The popularity of ultrasound-assisted lipoplasty dwindled in the late 1990s. In 2001, Sound Surgical Technologies introduced a third-generation device that was designed to improve safety by reducing the power delivered to the tissues while maintaining efficacy. The smaller-diameter solid probes (2.2–4.5 mm) and unique grooved tip design emulsify fat efficiently at 36 kHz while preserving surrounding tissues and structures. The tunable nature of the system allows almost all body areas to be treated safely and effectively [12]. VASER® is currently the gold standard for use in high-definition body contouring. Figure 6.1 shows the difference between the smaller-diameter VASER® probes and the previous-generation large-diameter hollow cannula.

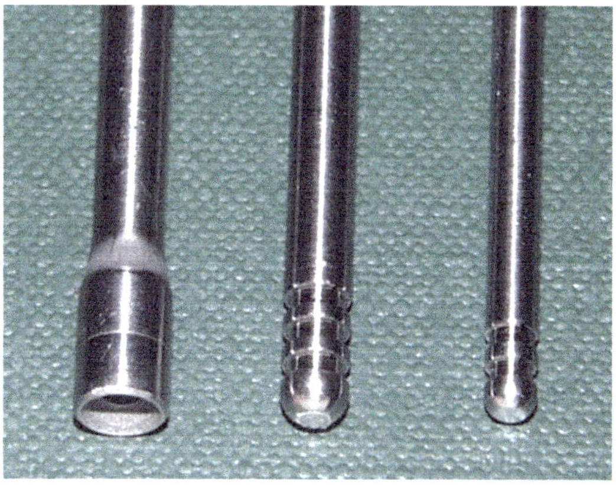

Fig. 6.1 A comparison of the third-generation VASER solid probes and the Lysonix 2000 hollow ultrasonic cannula

A.E. Hoyos, P.M. Prendergast, *High Definition Body Sculpting*,
DOI 10.1007/978-3-642-54891-8_6, © Springer-Verlag Berlin Heidelberg 2014

VASER® technology is fairly different from previous generations of ultrasound in the sense of better results and less complication rates. The key is in how it works: the resonance. Resonance is a physical effect seen in nature. It is not a laboratory reaction or an invention. The main description of what resonance is lies in music. Famous singers like Ella Fitzgerald were known for reaching a specific note breaking glass. How could a simple wave of sound do that? There is a specific frequency of natural vibration. The glass and other materials have a vibration frequency in which they start vibrating by themselves, increasing the vibration in a logarithmical way until reaching a break point.

The concept of resonance in VASER® is based in two notions: One is that the frequency of the VASER® (36 mHz) is closest to the resonance of fat. While fat vibrates, it gets emulsified with less power delivered. The second notion is the cell size: comparatively, the fat cells are ten times bigger than the other cells around (blood vessels, nerves, connective tissue), making fat more sensitive to the ultrasonic energy than the other tissues.

Principles of UAL and VASER

Vibration amplification of sound energy at resonance (VASER®) is a third-generation of ultrasound-assisted liposuction (UAL) that uses ultrasonic energy as a means to eliminate fat. Ultrasound technology emulsifies the fat for removal in such a delicate way that preserves as much of the tissue matrix as possible while emulsifying the desired amount of fatty tissue [3].

Third-generation ultrasound-assisted lipoplasty (UAL) requires three main steps: infiltration of tumescent fluid, emulsification of adipose tissue with solid probes, and aspiration of the fatty emulsion. The solid metal probes are made to vibrate at ultrasonic frequencies (above 20 kHz) in order to induce their effects on the subcutaneous fat. The basic physics of UAL, tissue interactions, and advantages of third-generation UAL in high-definition body sculpting are described in this section [3].

The UAL system comprises an electronic generator and an ultrasonic handpiece. Within the handpiece, electrical energy is converted to mechanical energy in the form of vibration through a piezoelectric transducer. This vibratory motion is channeled through the handpiece to the attached titanium probe. As such, the metal probe is made to vibrate at ultrasonic frequencies; this is 36 kHz with the VASER® system. At this resonant frequency, probes of certain lengths vibrate longitudinally with the handpiece. The forward and back movement of the probe is maximal at the tip where energy is focused. Although the displacement of the tip of the probe is only in the order of microns, it is sufficiently powerful to exhibit its effects on the surrounding tissues. By increasing the amplitude on the generator, the displacement becomes greater and the power increases. It is the interaction of the tip of the probe with the surrounding tissues that determines the efficacy of the system. The unique grooved design of the VASER® probes plays a significant role in the coupling of power to the tissues.

The tissue interaction between titanium ultrasonic probes and wet adipose tissue that leads to disruption and emulsification can be broadly divided into three mechanisms: cavitation, mechanical, and thermal [3, 13]. Although it is not certain which mechanism prevails, it is likely that cavitation and mechanical disruption of the adipose tissue are important, whereas thermal destruction of fat is undesirable and may lead to burns. Cavitation occurs when microscopic air bubbles in the tumescent fluid surrounding fat expand due to the compressive and rarefactive forces caused by the vibrating ultrasonic probe (Fig. 6.2). The bubbles (not the adipocytes) get larger and larger until they finally implode, releasing energy that disrupts the adipocytes from their architectural support within the lobules. The fat cells themselves do not burst or implode. It is important to remember that the cavitation process occurs close to the tip of the probe, in a halo region within a few millimeters of it. It does not occur in a spray gun fashion. As such, the probe must pass methodically in every proposed treatment area.

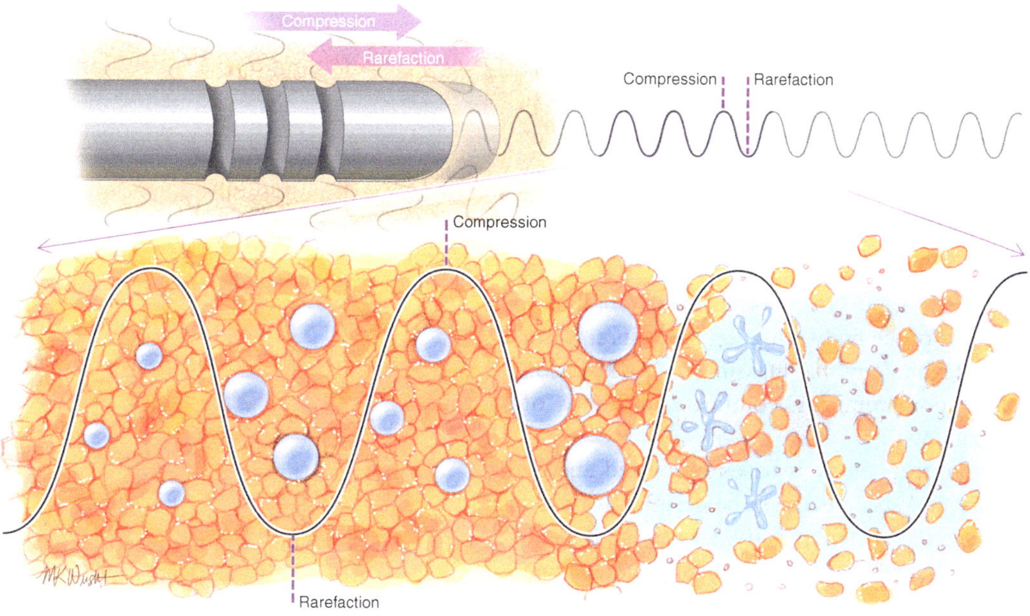

Fig. 6.2 The cavitation effect. The VASER® probes vibrate at ultrasonic frequencies creating compressive and rarefactive forces around the grooved tip. Cavitation microbubbles expand and then implode, releasing energy that disrupts the adipocyte architecture until an emulsion of fat and fluid is formed

Mechanical disruption of fat occurs at the tip of the probe, where the vibrating metal surface comes in contact with the adipocytes. If the probe is not in constant to-and-fro motion within the tissues, the high-frequency vibration begins to heat the tissues. This thermal energy is not the desired mechanism of action of UAL and only serves to increase the incidence of burns and seromas. Cavitation and mechanical disruption of adipose tissue occurs due to the relative fragility of this tissue compared to other tissues such as vessels, muscle, and nerves.

The main advantages of the VASER® third-generation UAL system relate to its safety, smoothness, and ability to treat the superficial tissues. VASER® is safer than previous UAL technologies for a number of reasons. Firstly, solid probes are used so the protective tumescent fluid is not withdrawn during ultrasound delivery to the tissues. Ultrasound energy should never be delivered to dry tissues. Secondly, the probes are smaller in diameter compared to its predecessors. Since the amount of energy delivered to tissues is approximately proportional to the square of the diameter of the probe, narrower probes deliver much less energy and are safer. The efficiency of the narrower VASER® probes is not just preserved but increased due to the grooves at the tip of the probes. The grooves increase surface area and increase coupling with the surrounding tissues. Cavitation occurs in front of as well as to the sides of the grooved tip, increasing efficiency and reducing the amount of total energy required to disrupt a given volume of adipose tissue. Thirdly, ultrasound energy delivered to the tissues is selective for lobules of fat bathed in tumescent solution, such that collateral damage to the tissue matrix, lymphatics, nerves, and vessels is minimized. This translates to an easier recovery for the patient with less bruising, swelling, and pain. The ability to halve energy delivered to the tissues using the pulsed (VASER) mode is important during the very superficial work required for high-definition lipoplasty. Fourthly, the unique vented cannulae and small port holes featured with the VentX design facilitate refined contouring in delicate and superficial tissues and reduce avulsion and trauma to tissues. Finally, VASER®-assisted lipoplasty has shown to reduce blood loss and improve skin retraction compared to suction-assisted lipoplasty [14]. This has important implications in high-definition contouring where large surface areas are often treated in a single procedure and where excellent skin retraction is essential in order to reveal underlying muscular anatomy.

VASER® Lipo System is designed to optimize all phases of the body sculpting procedure. It is a unique technology that maximizes fat extraction without compromising comfort and safety of their patients.

As the technology is based on pulsed energy delivery and specialized probe designs, we need to know the different fatty tissues and some other technical aspects to actually understand why VASER® is by now the gold-standard in liposculpture.

VASER® Technology and Instrumentation

The VASER® (Valeant Pharmaceuticals North America LLC, Bridgewater, NJ) third-generation ultrasound-assisted lipoplasty console consists of an integrated system including all the elements required for flow rate-controlled tumescent infiltration, tissue-selective destruction of fat, negative pressure aspiration, and collection of emulsified fat in disposable canisters. Foot pedals control infiltration and ultrasound delivery, and dials on the digital display component adjust flow rate and ultrasound power output (Fig. 6.3). The amplitude of energy can be adjusted at the console in increments of 10 %, from zero to 100 %. The solid titanium probes are attached to the ultrasonic handpiece using an attachable wrench to ensure a snug fit (Fig. 6.4). The probes are used to emulsify fat in an extra step before aspiration, thus preserving the fluid medium required to protect tissues from excessive ultrasound energy.

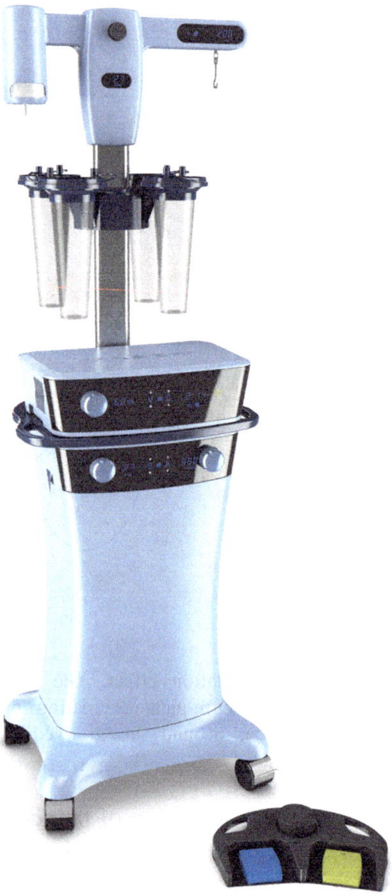

Fig. 6.3 The VASER® (Valeant Pharmaceuticals North America LLC, Bridgewater, NJ) console

Probes are small in diameter (2.2, 2.9, 3.7, and 4.5 mm) and contain grooves at the distal ends in such an arrangement that ultrasound energy is delivered both from the tip and from the sides of the probe in varying ratios depending on whether a one-, two-, or three-grooved probe is used (Fig. 6.5). The 2.2 mm probe is used for facial applications and the others for body applications depending on the volume of tissue treated. The result of the grooved probe design is improved efficiency of emulsification of fatty tissues using less energy than would be required with previous instruments. In general, a probe with fewer grooves is used for disrupting more fat in fibrous areas and a probe with more grooves is used for debulking softer fat. A specialized "arrow" probe is also available for treating gynecomastia (Fig. 6.5).

Previous ultrasound systems delivered energy to the tissues continuously once

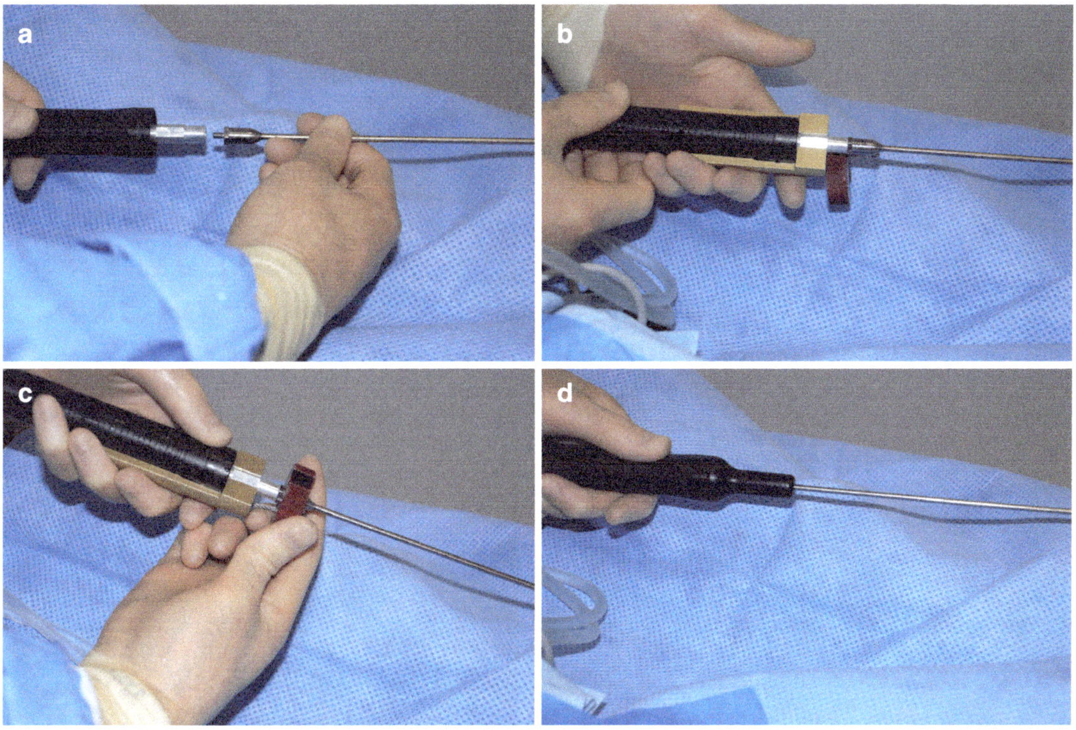

Fig. 6.4 (**a**) The solid titanium VASER® probe is screwed into the ultrasonic handpiece. (**b**) The handpiece fits snugly into the housing of the wrench. (**c**) The wrench is used to gently tighten the root of the probe. (**d**) An appropriately sized plastic casing covers the hub of the probe

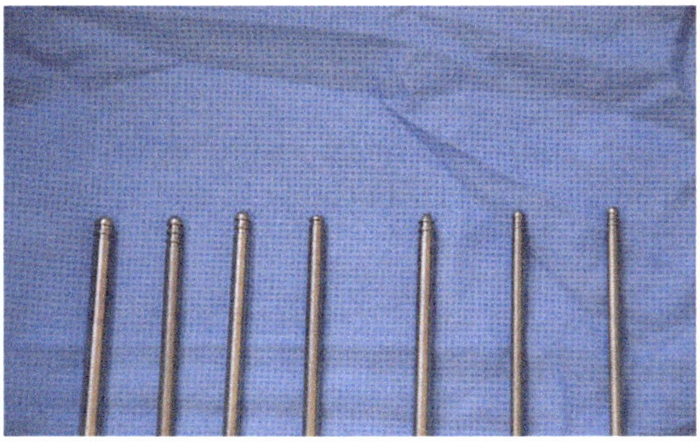

Fig. 6.5 VASER® ultrasonic probes. From left to right: 4.5 mm probe, 3.7 mm 3-groove probe, 3.7 mm 2-groove probe, 3.7 mm 1-groove probe, arrow probe, 2.9 mm probe

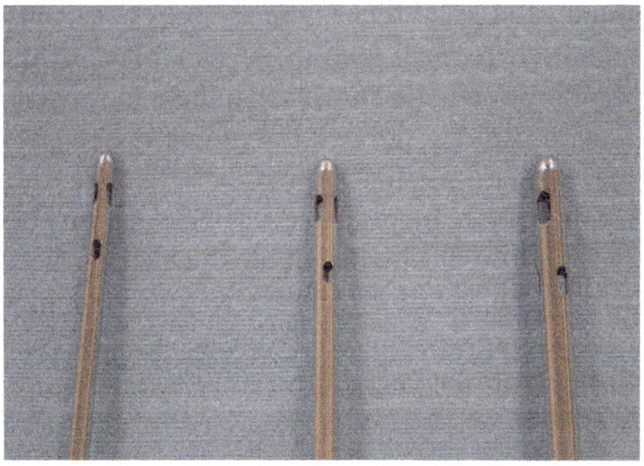

Fig. 6.6 VentX cannula tips. From left to right: 3.0, 3.7, and 4.6 mm cannulae. The total area of the ports is balanced with the cross-sectional area of the cannula to improve efficiency and reduce trauma

activated. With the VASER® system, the option to deliver energy continuously or in a pulsed mode is available. Pulsed, or VASER®, mode delivers 10 bursts of energy per second, roughly halving the total energy delivered to the tissues while maintaining efficiency. VASER® mode is utilized in delicate areas or during high-definition work very close to the dermis. The VentX cannulae were designed for use with VASER® and have smaller port holes than standard liposuction cannulae of the same diameter (Fig. 6.6). This feature reduces avulsion and

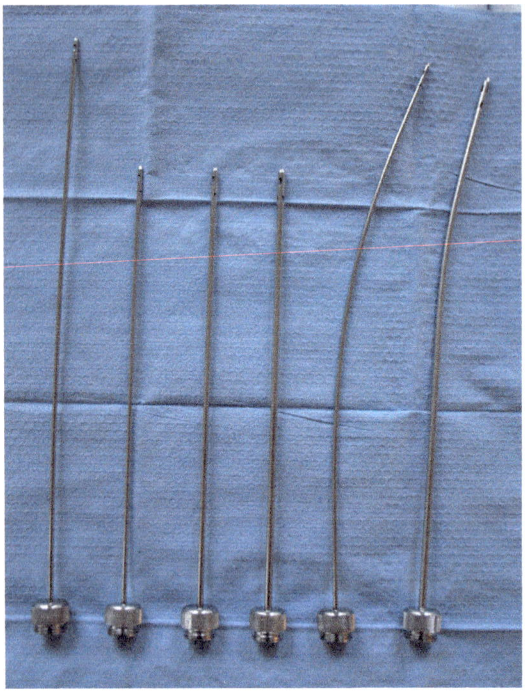

Fig. 6.7 Straight, long, and curved cannulae designed for body contouring. Long and curved cannulae are important when utilizing hidden (stealth) incisions in high-definition lipoplasty

trauma to tissues during the aspiration of emulsified fat. A small hole in the handpiece of the aspiration cannula ensures that there is constant flow of aspirate through the tubing, even when the cannula is in the patient. The venting through the cannula reduces the vacuum and reduces trauma to the tissues. This has been termed the VentX effect. The various cannulae used for high-definition lipoplasty are designed to improve efficiency, treat superficial tissues, minimize trauma, and access entire aesthetic units from hidden incisions. VentX cannulae optimize efficiency and ensure continuous even suction even when the cannula is in the tissues. These include 3.0, 3.7, and 4.6 mm cannulae and are available in straight, angled, or curved designs (Fig. 6.7) [15]. Powered cannulae that are relatively atraumatic may also be used during the aspiration phase following VASER® emulsification to accelerate the process (Fig. 6.8). A 4 mm blunt tip basket cannula is utilized for releasing fibrous tissue and improving unwanted contour irregularities and cellulite (Fig. 6.9).

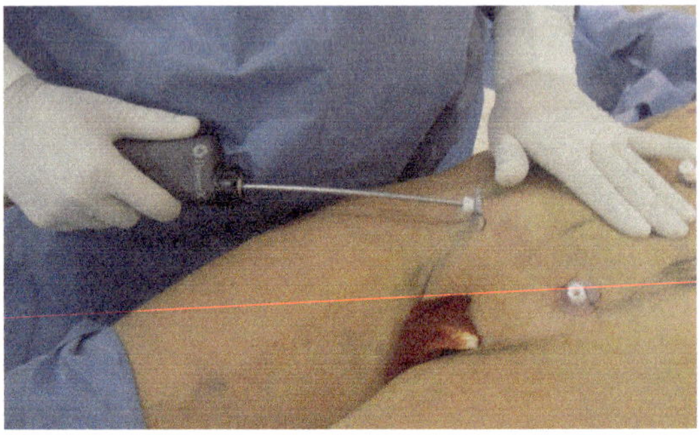

Fig. 6.8 The PowerX power-assisted handpiece and cannula

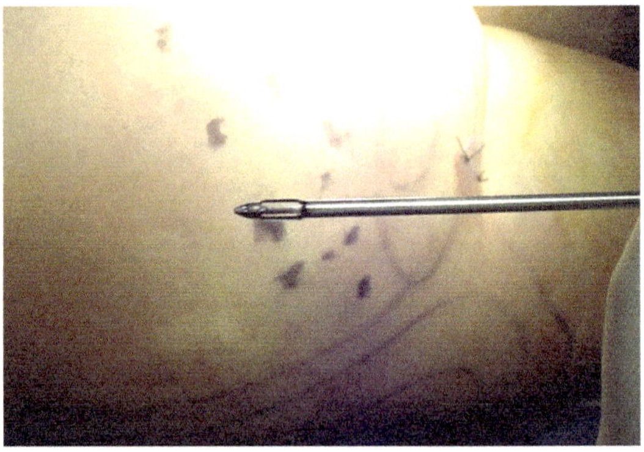

Fig. 6.9 Basket cannula for releasing fibrous bands and treating cellulite

VASER® Technique

The tumescent technique is described in Chap. 5. Once sufficient time has elapsed for vasoconstriction following tumescence, an appropriately sized and grooved VASER® probe is selected depending on the volume of fat present and whether the tissues are soft or fibrous (Table 6.1). For high-definition sculpting, the superficial subdermal subcutaneous fat should be treated first in VASER® mode. The author usually commences here with a 3.7 mm two-grooved probe using amplitude of 80 %. Gentle but deliberate,

Table 6.1 Author's preferred VASER® probe selection according to the volume of fat and density of tissues for high-definition lipoplasty

Density	Volume	Probe	Mode[a]	Energy (%)
Soft	Medium–large	3.7 mm (3 grooves)	Continuous	70–80
Soft	Small	2.9 mm (3 grooves) or 3.7 mm (2 grooves)	Continuous or pulsed	70–80
Slightly fibrous	Medium–large	3.7 mm (2 grooves)	Continuous	80–90
Slightly fibrous	Small	2.9 mm (3 grooves) or 3.7 mm (1 groove)	Continuous	80–90
Very fibrous	Medium–large	3.7 mm (2 grooves) or 3.7 mm (1 groove)	Continuous	80–90
Very fibrous	Small	2.9 mm (3 grooves)	Continuous	80–90

[a]All superficial ultrasound delivery within 10 mm of the dermis should be performed on pulsed mode

long to-and-fro strokes are made with the operating hand like the bow movements of a cellist. Movements should be graceful and continuous with no torquing which could conduct excessive heat through the skin port and result in a burn. Although the skin port protects the skin around the incision to some degree, wet towels folded twice should be placed adjacent to the port during ultrasound delivery to protect the skin from contact with the probe. The probe should be parallel to the skin and guided by the nondominant hand. Some resistance is felt as the probe gently creates tunnels through the fat, but it should not stop the probe in its path or require grasping and pushing of the probe with the operating hand. If excessive resistance is encountered, energy is increased to 90 %, or an alternative probe is selected. The author continues emulsification until no resistance is encountered in the treatment area so that the skin is undermined and allowed to redrape during the postoperative period. Ultrasound is only delivered inside the patient and in an area where there is sufficient wetting solution. Since tumescence is a temporary state, some reinfiltration of tumescent fluid may be required in the superficial plane immediately prior to emulsification. As well as emulsifying fat in the ipsilateral side, the probes are long enough to pass to the contralateral side and this criss-crossing maneuver is important for smooth, even results. As well as emulsifying all marked areas to a point of minimal or no resistance, feathering should be done by emulsifying to a lesser degree in border areas to create smooth transitions between contours. After the superficial fat is treated, continuous mode is used to emulsify the deeper fat. A total of 60–90 s of ultrasound delivery per 100 ml of tumescent fluid infiltrated is usually used, but the endpoint is predominantly determined by the feel of the tissues rather than timing. Once emulsification is complete, skin ports are removed and a suitably sized suction cannula is inserted. In general, smaller cannulae are less likely to create post-liposuction defects and irregularities. The author uses 3.7 and 3.0 mm VentX cannulae which have port sizes smaller than those on 3.0 and 2.4 mm Mercedes cannulae, respectively. Aspiration of emulsified fat is easy and requires little force. To increase efficiency further, the PowerX system is employed. This generates up to 360° of alternating clockwise and anticlockwise rotation of the cannula at a rate of up to 420 times per minute. Various aspiration orifice patterns are used with the PowerX system, including standard, Mercedes, Spiral, and Mendieta. During aspiration, the operating hand moves forward and backward radially like the spokes of a wheel while the other hand stabilizes the skin over the tip of the cannula. As suction continues, the pinch test is performed intermittently to assess symmetry and reduction in thickness of the fat layer. In traditional body contouring, the endpoint is reached when the desired amount of debulking and improvement in body contour has been achieved based on the pinch test and careful inspection from different vantage points in the operating room. In high-definition body sculpting, additional very superficial lipoplasty is performed with small cannulae in order to create controlled irregularities and negative spaces. These techniques are described elsewhere in this book.

Advantages

Since the advent of ultrasound-assisted liposuction, many different affirmations have been down around its convenience or its avoidance. This is the time where evidence-based medicine could support different statements around VASER® and liposculpture.

Different studies have been published supporting the use of ultrasound in cosmetic surgery and VASER® is not the exception. In a multicenter single-blinded study was demonstrated the safety use of VASER® in a vast amount of procedures. No major complications were reported with its use and advantages were mentioned as surgery time was shorter than standard liposuction; this is associated with the easier way to extract the fatty tissue after ultrasound emulsification [16]. Moreover, surgeons around the world have experienced its particularly advantageous for tight, fibrous areas such as the back and posterior flanks, areas where increased blood loss would be expected with standard liposuction. Following this idea, they have also concluded that VASER® reduces the surgeon effort [16].

In our experience we can infer that surgery length might be shortened and surgeon efficiency improved due to the minor trauma over tissues and the easy way to perform liposuction as the fat emulsification softens the aspirate technique. Also, we have noticed that smaller incisions had to be made to access the different zones for lipo.

Although, VASER®-assisted lipoplasty typically takes longer than standard suction-assisted lipoplasty due to the extra step required for emulsification of adipose tissue before aspiration, the technology has several advantages. Fine probes and tunable power allow delicate and superficial tissues to be treated without causing unwanted irregularities. The unique pulsed (VASER®) mode also halves the energy delivered to the tissues and represents an important feature for subdermal clearance of fat without causing complications. In order to treat fibrous tissue such as the back or male breasts, the power output is increased, continuous ultrasound is selected, and a more aggressive probe, such as the one-grooved or arrow probe, is selected. The cavitation and mechanical forces that are produced with the VASER® probes vibrating at ultrasonic frequencies disrupt relatively weak adipose tissue much more readily than more dense tissue such as vessels, nerves, and fibrous septae. As a result, there is a selective emulsification of fat with sparing of surrounding tissues. This translates to less bleeding, less bruising, and an easier and more rapid recovery for the patient than suction-assisted lipoplasty. The majority of fat aspirated following treatment with VASER® is viable. This is particularly important for high-definition body sculpting where large volumes of fat may be used to contour the buttocks, hips, or breasts.

References

1. Cimino WW (2010) History of ultrasound-assisted lipoplasty. In: Shiffman MA, Di Giuseppe A (eds) Body contouring: art, science, and clinical practice. Springer, Berlin, p 399
2. Panetta NJ, Gupta DM, Kwan MD, Wan DC, Commons GW, Longaker MT (2009) Tissue harvest by means of suction assisted or third-generation ultrasound-assisted lipoaspiration has no effect on osteogenic potential of human adipose-derived stromal cells. Plast Reconstr Surg 124(1):65–73
3. Cimino WW (1999) The physics of soft tissue fragmentation using ultrasonic frequency vibrations of metal probes. Clin Plast Surg 26:447–461
4. Kelman C (1967) Phacoemulsification and aspiration. A new technique of cataract removal. A preliminary report. Am J Ophthalmol 64(1):23–25
5. Ogawa T, Hattori R, Yamamoto T, Gotoh M (2011) Safe use of ultrasonically activated devices based on current studies. Expert Rev Med Devices 8(3): 319–324
6. Scuderi N, Devita R, D'Andrea F, Vonella M (1987) Nuove prospettive nella liposuzione la lipoemulsificazone. Giorn Chir Plast Ricostr ed Estetica 2(1):33–39
7. Zocchi ML (1993) Clinical aspects of ultrasonic liposculpture. Perspect Plast Surg 7:153–174

8. Zocchi ML (1996) Ultrasonic assisted lipoplasty. Clin Plast Surg 23(4):575–598
9. Troilius C (1999) Ultrasound-assisted lipoplasty: is it really safe? Aesthet Plast Surg 23(5):307–311
10. Baxter RA (1999) Histologic effects of ultrasound-assisted lipoplasty. Aesthet Surg J 19:109–114
11. Grolleau JL, Rouge D, Chavoin JP, Costagliola M (1997) Severe cutaneous necrosis after ultrasound lipolysis. Medicolegal aspects and review. Ann Chir Plast Esthet 42(1):31–36
12. Cimino WW (2001) Ultrasonic surgery: power quantification and efficiency optimization. Aesthet Surg J 21(3):233–240
13. Cimino WW (2010) Ultrasound-assisted lipoplasty: basic physics, tissue interactions, and related results/complications. In: Shiffman MA, Di Giuseppe A (eds) Body contouring: art, science, and clinical practice. Springer, Berlin, p 392
14. Nagy MW, Vanek PF Jr (2012) A multicenter, prospective, randomized, single-blind, controlled clinical trial comparing VASER-assisted lipoplasty and suction-assisted lipoplasty. Plast Reconstr Surg 129(4):681e–689e
15. Cimino WW (2006) VASER-assisted lipoplasty: technology and technique. In: Shiffman MA, Di Giuseppe A (eds) Liposuction principles and practice. Springer-Verlag Berlin Heidelberg, pp 239–244
16. Jewell ML, Fodor PB, de Souza Pinto EB, Al Shammari MA (2002) Clinical application of VASER–assisted lipoplasty: a pilot clinical study. Aesthet Surg J 22(2):131–146

Fat Anatomy, Metabolism, and Principles of Grafting

7

Liquid Gold

In the 1999 movie *Fight Club*, Tyler Durden, played by Brad Pitt, makes a living stealing fat from plastic surgery clinics and turning it into bars of soap. Who could foresee that the waste we throw away after every liposuction procedure could be recycled for another use?

Recycling industrial and human effluence has become an industry in itself. Fat is no exception. Some restaurants donate used animal and vegetable fat for use as biofuel for cars. Why not human fat? Although the prospect of using human adipose tissue as an energy source in industry seems bizarre, its use as an autotransplant in aesthetic surgery for beautification has been broadly accepted. To many surgeons, it has become liquid gold, allowing natural contouring of the body—even large surface areas—without many of the risks associated with silicone implants.

In 1893 Gustav Adolf Neuber first reported fat grafting as a surgical procedure at the 22nd meeting of the "Deutschen Gesellschaft für Chirurgie" in Berlin. The proceedings of this meeting were published in German only, and this limited the dissemination of fat grafting as an innovative technique to the non-German speaking world. In the 1980s, almost a century later, the idea of fat grafting gained new interest, particularly when liposuction techniques were popularized.

In the early 1980s, the Argentinian plastic surgeon Abel Chajchir conducted pioneering fat grafting procedures in humans [1, 2]. He designed instruments to aspirate fat, systems to freeze the fat, and techniques for subsequent grafting. This idea of volume replacement using one's own fat was explored by only a few pioneers at the time, and generally disregarded or ignored by the rest of the medical community. Another visionary surgeon, Sydney Coleman, developed his technique of lipostructure and transformed fat grafting from an unreliable procedure to one that is safe, effective, and generally regarded as the gold standard in autologous fat transfer [3, 4]. Tiny pearls of fat are grafted using special blunt cannulae.

Zuk et al. reported the presence of stem cells in human adult fat in 2002 [5]. Since stem cells can differentiate into almost any type of cell, the promise of tissue regeneration from adipose-derived stem cells has become the subject of international research efforts. The fat that was once discarded after liposuction may be employed to restore damaged, aged, or atrophied tissues. Conditions such as diabetes, degenerative diseases, and even normal aging may be ameliorated by processing harvested lipoaspirate.

On the one hand, adipose tissue is regarded as undesirable and its excess is evident as the problem of obesity continues to grow worldwide. On the other hand, adipose tissue is acknowledged as essential for hormonal and metabolic processes and thermoregulation and for contributing to the beautiful curves and contours of the human

A.E. Hoyos, P.M. Prendergast, *High Definition Body Sculpting*,
DOI 10.1007/978-3-642-54891-8_7,

form. International organizations, such as the International Federation for Adipose Therapeutics and Science, run dedicated educational and scientific activities devoted to fat.

Fat Metabolism and Endocrinology

Fatty tissue is the largest energy reserve in the body. At birth, fat represents about 17 % of bodyweight; in adolescence, around 20 % in women; and 10 % in men with some phenotypic variations. In normal adults, fat approaches 15–20 % in men and 25–30 % in women. Two types of fat are described in the human body: white adipose tissue and brown adipose tissue.

The distribution of body fat varies between populations in different countries. However, fat excess in the upper body is often associated with certain disease states, especially metabolic disorders. Fat distribution is determined by a complex interplay between central regulation in the hypothalamus, receptors in the adipose tissue, and the various molecules that interact with these receptors. Catecholamines, insulin, growth hormone, steroids, and diverse neuropeptides modulate activity at these receptors. Lipogenesis and lipolysis are regulated by lipase lipoprotein and hormone-sensitive lipase, respectively. This system is regulated mainly in the hypothalamus where an assemblage of regulatory centers governs homeostasis. The ventromedial nucleus of the hypothalamus serves as a satiety center and the lateral hypothalamic area serves as a feeding center. They coordinate the processes that govern eating behavior and the subjective perception of satiety. Further, the secretion of hormones from the thyroid gland, adrenal gland, and pancreatic islet cells is influenced by these areas in response to metabolic stress.

The hypothalamus regulates caloric intake, utilization, and storage in a manner that tends to maintain the body weight in adulthood. Although the biochemical mechanisms that control fat deposits are well recognized, the presumptive set point around which it attempts to stabilize body weight is poorly defined or maintained, as it changes readily with changes in physical activity, composition of the diet, emotional states, stress, pregnancy, and so on. Carbohydrate metabolism is functionally related to lipogenesis in the adipose tissue. Both processes are regulated in the liver in order to obtain the energy from glucose the body needs in different metabolic situations.

Mechanisms involved in obesity-related pathologies include increased fatty acid input to the portal circulation, tumor necrosis factor and angiotensin II production, and steroidogenesis. Adipocyte insulin resistance may be implicated in the complex pathogenesis of obesity.

White fat cells (adipocytes) produce leptin, a key hormone in the regulation of body weight. Starvation corresponds to low leptin levels, while obesity corresponds to high levels of leptin. The hypothalamus specifically controls the feeding process depending on the signals received from the cells in the gastrointestinal tract and on the leptin levels.

Primarily, brown fat cells play a thermoregulatory role in mammals. However, thermogenic defects observed in some obesity models in animals do establish a link with the development of obesity. In humans, brown fat cells play an important role in heat production, at least in the perinatal period. However, the complete role of brown fat is not fully understood. The possibility to pharmacologically stimulate these fat cells makes them a potential target for therapeutic intervention in obesity.

Fatty tissue also plays an important role as an energy source during exercise. Fat, the major energy store in the body, is mobilized from adipose tissue as free fatty acids to provide metabolic fuel. At lower exercise intensities, fats may provide 50–60 % of the energy for muscle contraction, but this process cannot keep pace with the high demands for energy that occur during heavy exercise. Energy liberation from fat is slower than the liberation of glucose from glycogen. Moderate activity, in fact, favors the consumption of fat as muscle fuel. The depletion of body fat reserves is almost never a limiting factor in muscle activity. In the absence of other fuels, proteins can serve as an energy source for contraction, particularly as it occurs during heavy, prolonged, or intense exercise.

Fat Anatomy: The Subcutaneous Tissue and Superficialis Fascia

The subcutaneous tissue is an organ that has received limited attention by anatomists. Is has been widely known as a three-layer system divided by a membranous tissue. This tissue layer has received many names such as superficial fascia, Scarpa's fascia, Colles' fascia, and Camper's fascia [6–9]. The varied nomenclature can be somewhat confusing.

Current classification divides this structure into three layers: a superficial adipose tissue layer (SAT), an intermediate membranous layer (superficialis fascia), and a deep adipose tissue layer (DAT) (Fig. 7.1) [8, 9].

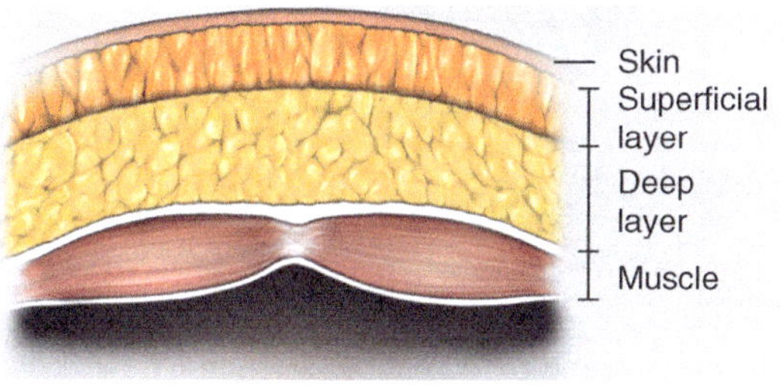

Fig. 7.1 Fat anatomy. Composed of two main layers: superficial and deep. A third intermediate layer is composed of the superficial fascia

The SAT layer is characterized by fibrous septa that define polygonal lobes of fat tissue. The thickness of this layer is relatively constant throughout the body. It is this layer that correlates with the pinch test that is commonly used to gauge the depth of insertion of the cannula for suction lipectomy.

The intermediate membranous layer is a continuous fibrous membrane rich in elastic fibers.

In the DAT layer the obliquely oriented fibrous septa define large and flat lobes of fat tissue. The boundary between this layer and the muscle consists of a filmy membranous sheet called the innominate or Gallaudet's fascia. This fascial layer is tightly adherent to and often undistinguishable from the underlying muscle fascia. This layer varies significantly according to anatomic region; it is usually thicker in the periumbilical region over the rectus abdominis muscle sheath and tapers laterally as it approached the external oblique muscle.

The thickness and proportion of these layers varies throughout the body depending on the anatomic region (Fig. 7.2) and on the characteristics of the patient. These variations have been studied and clearly characterized for some areas:

- The abdominal area has a prominent fascial plane, making it easier to distinguish between the two fatty layers. The SAT is thicker in the

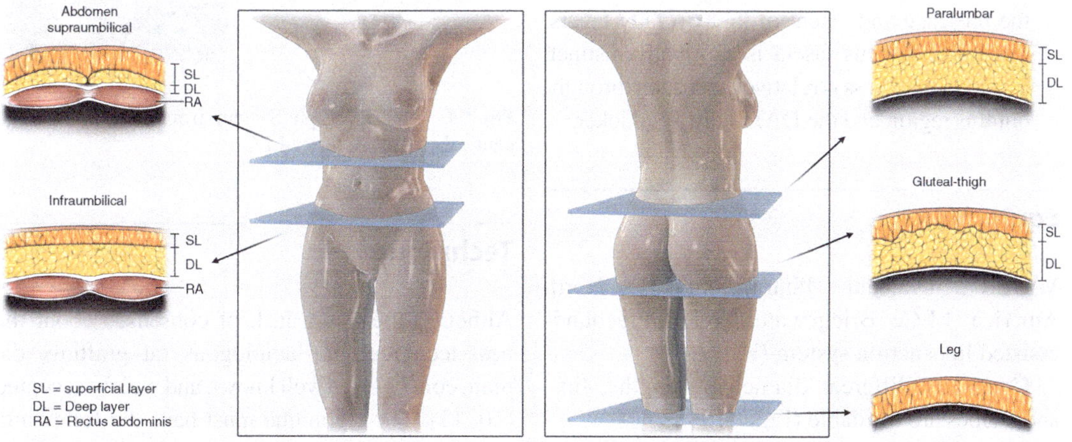

Fig. 7.2 Relationship of fat layer thickness with anatomic area thoughout the body

upper abdomen and thinner in the lower abdomen. The DAT is always thicker in the periumbilical region over the rectus sheath and tapers laterally as it approached the external oblique muscle.

- In the leg the SAT/DAT division is not clear. There is an attenuated fibrous membrane barely discernible beneath a single layer of subcutaneous fat and separating it from the underlying muscle fascia. The adipose tissue is similar to the superficial fatty layer of the trunk in gross appearance, density, and structure.
- In the gluteus and thighs the subcutaneous fascia fuses with the gluteal crease and infragluteal fold medially and with the iliac crest superiorly. Laterally and inferiorly the subcutaneous fascia continues uninterrupted into the thigh where it merges with the iliotibial tract. The SAT depth is quite constant throughout the buttocks, while the DAT is more prominent over the gluteal muscles and iliotibial tract having a maximal thickness of about 5 cm below the iliac crest. It is thinner over the trochanter, and thinner again as it proceeds distally down the thigh. This layer appears dense and rather compact, with regularly spaced fat lobules bound by sturdy fibrous septa. It is often indistinguishable from the superficial layer.
- The paralumbar subcutaneous adipose tissue resembles that of the abdomen with respect to the presence and extent of the two fatty layers. The subcutaneous fascia is especially distinct. The SAT thickness is relatively constant throughout this region and the DAT is always thicker.

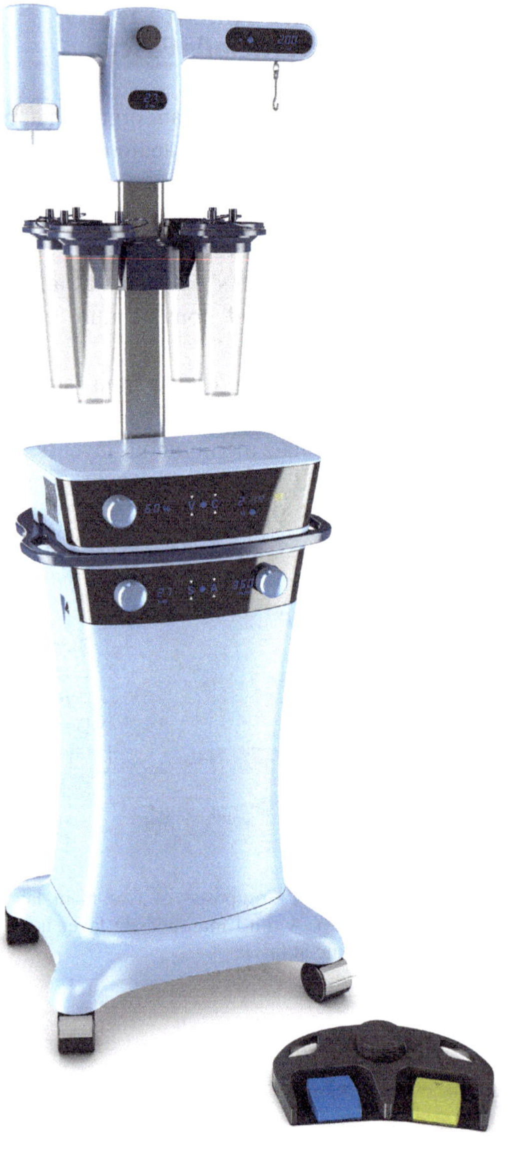

Fig.7.3 VASER® Lipo System from Valeant Pharmaceuticals North America LLC

Equipment

VASER® (Valeant Pharmaceuticals North America LLC, Bridgewater, NJ) ultrasound-assisted liposuction system (Fig. 7.3)

Cannulae: different diameters, lengths, tips, and shapes are available (Fig 7.4).

Fat collection and separation systems (Fig. 7.5)

Syringes (Fig. 7.6)

Centrifuge (Fig. 7.7)

Technique

Although there is a lack of consensus about the best technique for autologous fat grafting, the main concepts are well known and widely accepted [10, 11]. The technique must have the following: (1) a properly selected donor site, (2) a relatively atraumatic method for harvesting, (3) suitable post-extraction management of the graft and, and

(4) an injection procedure that maximizes structural integrity, nutrition, and survival of the fat.

Donor Site

The selection of the donor site is either based on the surgeon's preference, chosen because of ease or accessibility, or chosen by the patient. The most commonly used sites for large volume fat harvesting are the abdomen, thighs, flanks, buttocks, and breast. Whether one site yields fat that is more viable when grafted over another is not known. However, recent work has shown that adipose-derived stem cells can improve the longevity and volume of the fat graft [12]. These cells are predominantly found in the lipoaspirate from the inner thigh and lower abdomen and therefore make these areas ideal sites for harvesting (Fig. 7.8).

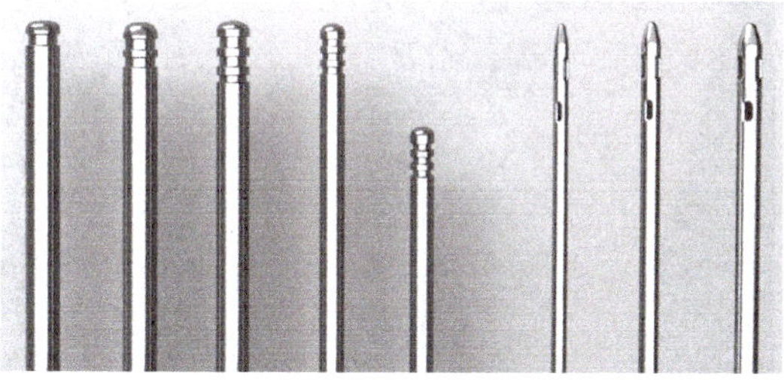

Fig. 7.4 VASER® probes and cannulae. VASER® probes have a different number of rings to efficiently emulsify fat of varying degrees of fibrousness: 3-ring probe for soft fat, 2-ring probe for moderate fat, 1-ring probe for hard fatty or fibrous tissue. The "SST" cannulae used with the VASER® system have smaller holes than other cannulae. The surface area of the holes allows improved efficiency while minimizing trauma during aspiration

Harvesting

Debate continues over the optimal harvesting technique for autologous fat grafting. The two main techniques employed are machine liposuction and syringe aspiration. In both, the histological structure is preserved, but it seems that the cellular function of adipocytes is better preserved following syringe aspiration. What is clear is that controlling the vacuum pressure is essential. When the vacuum exceeds 700 mmHg, the tissue is damaged and the cell viability is significantly compromised. The Coleman technique appears to achieve a superior level of cellular function

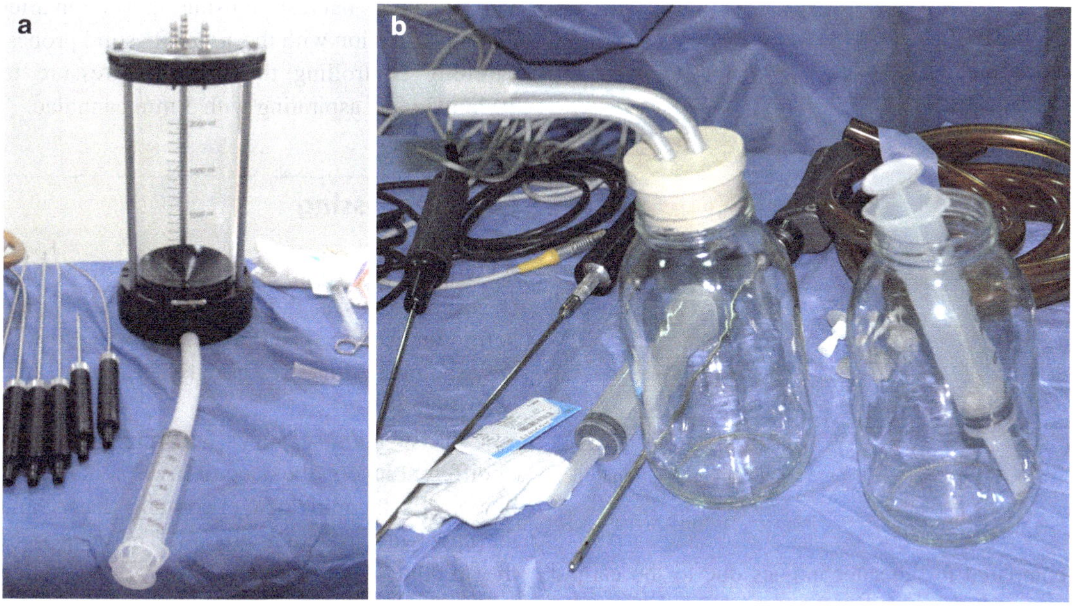

Fig. 7.5 Fat collector systems: (**a**) closed (**b**) open system

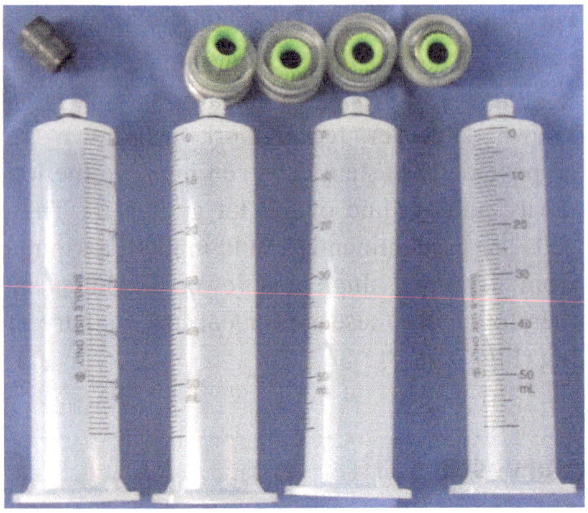

Fig. 7.6 Syringes used for centrifugation and fat injection (Lipokit® system)

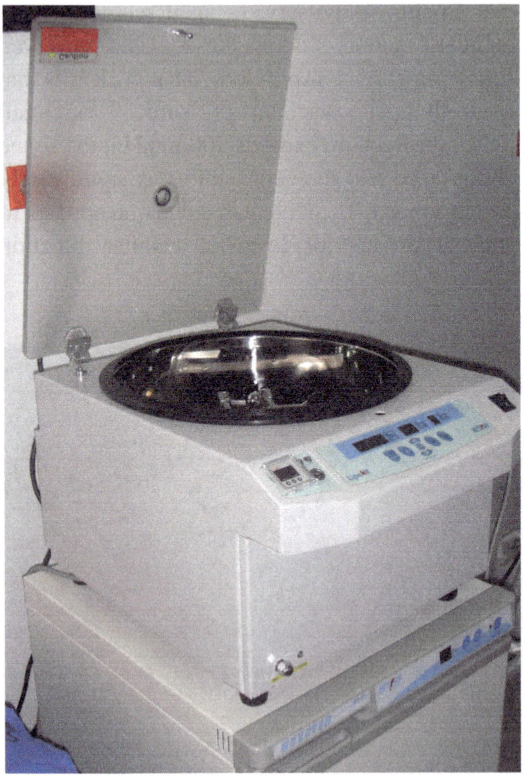

Fig. 7.7 Lipokit® Centrifuge (Medikan International Inc.)

compared to other techniques due to the careful management of the graft with small cannulae. This technique is mainly used for facial procedures.

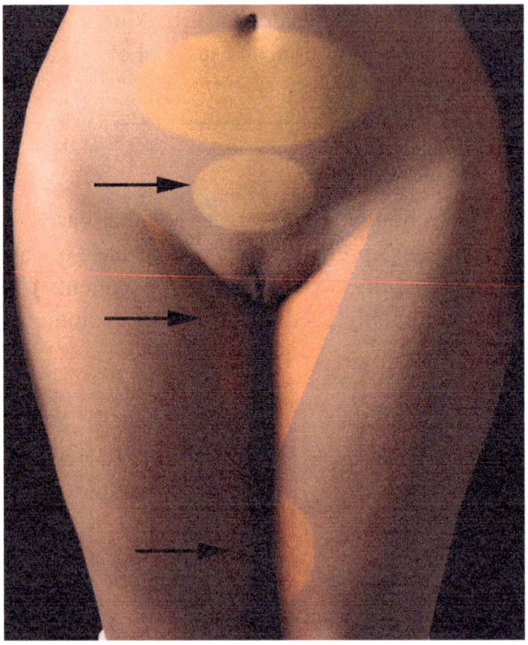

Fig. 7.8 Ideal harvesting sites for stem cell-rich fat (*arrows*)

The ideal cannula for harvesting was initially believed to be the one with the largest diameter. However, it is now known that the most important consideration is to control the negative pressure and keep it to a minimum.

The authors harvest fat using liposuction after fat emulsification with the VASER® solid probes, carefully controlling the negative pressure to 10 mmHg and aspirating with 3 mm cannulae.

Graft Processing

As with the previous steps in fat harvesting, there is no consensus in the best way to process fat before reinjection. The three main methods used are sedimentation by gravity, filtering, and centrifugation.

Centrifugation separates fat, lipids, and cells in different layers: the deepest layer contains the blood cells, the middle layer contains the fat, and the upper layer contains the oil. The deepest of the middle layer contains most of the viable adipose cells and many angiogenic growth factors (Fig. 7.9). The speed of centrifugation is

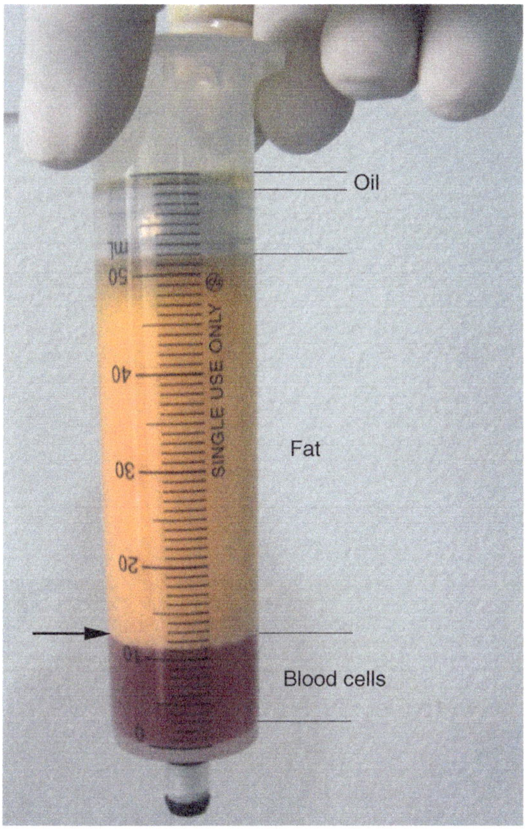

Fig. 7.9 Decantation layers after centrifugation: blood cells, fat, and oil. The lowest fat layer (*arrow*) contains most of the viable adipose cells and angiogenic growth factors

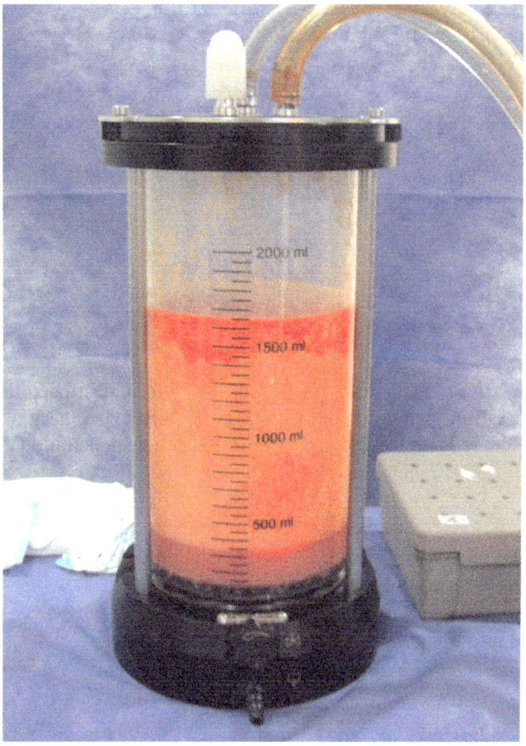

Fig. 7.10 Fat collection after gravity decantation

important in order to yield the most viable cells. The best survival rate is achieved by centrifuging between 1,500 and 3,000 rpm for up to 5 min; if centrifugation is employed, we recommend 3,000 rpm for 3 min or the use of 1,200 G of optimal centrifugal force. The graft obtained by this means has also a higher density, which has a better survival rate.

When the harvested tissue is decanted, more viable adipocytes are found compared to centrifugation but there are less stem cells and more contamination with blood cells. The centrifugation may damage more adipocytes but holds a higher amount of stem cells.

We use the decantation process for most cases, by removing the infranatant and adding antibiotic (Fig. 7.10). In small-volume fat grafting, we prefer to use centrifugation to maximize the fat survival. This is used for fat grafting to deltoids, breasts, and calves.

Injection Procedures

It is generally accepted that using a single-bolus injection with large volumes of fat produces unwanted results and even complications. The thicker the graft, the higher the risk of failure because the graft survival depends on the nutritional support, vascularization, and oxygenation from surrounding tissues [13–15].

The graft can be placed in multiple layers. However, when placed in the muscular layer, the survival is improved.

The grafts are placed using a 3 mm cannula (Fig. 7.11) in small amounts injected as the cannula is withdrawn in a retrograde motion. This must be performed in multiple threads, through multiple tunnels, and at different tissue planes (Fig. 7.12). The details of anatomical placement will be discussed in each specific chapter on technique.

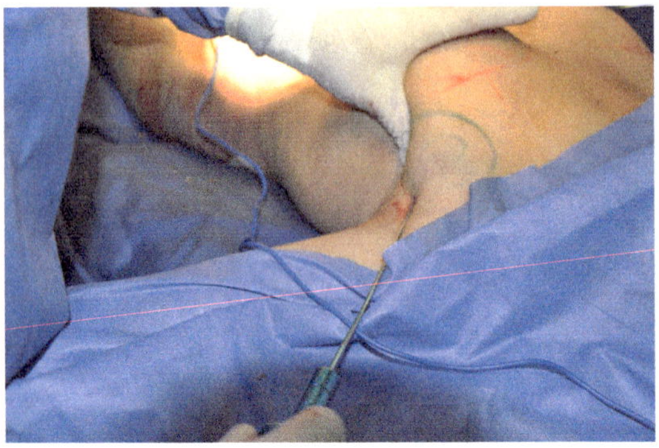

Fig. 7.11 Curved 3 mm cannula used for breast-pectoral grafting helps the surgeon to adequately place the graft and reduces the risk of inadvertent thoracic penetration

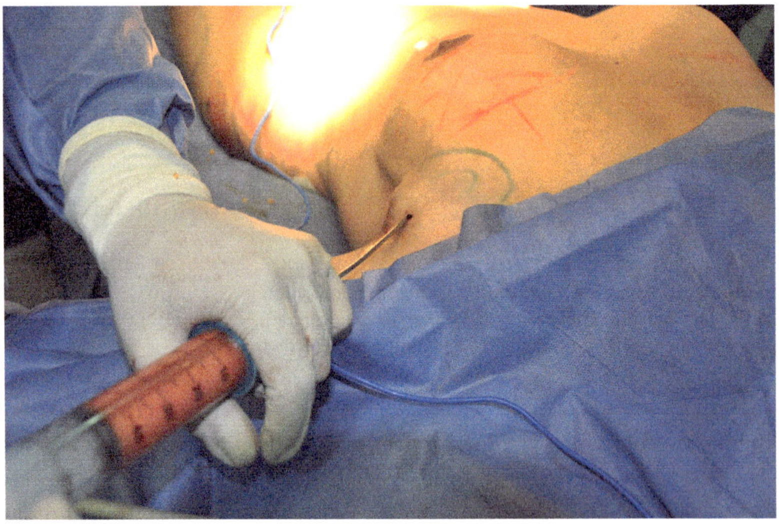

Fig. 7.12 Grafting technique for the breast. Fat injection performed through the anterior axillary incision

References

1. Chajchir A, Benzaquen I (1989) Fat-grafting injection for soft-tissue augmentation. Plast Reconstr Surg 84(6):921–934; discussion 935
2. Chajchir A (1996) Fat injection: long-term follow-up. Aesthetic Plast Surg 20(4):291–296
3. Coleman SR (2001) Structural fat grafts: the ideal filler? Clin Plast Surg 28(1):111
4. Coleman SR, Saboeiro AP (2007) Fat grafting to the breast revisited: safety and efficacy. Plast Reconstr Surg 119(3):775–785; discussion 786–787
5. Zuk PA, Zhu M, Ashjian P, De Ugarte DA, Huang JI, Mizuno H, Alfonso ZC et al (2002) Human adipose tissue is a source of multipotent stem cells. Mol Biol Cell 13(12):4279–4295
6. Avelar J (1989) Regional distribution and behavior of the subcutaneous tissue concerning selection and indication for liposuction. Aesthetic Plast Surg 3: 155–165
7. Markman B, Barton FE Jr (1987) Anatomy of the subcutaneous tissue of the trunk and lower extremity. Plast Reconstr Surg 2:248–254
8. Lancerotto L, Stecco C, Macchi V, Porzionato A, Stecco A, De Caro R (2011) Layers of the abdominal wall: ana-

tomical investigation of subcutaneous tissue and superficial fascia. Surg Radiol Anat 33(10):835–842
9. Stecco C, Macchi V, Porzionato A, Duparc F, De Caro R (2011) The fascia: the forgotten structure. Ital J Anat Embryol 116(3):127–138
10. Etzkorn JR, Divine JM, Lopez JJ, Cohen G (2011) Autologous fat transfer: techniques, indications, and future investigation. Cosmet Dermatol 24:470–476
11. Shiffman MA (ed) (2010) Autologous fat transfer: art, science, and clinical practice, 2010th edn. Springer, Berlin/Heidelberg
12. Kamakura T, Ito K (2011) Autologous cell-enriched fat grafting for breast augmentation. Aesthetic Plast Surg 35(6):1022–1030
13. Gutowski KA, ASPS Fat Graft Task Force (2009) Current applications and safety of autologous fat grafts: a report of the ASPS fat graft task force. Plast Reconstr Surg 124:272–280
14. Pu LLQ (2011) Towards more rationalized approach to autologous fat grafting. J Plast Reconstr Surg 65(4):413–419
15. Xie Y, Zheng DN, Li QF, Gu B, Liu K, Shen GX, Pu LLQ (2010) An integrated fat grafting technique for cosmetic facial contouring. J Plast Reconstr Aesthet Surg 63(2):270–276

Part II

The Male Patient: Technique

8 Male Abdomen and Torso

Introduction

In the past, liposuction was a procedure dedicated only to removing unwanted fat. There was no surgical option for slimming or creating an athletic form. In men, the "six-pack" abdomen defines an athletic and masculine appearance. In reality, few men have the combination of genes, dietary habits, and exercise required to develop and reveal the bellies of the rectus abdominis that produce the "six-pack."

The most common request from men who seek body contouring is a well-defined "six-pack" abdomen. Women desire a flat abdomen and occasionally seek limited definition of the anterior abdominal wall. Even athletes with intensive physical training regimens become frustrated with their inability to lose unwanted fat in certain areas. In these individuals, a genetic predisposition to storing fat in areas that obscures muscular definition makes it almost impossible to develop a highly defined muscular appearance.

The approach to high-definition body sculpting depends on the patient's body type and body mass index [1–5]. If the patient is overweight, the main focus of the surgery will be to remove as much fat as possible first and then reveal the anatomy. If he is already slim or athletic, the fat removal will serve to reshape and not to "debulk." For those slim patients, we use intramuscular autologous fat grafting to augment poorly defined muscles [3, 6]. Regardless of preoperative body type, the singular goal of high-definition body sculpting in the male patient is to produce an athletic, muscular appearance (Fig. 8.1) [3]. Once patients see the results of the procedure, they are more inclined to lead a healthy lifestyle to maintain their new appearance. As results improve with diet and exercise, a cycle of positive feedback is created that motivates the patient further and continues to improve results over time.

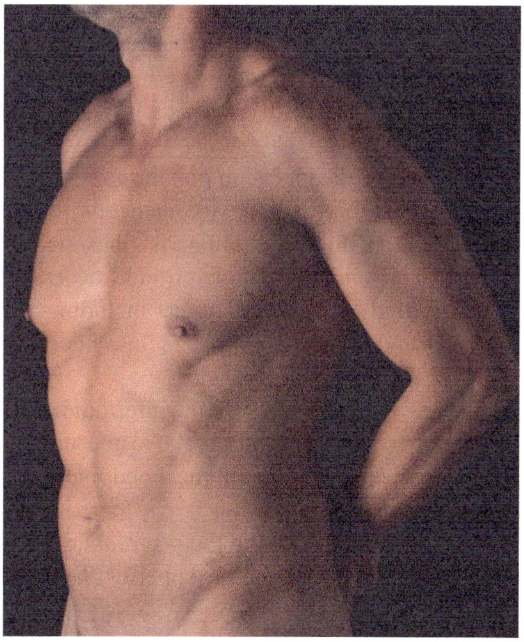

Fig. 8.1 Athletic abdominal muscles in male

A.E. Hoyos, P.M. Prendergast, *High Definition Body Sculpting*,
DOI 10.1007/978-3-642-54891-8_8, © Springer-Verlag Berlin Heidelberg 2014

Stealth Incisions

Numerous incisions are required in order to perform high-definition lipoplasty. Consideration must be given to the location of these incisions. As surgeons, the balance lies between operating comfortably from easy access sites that leave visible scars and hiding incisions in concealed folds or creases, at the cost of working from awkward positions that may necessitate additional incisions to reach all contours anyway.

Even small incisions can leave conspicuous scars, particularly if they are hyperpigmented or hypertrophic. Various factors influence the healing process, including age, race, presence of body hair in men, and the suturing method. When closure is indicated, the author prefers subdermal continuous sutures. The ideal access points should not leave visible scars over the abdomen or the back and should be hidden in the underwear or in the natural folds of the skin. This avoids stigmata of lipoplasty surgery, such as visible or symmetric linear scars. Even with good contouring results, some patients are reluctant to wear a bikini or sunbathe if noticeable scars are present.

The author has perfected the use of hidden or "stealth" incisions and developed various long and curved cannulae to comfortably access the entire body.

In men, the ideal incision points should be:

Pubis: below the hairline, two incisions in line vertically with the semilunaris lines (lateral rectus abdominis). These provide access to most of the abdominal area, including the flanks and waistline, and the rectus abdominis bellies.

Umbilical: provides access to the inferior abdominal area, vertical midline above the umbilicus, and central supraumbilical abdomen.

Nipple: in men this incision is the most hidden one, providing access to the pectoral area, the superior abdomen, and the superior flank and axillary areas.

Anterior axillary fold: provides access to the arm, pectoral area, and lateral chest. This site is essential for fat grafting in pectoralis major and minor and gynecomastia removal.

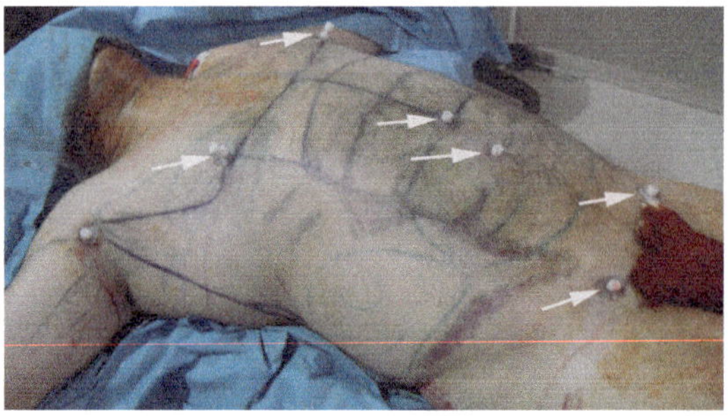

Fig. 8.2 Abdominal incisions (*arrows*) with ports stitched in place

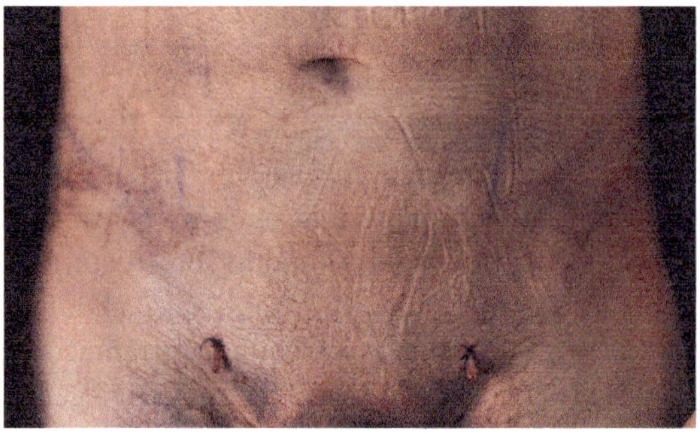

Fig. 8.3 Postoperative drains in the pubical area in men

In the abdominal area, stealth incisions are always preferable. However, if additional access sites are necessary to define the horizontal tendinous intersections of the rectus abdominis, asymmetric incisions can be placed along the abdomen. The stealth incision sites are shown in Fig. 8.2.

The Use of Drains

After treating the male abdomen and torso, drains should be placed in the inguinal area. The use of drains is necessary since aggressive liposuction of the flank area increases the risk of fluid collection in this area with gravity. Two drains are placed at the end of the procedure through the pubic incisions (Fig. 8.3). Either open or closed drains are acceptable, depending on the preference of the surgeon and patient.

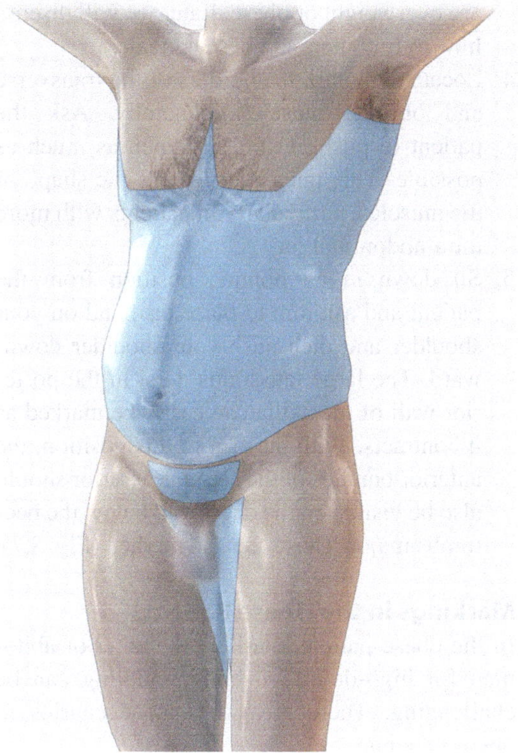

Fig. 8.4 Common areas for deep fat extraction in men (blue)

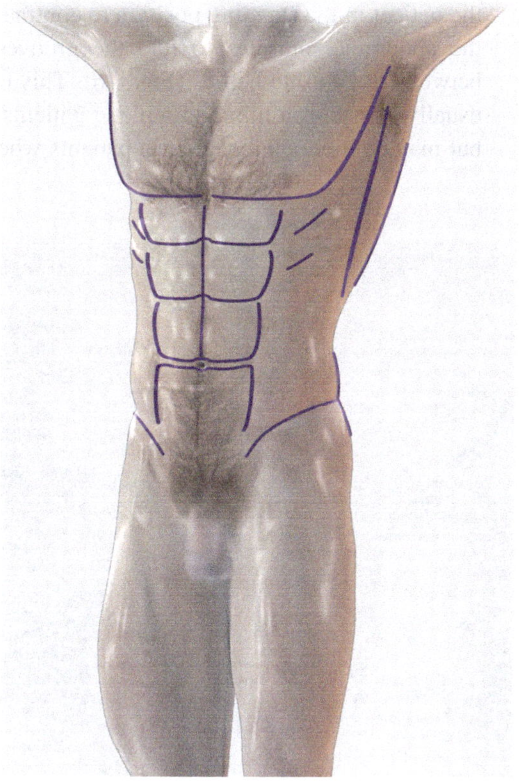

Fig. 8.5 Illustration showing the areas for superficial framing

Markings

The preoperative markings are done in three steps with the patient in the standing position. It is recommended to use different color markers for different stages.

Deep Markings

First, the typical liposuction markings are made in the areas where extra fat is located: usually on the abdominal area, mostly infraumbilical, the "love-handles," the flanks, the pectoral area, and lateral to it toward the axilla (Fig. 8.4).

Framing

The framing is the marking that represents the actual position of the muscles and other superficial anatomical landmarks (Fig. 8.5). The location of these landmarks might be defined by palpation with the patient at rest only but may require the patient to contract the muscles in specific areas. Sonographic guidance is particularly useful in most cases.

The initial assessment of the position of the muscles and tone has to be done with the patient in the standing position:

1. Ask the patient to inhale deeply until the costal margin is visible. Mark the costal margin bilaterally to define the cartilaginous thoracic arch.
2. Palpate and mark the linea alba in the midline from the supraumbilical area to just below the xiphoid process. Remember that no midline should be marked below the umbilicus.
3. Feel for the lateral borders of the rectus abdominis. If possible, try also to locate the transverse tendinous intersections by carefully palpating with the tips of the fingers. Ask

the patient in the standing position to contract the abdominal muscles to find the grooves between the muscle bellies (Fig. 8.6). This is usually possible in thin and athletic patients, but may be more challenging in patients who are overweight or obese. Later we will discuss how to find them in obese patients.

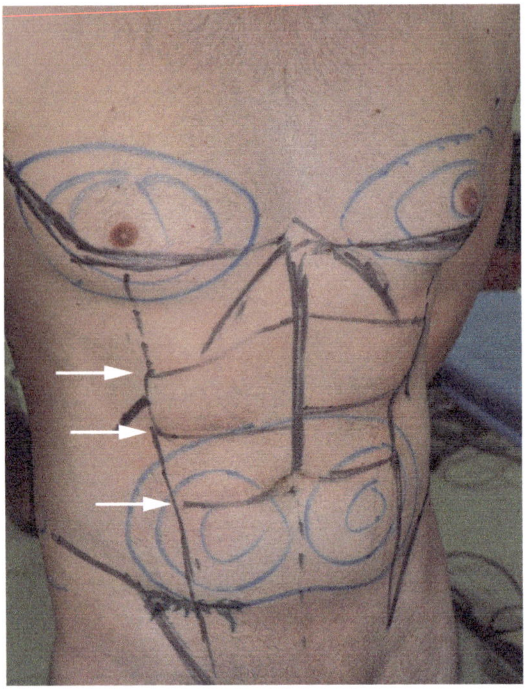

Fig. 8.6 Markings on the patient. *Arrows* showing the transverse inscriptions of the rectus abdominis muscle

4. Locate and mark the borders of the transverse and oblique muscles bilaterally. Ask the patient to push out the abdomen as much as possible. This maneuver reveals the shape of the muscles, particularly in patients with more intra-abdominal fat.
5. Sit down in an oblique position from the patient and ask him to place his hand on your shoulder and then push your shoulder downward. The large latissimus dorsi in the posterior wall of the axilla can easily be marked as it contracts. With the arm in this position, the anterior bundles of the serratus anterior should also be visible on the chest wall below the pectoralis major. These are also marked (Fig. 8.7).

Markings in the Obese Patient

In the obese patient, marking the anterior abdomen for high-definition body sculpting can be challenging. There are two main scenarios in obese patients:

1. Predominantly intra-abdominal fat content: while this kind of patient is more challenging in terms of results, the markings are straightforward.
2. Predominantly extra-abdominal fat content: this is the most challenging patient to mark and to obtain good results. While the pectoralis

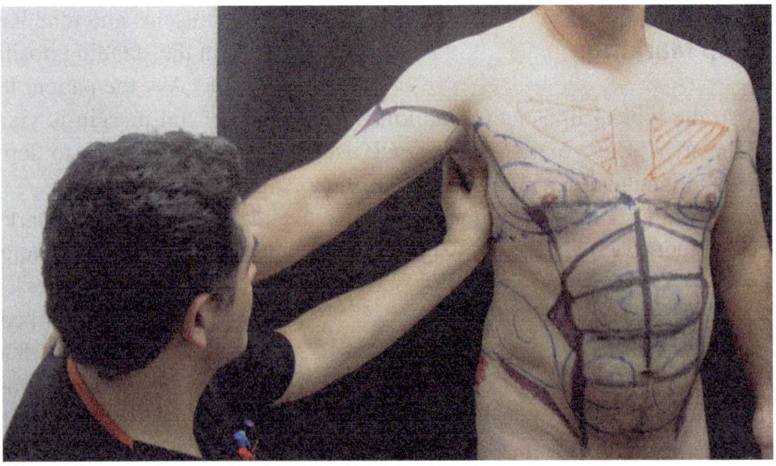

Fig. 8.7 Pushing down the arm against the surgeon's shoulder. By this maneuver, the latissimus dorsi muscle and serratus muscles are contracted and easily seen for marking

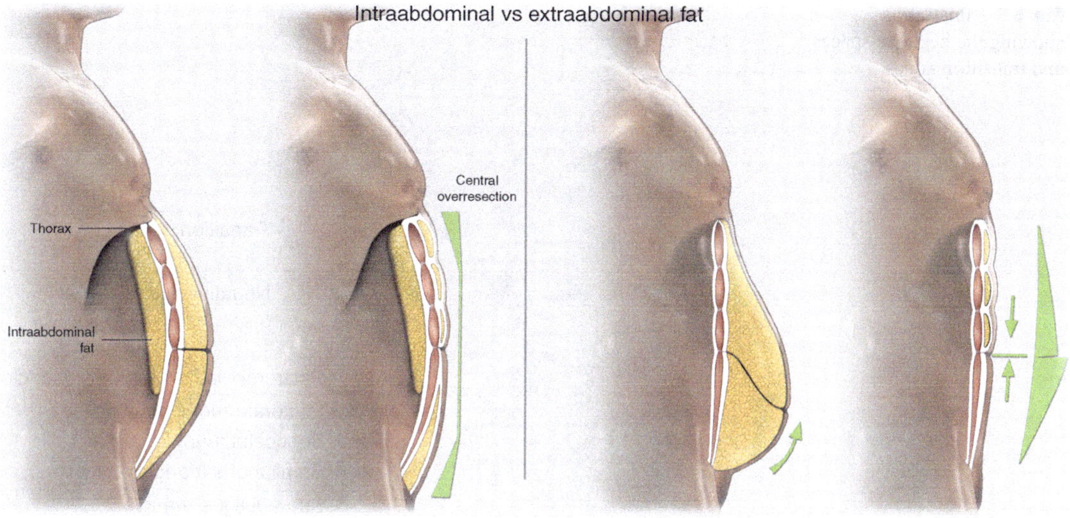

Fig. 8.8 Illustration showing fat distribution in the male abdomen. Fat is resected according to the shape of the abdomen in order to provide a flattened appearance

markings are never a problem, excessive fat obscures the rectus abdominis landmarks. There are additional positions to mark the rectus abdominis:

(a) In the supine position, ask the patient to perform an upper abdominal crunch and mark the lateral borders of the rectus during contraction. The upper tendinous intersections are often also palpable in this position.
(b) Next, ask the patient to do a lower abdominal crunch while raising the legs. During this maneuver, the lower insertions of the rectus abdominis should be palpable or even visible.

The main fat extraction in male obese patients varies according to the presence of intra-abdominal vs. extra-abdominal fat (Fig. 8.8). In patients with extra-abdominal fat, the resection is focused on the lower abdomen and retraction is highly encouraged by performing thorough superficial fat resection.

In patients with mostly intra-abdominal fat, fat is resected more thoroughly over the central abdomen in order to diminish the curvature of the anterior abdomen. As the intra-abdominal fat cannot be reached by liposuction, a strict low-carbohydrate diet after the surgery should be followed to reduce body fat.

Negative Spaces

The negative spaces represent the areas that form the shadows of the superficial anatomy (Fig. 8.9). As we have already marked the areas of superficial (framing) and deep lipoplasty, connecting these two layers would make this an intermediate layer of markings. The negative spaces are specific areas as follows:

1. Area below the external oblique and transverse muscles, leaf shaped
2. Area below the rib cage, triangular
3. Supraumbilical area following the midline, oval
4. Areas between the transverse inscriptions of the rectus muscle, small triangles following the lateral border of the indentations
5. A triangular-shaped area between the superolateral border of the rectus abdominis and the lower border of the pectoralis major
6. A large triangular area between the lateral border of the pectoralis major and the lateral aspect of the latissimus dorsi

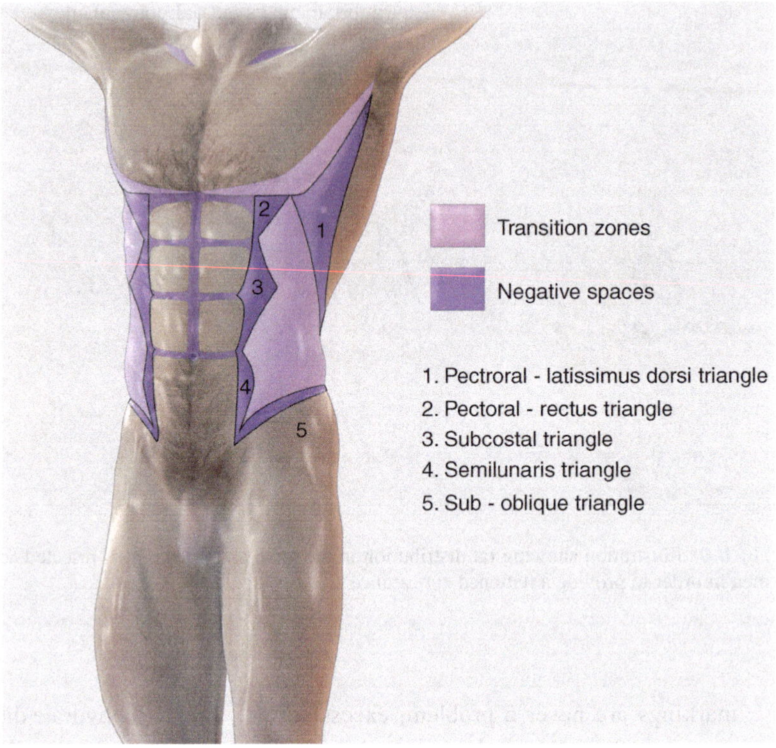

Fig. 8.9 Illustration showing the negative spaces and transition zones

Procedure

The procedure initiates with the infiltration. When we use general anesthesia, the solution consists of 1,000 cc Ringer's lactate and 1:100,000 epinephrine and lidocaine 20 cc of 1 % solution.

Infiltration

Following a 2:1 ratio, the idea is to infiltrate half of the volume in the superficial layer and half in the deep layer. Infiltration should begin in the deep layer and then proceed to the superficial layer. The rationale for infiltrating superficially last is to ensure that there is wetting solution in this layer during ultrasound delivery. If the superficial layer is infiltrated first, migration into deeper layers as time elapses may leave the skin unprotected from the VASER probe energy.

Emulsification

Unlike infiltration, the emulsification process begins in the superficial layer and later moves to the deep layer (Fig. 8.10). Although it is important to wait at least 12 min for the epinephrine to cause adequate vasoconstriction, prolonged delay should be avoided to prevent the migration of fluid to the inferior layers. The probe movement is smooth, and the VASER system is tuned to pulsed mode to prevent excessive heat generation. Additional VASER time may be applied to the framing areas, and the marked areas of negative spaces.

Once the superficial layer has been fully treated, proceed to the deep layer. Begin with the deepest areas to ensure full emulsification, rubbing the probe against the muscular layer. This will ensure to emulsify almost all of the fat in this layer. Once there is loss of resistance in the deeper layers, the probe moves again toward the superficial layer until all layers are treated adequately.

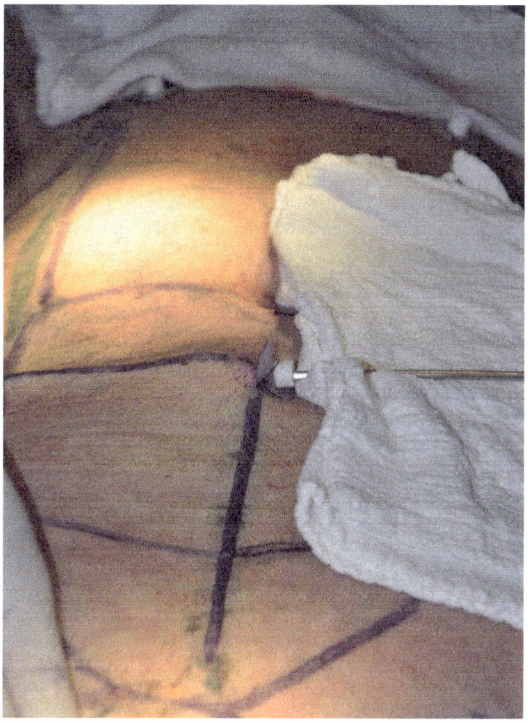

Fig. 8.10 Emulsification via VASER. The VASER probe is inserted through the umbilical incision

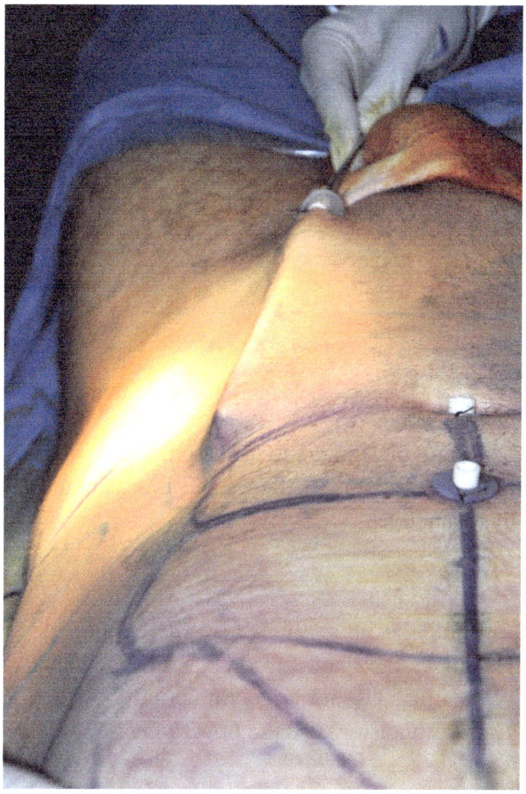

Fig. 8.11 Superficial framing of the rectus abdominis in the lower abdomen

Extraction

Deep Extraction

Start with the deep layer focusing on the infraumbilical area. Try to empty the whole anterior abdomen until only a 1 cm thickness flap remains. Proceed with the deep area of the flanks, this time leaving a flap of just 0.5 cm. Once this area is complete, start with the deep layer in the supraumbilical anterior abdomen. Determine first how much of the fat is actually extra-abdominal versus intra-abdominal fat. It is important to remember that most of the thickness in the upper abdomen is superficial fat, so the extraction should be performed using small cannulae. Start using a 3.7 mm cannula in the deep layer and do not over-extract in this area. A 1 cm flap should remain.

Proceed next to the pectoral area. Remove the deep fat over the pectoral muscles, including glandular tissue if the patient has gynecomastia. However, the upper poles should not be over-resected. Then empty the deep fat of the pectoralis–latissimus triangle from the nipple and axillary fold incisions.

> **Warning!**
> For safety reasons try to avoid resecting the upper abdominal fat from the lower incisions. When working in the upper abdomen, use the incisions placed in the areolae. In the flanks, too, use the axillary fold and areolar incisions to work over the rib cage area. When suctioning the central abdomen, use smooth, non-forced criss-crossing movements.

Superficial Framing

Start the process of superficial framing by defining the rectus abdominis in the lower abdomen (Fig. 8.11). Pinch the skin and use the cannula

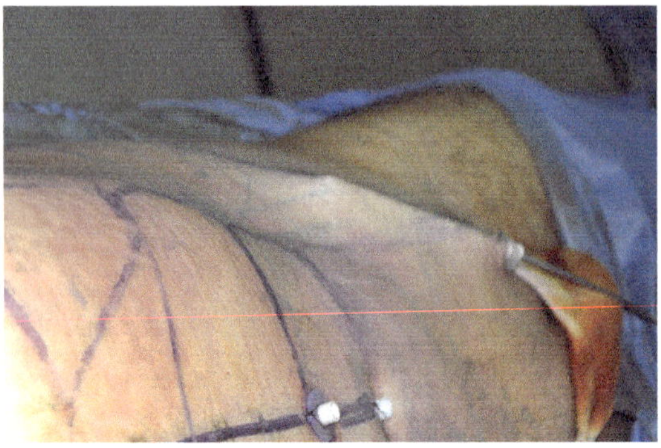

Fig. 8.12 Transverse–oblique muscle line framing

between your fingers to thin the flap and obtain a ridge or indentation. Use a 3.7 mm cannula for this maneuver.

Warning!
Mark the point of the costal margin that crosses the line of the rectus in the supine position. Do not cross this point from the lower incision, use the upper ones.

Use the 3.0 mm cannula and work over the transverse–oblique muscle line. You can also pinch the tissue and work very superficially here to create a flap as thin as the skin (Fig. 8.12).

Superficial framing continues from the nipple incisions. Using a 3.7 mm cannula, the lateral border of the rectus abdominis is defined by suctioning superficially exactly below the preoperative markings (Fig. 8.13). Since this area is very sensitive to liposuction, it is important to stop and check the appearance of the tissues frequently to avoid overdoing the resection. Remember that the lateral lines of the rectus, especially on the upper abdomen, follow the curvature of each indentation of the muscle; hence the linea semilunaris is not a straight line. Follow the real curvature of the rectus to ensure a realistic and natural result.

Warning!
If you are not sure where the semilunar line is, it is better to go a little lateral than its predicted location. You can always go back and re-do this line, but if it is defined too medially, the correction would be impossible.

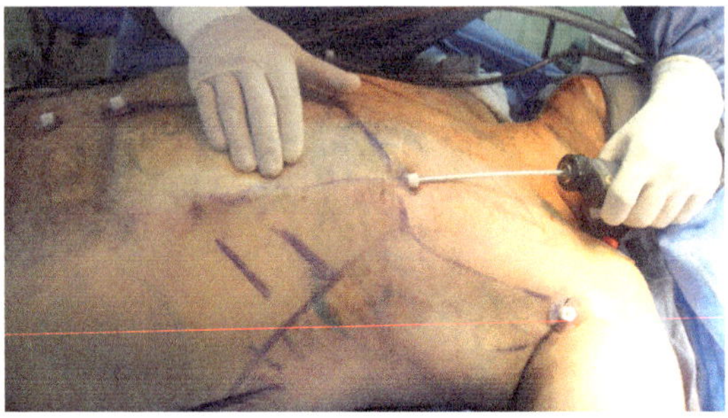

Fig. 8.13 Fat extraction through the sub-nipple incision. Note that the cannula is following the lateral lines of the rectus abdominis muscle. Remember to follow the contour of the muscle and not a straight line

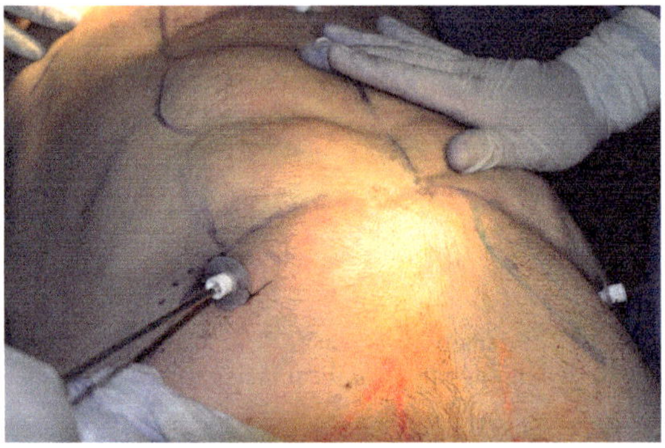

Fig. 8.14 Muscular line framing, through the sub-nipple contralateral incision

Defining the pectoralis major and latissimus dorsi is achieved by emptying the triangular space between the two muscles. The inferior and lateral borders of the pectoralis major are defined first by suctioning superficially using a 3.0 mm cannula from the anterior axillary incision, followed by a 3.7 mm cannula. Use the same incision for marking the line of the latissimus dorsi. Empty the triangle again in a superficial way. The sub-nipple access site is used to further define the pectoralis line between the inferior margin of the pectoralis major and rectus abdominis (Fig. 8.14).

Defining the Rectus Abdominis

This is the most rewarding, but also the most challenging, area to work. The horizontal inscriptions are created to define the horizontal

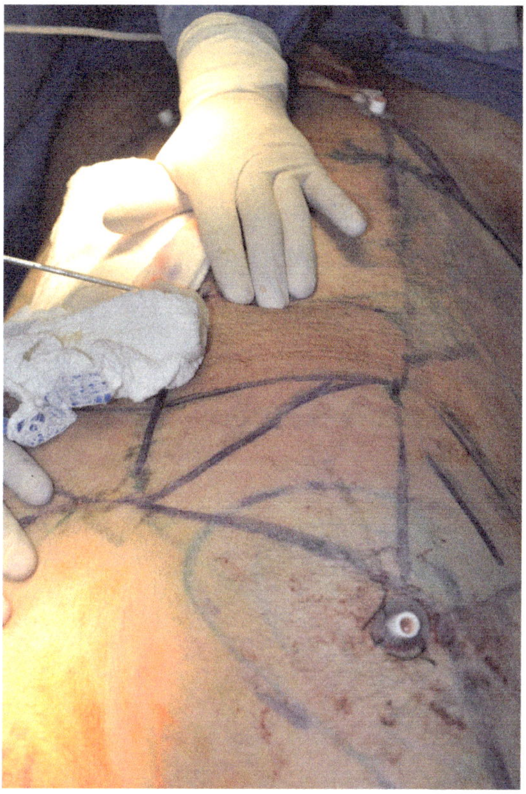

Fig. 8.15 Rectus abdominis contouring, parallel to the incision point

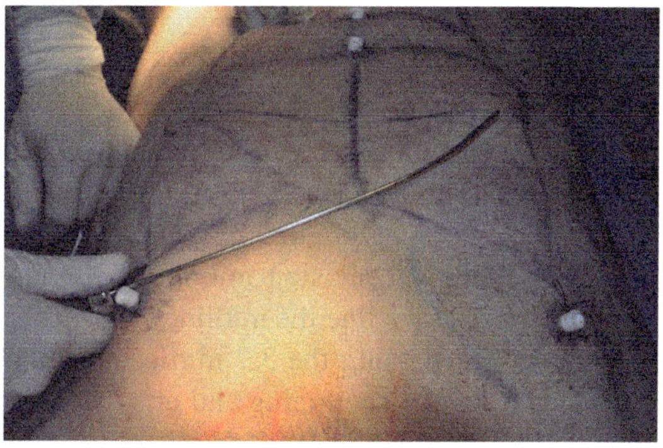

Fig. 8.16 Curved cannulae allows easy access to the framing sites

tendinous intersections of the rectus abdominis m. There are three main ways to create the horizontal inscriptions:

1. Directly, parallel to the incision point. This requires an incision at every level in line with the horizontal inscription. For most patients, this requires at least three incisions (Fig. 8.15).
2. Directly, using curved cannula (Fig. 8.16). This obviates the need for incisions at every level of inscription.
3. Indirectly, by creating the inscription perpendicular to the incision point. Using compression over the marked tendinous intersections, the linear depressions are gradually formed by repeatedly passing the 3.0 mm cannula below the focally compressed tissue. This is more difficult than the other techniques and may be used alone or as an adjunct to the other methods.

Warning!

Always follow the real anatomy of the patient, no matter how awkward it may seem. If you fail to find and achieve the rectus inscriptions, when the patient starts dieting and/or exercising, they will observe double inscriptions and a failed result.

Always start with a small cannula (3.0 mm), either straight or curved. Begin from the umbilical incision. Start in the very superficial layer and later proceed more deeply, until the groove is formed. Once the lower inscription is created, proceed to the upper ones. They can usually be completed through the nipple incisions. If not, an extra incision can be made over the line of the lower 2nd horizontal inscription.

If a further incision is required for access over the 3rd horizontal inscription, it is better to place this incision on a lateral point rather than in the midline. Visible incisions should always be placed asymmetrically to avoid leaving the patient with obvious signs of having had aesthetic surgery. In order to produce a natural, rounded depression, the inscriptions should be sculpted from several access points. Criss-crossing from three access sites produces a natural tonal progression from the grooves to the convex surfaces of the rectus abdominis bellies.

Midline

Always leave the midline for last. The idea is not to overdo the midline when doing the horizontal inscriptions. The horizontal inscriptions should be completed first before defining the linea alba. From the umbilical incision initially, a 3.0 mm cannula is used to define the midline. The groove is then deepened using the 3.7 mm cannula and rounded by further suctioning and criss-crossing from the superior access incisions (Fig. 8.17).

The Intermediate Layer

The secret of an exceptional result in high-definition lipoplasty belongs in this step of the surgery. The artistry of transforming carved fat into shapes that look and feel natural takes its origins in the interaction of light and form [3]. Follow two simple rules and your results will be better than expected:

1. Turn lines into curves.
2. Create shadows along the natural ones in the anatomy.

Start with the lower negative space, just below the line of the oblique–transverse muscle. Start every negative space with a full extraction just next to the line and make it smoother as you go further distally from the line.

Proceed with the semilunar lines and pass from the upper incisions to meet the lower semilunar lines. Remember that the lateral borders of the rectus abdominis form curves, not straight lines along the way.

The negative space in the subcostal region is created by suctioning inferior to the costal margin from the sub-nipple incisions. This area always moves from the standing position to the supine position, so be guided by the previous markings made with the patient standing.

From the nipple and anterior axillary incisions, proceed to the space below the pectoralis major. Depending on the anatomy, this space may appear as a linear groove or as a broader triangle between the upper bellies of the rectus abdominis and pectoralis major.

Lastly, the triangular negative space between the pectoralis major and the anterior border of the latissimus dorsi is deepened.

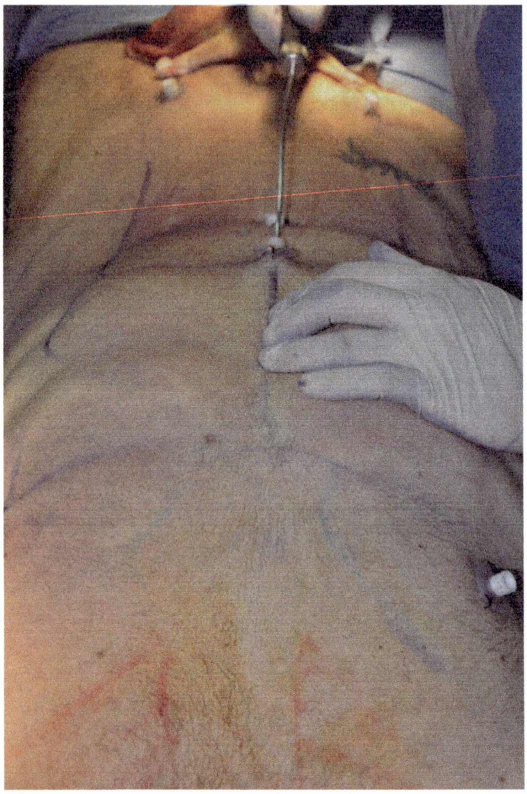

Fig. 8.17 Midline contouring

Before completion, the definition is assessed by careful inspection. The negative spaces and controlled irregularities can be deepened at this stage using a 3.0 mm cannula if more definition is required. However, it is important not to be excessively aggressive in the subdermal layer to prevent seromas, unwanted irregularities, and damaging the subdermal vascular plexus. Results are seen immediately after surgery, but final results are appreciated once edema resolves and the skin retraction is complete after about 6 months (Figs. 8.18, 8.19, and 8.20).

Postoperative Care

The superior incisions may be closed using subdermal sutures. Drains should be placed in the lower dependent incisions. The drains can be left open or closed. A compression foam vest and garment is applied immediately. The postoperative care is described in Chap. 20.

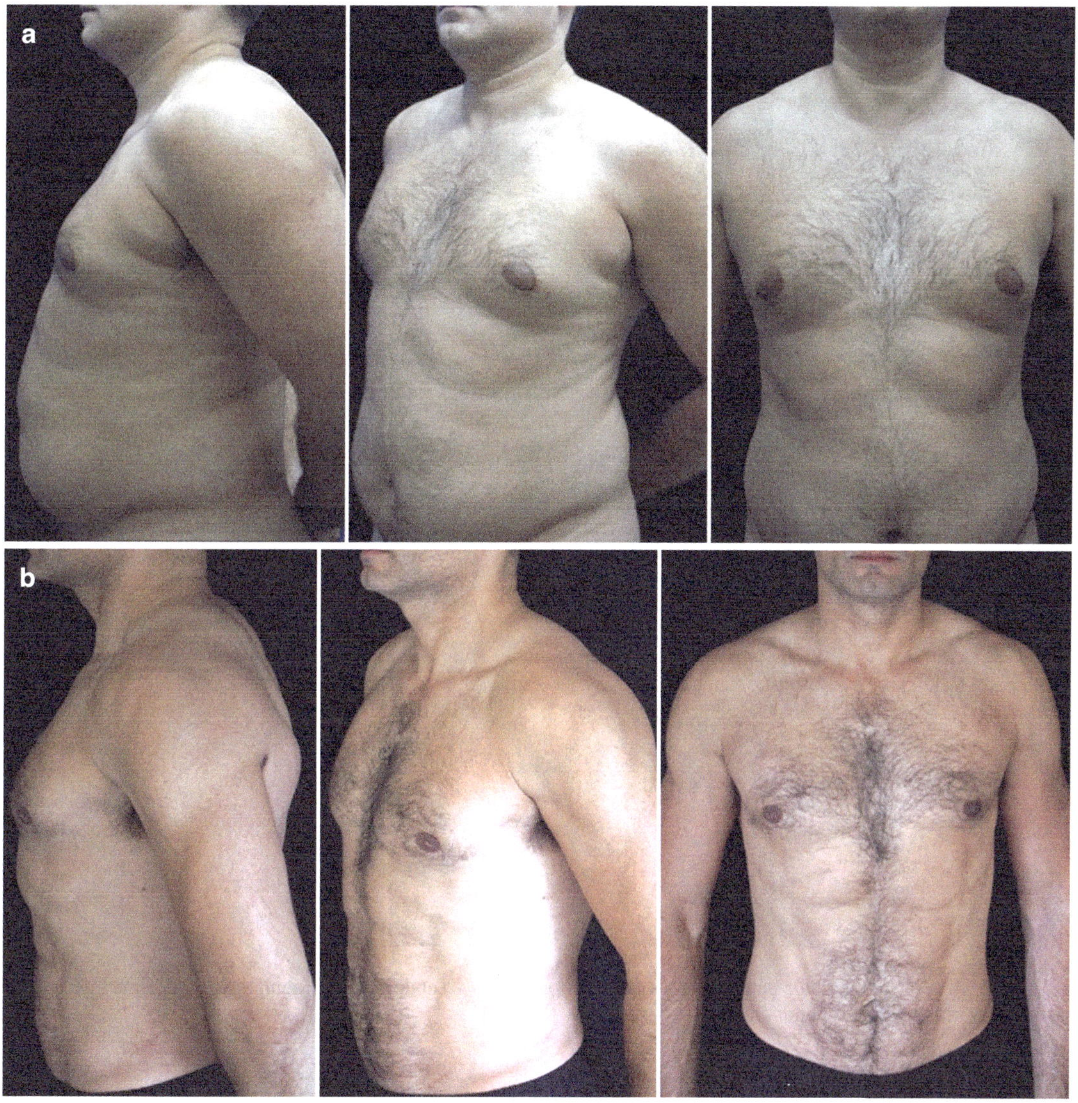

Fig. 8.18 42-year-old fat male patient preoperative (**a**) and 6 months after the liposculpture (**b**)

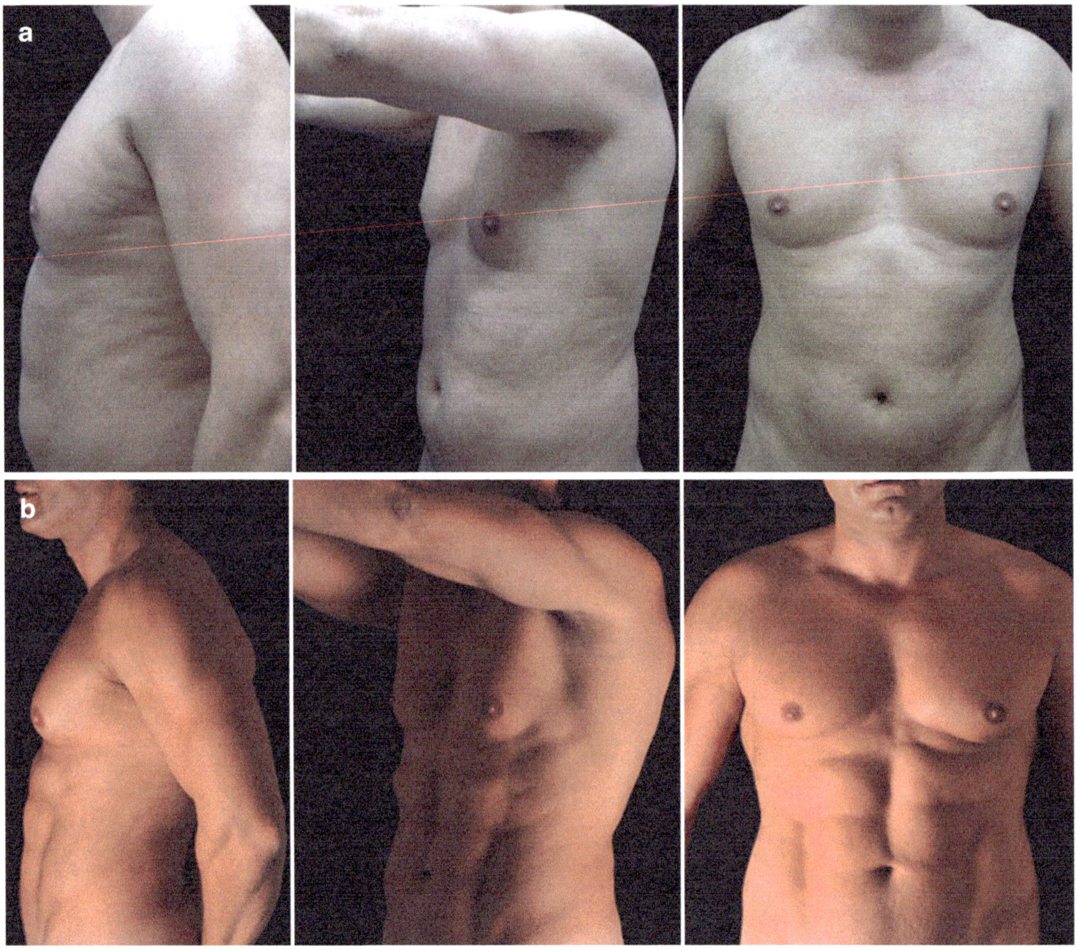

Fig. 8.19 42-year-old fat male patient pre- (**a**) and postoperative (**b**) abdominal liposculpture. Notice the high muscular definition of the rectus abdominis

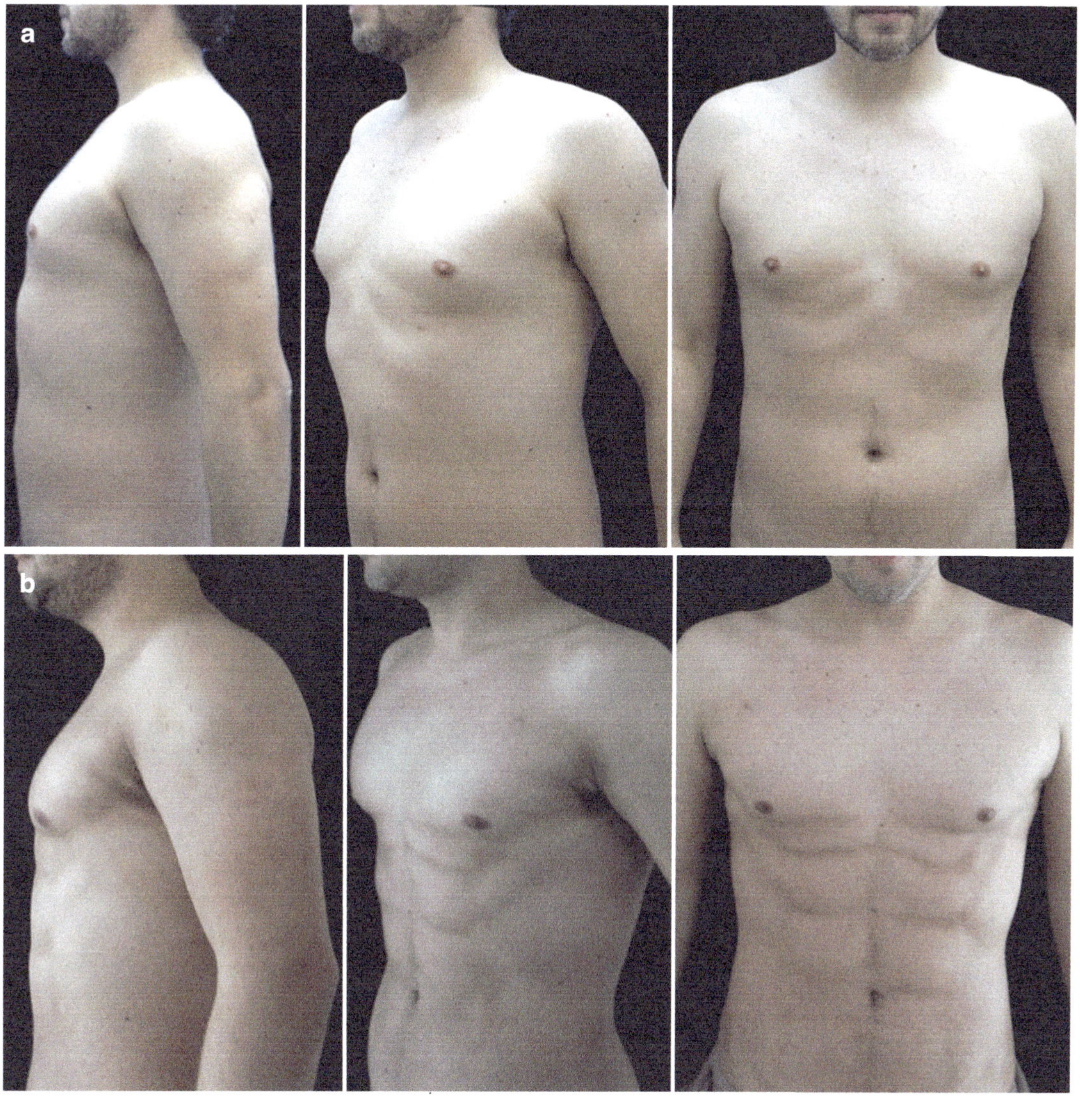

Fig. 8.20 26-year-old slim male patient pre- (**a**) and postoperative (**b**) abdominal liposculpture

References

1. Avelar J (1989) Regional distribution and behavior of the subcutaneous tissue concerning selection and indication for liposuction. Aesthet Surg J 13:155–165
2. de Souza Pinto EB, Indaburo PE, Da Costa Muniz A, Martinez YP, Gerent KMM, Iwamoto H, Marão Miziara AC (1996) Superficial liposuction: body contouring. Clin Plast Surg 23(4):529–548
3. Hoyos AE, Millard JA (2007) Vaser-assisted high definition Lipoplasty. Aesthet Surg J 27:594–604
4. Rochrich RJ, Beran SJ, Di Spaltro F et al (1998) Extending the role of liposuction in body contouring with ultrasound assisted liposuction. Plast Reconstr Surg 101:1090–1102
5. Zocchi ML (1996) Ultrasound-assisted lipoplasty. Technical refinements and clinical evaluations. Clin Plast Surg 23:575–598
6. Toledo L, Mauad R (2006) Fat injection: a 20-year revision. Clin Plast Surg 33:47–53

Male Chest

9

Introduction

One of the most appealing characteristics of an athletic male body is a well-defined pectoral area (Fig. 9.1). The aesthetic standards for the male chest are strongly correlated with the shape and development of the pectoralis muscles. Abnormal fat deposition in the chest, gynecomastia, trauma, and congenital abnormalities distort the normal anatomy and are a common motivation to perform reshaping surgery. In addition, underdevelopment of the male chest musculature seems to be a result of modern urban lifestyle choices, including increased calorie intake, lack of physical activity, and resistance exercises. Most of the treatment options are focused on correcting the chest deficiencies and deformities [1–3].

The ideal male chest is defined by the exposure of the surface anatomy, which is a reflection of the disposition and development of the pectoralis muscles. Although it is a reflection of the muscle mass itself, the surrounding areas must also be treated in order to produce optimal definition [4, 5].

The anatomy of the pectoral area is divided into specific zones to fulfill the goals of the technique (Fig. 9.2).

For years, implants have been considered the gold-standard method for treating pectoral deficiencies [2]. However, their shortcomings include expensive prostheses and potentially serious complications, including a poor aesthetic result and a "female"-like appearance. With fat grafting and superficial liposuction, we can produce superior results compared to these traditional methods, thus making it a good alternative for male chest reconstruction [6, 7]. For the purposes of fat grafting and planning, the pectoralis major is divided into upper and lower poles. Aesthetically, the upper pole should have a

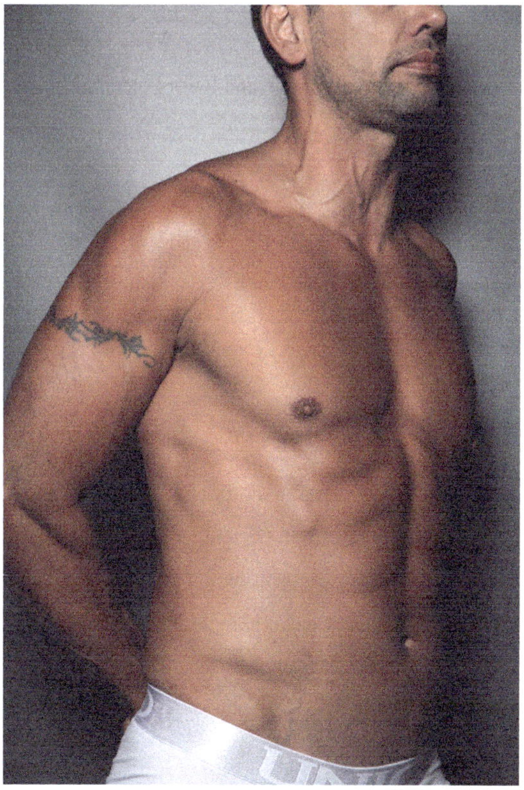

Fig. 9.1 Athletic male chest: notice the muscular shape of the pectoralis muscle in the superficial

A.E. Hoyos, P.M. Prendergast, *High Definition Body Sculpting*,
DOI 10.1007/978-3-642-54891-8_9, © Springer-Verlag Berlin Heidelberg 2014

greater volume than the lower pole, due to the greater muscle mass, so most of the fat will be grafted to this region.

The anatomical features surrounding the pectoralis muscle are divided into five "negative spaces": areas that should be concave in order to enhance the convexity of the pectoralis and surrounding muscles (Fig. 9.3).

The first negative space is a rhomboid between the inferior borders of the pectoralis major, the xiphoid process, and the origin of the rectus abdominis at the midline (interpectoral rhomboid).

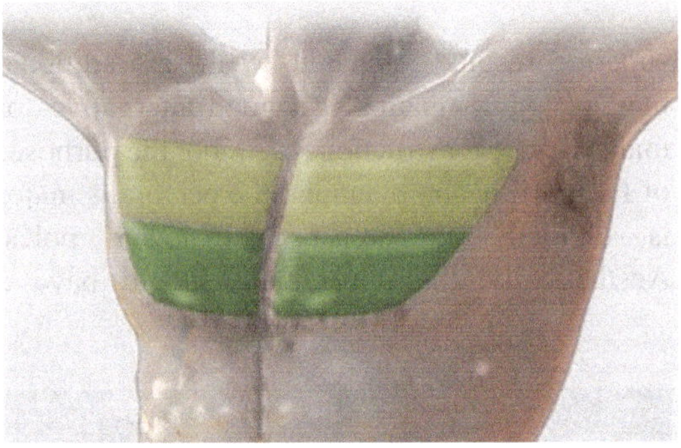

Fig. 9.2 Upper: *light green*, and lower pole: *dark green*

The second area is a triangle defined by the pectoral line and the lateral border of the rectus abdominis (subpectoral triangle). This area must be treated aggressively with subdermal and intermediate liposuction. It also links the definition of the pectoralis muscles with definition of the abdomen.

The third area is the triangular area between the lateral border of the pectoralis major and the lateral border of the latissimus dorsi (pectoralis–latissimus triangle). Even though this is beyond the pectoral area, in the contouring process it is important to expand the concavity to this limit.

The fourth area is defined as the triangular area bordered by the clavicle, deltoid, and clavicular portion of the pectoralis major (subclavicular or deltopectoral triangle).

The fifth area is a horizontal line along the inferior border of the pectoralis major, usually 1 cm below the nipple level (pectoralis line). This represents a negative space that softens along the lateral border of the muscle toward the upper pole.

Finally, a triangular area defined by three points: the inferolateral corner of the pectoralis major, the medial point of the pectoral line, and the

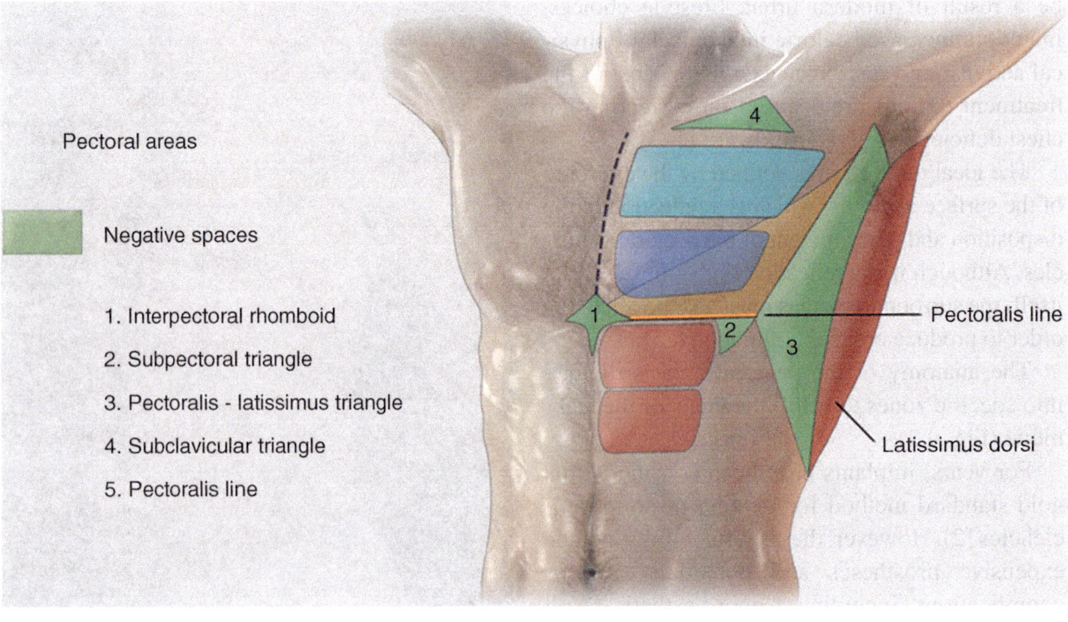

Fig. 9.3 Negative areas surrounding the pectoralis muscle (in *green*), upper pectoralis pole (in *light blue*), and lower pole (in *dark blue*)

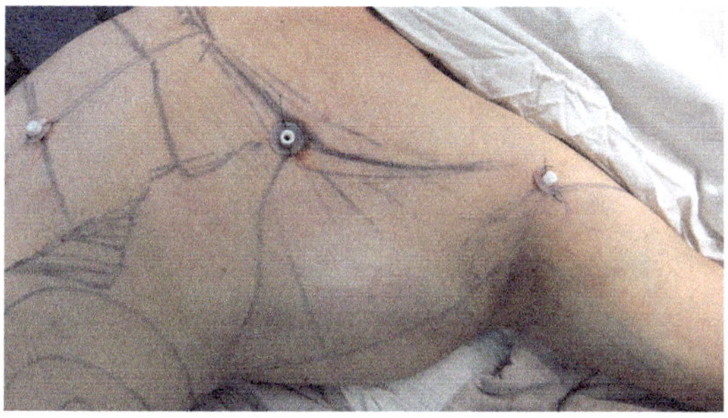

Fig. 9.4 Anterior axillary and sub-nipple incisions with ports stitched in place

lateral insertion of the pectoralis major. This area is essentially the lower lateral pole of the pectoral area. Deep liposuction should be performed in this area in obese and gynecomastic patients, sometimes extending to the limits of the fatty tissue beyond the underlying pectoral muscle [5].

Stealth Incisions

Ideally, the incisions should be placed with the patient in the supine position, with the arms abducted to 90°. Two 5 mm incisions are placed bilaterally, in the anterior axillary fold and in the areola just below the nipple. Silicone ports are placed into the incisions and sutured in place (Fig. 9.4).

The Use of Drains

The use of drains is not necessary in this area. In fact, the anterior axillary incisions are the preferred access sites for fat grafting. As such, it is mandatory to close these incisions to avoid retrograde fat leakage through the incision points.

Markings

Deep Markings

In the standing position, first mark the fat deposits to be removed with deep liposuction. Usually, there is extra fat around the nipples that extends beyond the border of the pectoralis muscles.

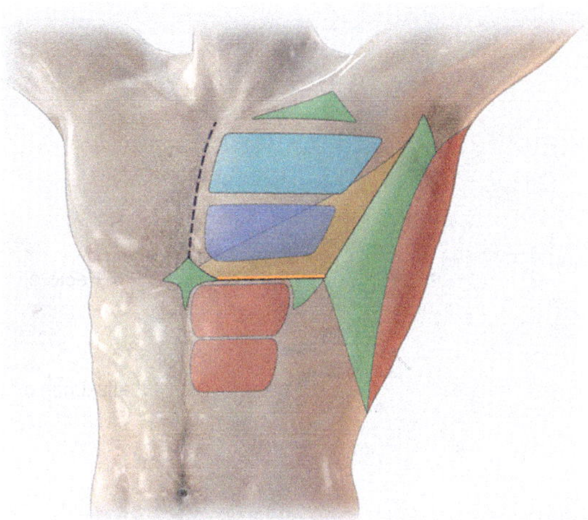

Fig. 9.5 Pectoral zones, negative spaces (in *green*). Deep extraction is shown as the triangular yellow zone, above it deep extraction should not be performed

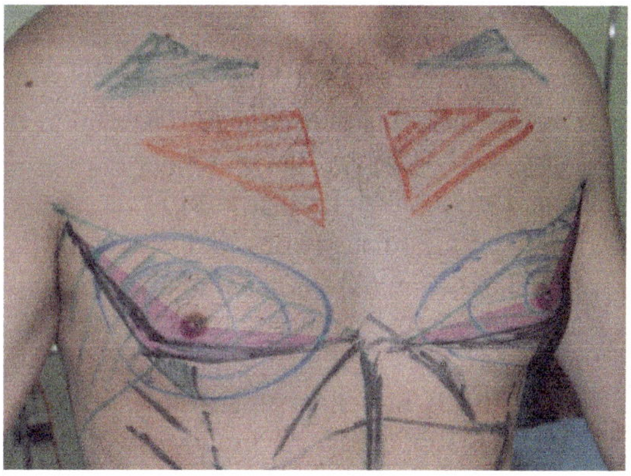

Fig. 9.6 Surface anatomy markings

Mark this area. For a clear upper limit, a triangular area between the inferomedial border of the pectoralis major and the anterior axillary fold is marked (Fig. 9.5).

Mark the depressions or areas that need more projection in the pectoralis, especially the upper pole. These areas will be treated with fat grafting.

Framing

Surface anatomy is marked in the areas of superficial liposculpture: the inferior and lateral margins of the pectoralis major are marked first. It is very important to mark these areas with the arms down (in adduction) for accuracy (Fig. 9.6).

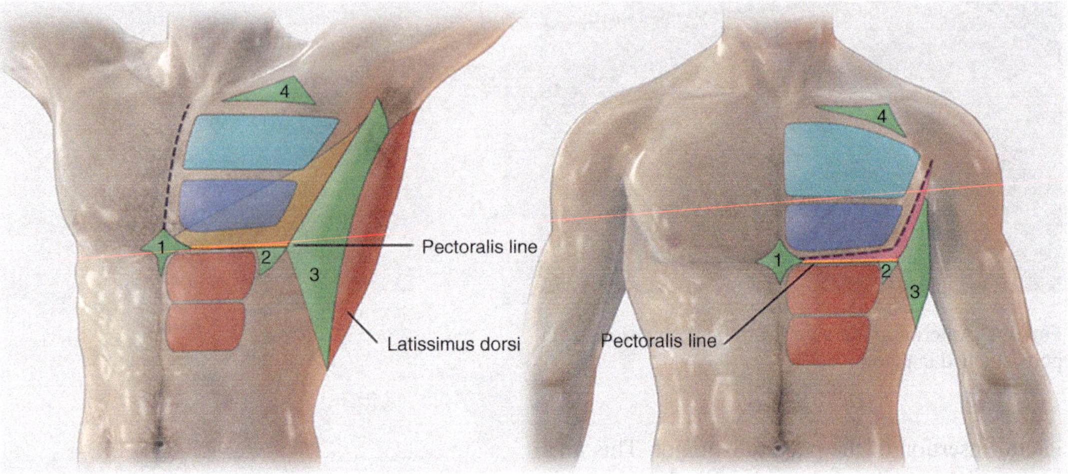

Fig. 9.7 Negative spaces marked in green: (*1*) interpectoral rhomboid, (*2*) subpectoral triangle, (*3*) pectoralis–latissimus triangle, (*4*) subclavicular triangle and pectoral line. The pink color describes a transition zone where smooth framing must be done

Warning!

One of the most common mistakes is to mark the borders of the pectoralis muscle in abduction of the arm (arms up), since we are marking other regions of the anatomy in this position. Also, mark accurately the areas of true gynecomastia behind the nipple (mammary disc) that require extensive resection. If resection of glandular tissue here is suboptimal, a deformity results due to interruption in the continuity of the pectoralis muscle line. This inadequate shape is called "sad pectoral."

Negative Spaces

The negative spaces are marked as follows:

1. The pectoralis–latissimus triangle, between the anterior limit of the latissimus dorsi and the lateral border of the pectoralis major
2. The inferior pectoral triangle, between the lower border of the pectoralis and the lateral border of the rectus abdominis
3. The pectoral line, following the lower border of the pectoralis major
4. The interpectoral rhomboid, bordered by the medial attachments of the inferior pectoralis muscles and the two bundles of the rectus abdominis toward the midline
5. The subclavicular triangle, between the clavicle and the upper limit of the pectoralis major (Fig. 9.7)

In patients with gynecomastia, the entire gland bud is marked and its area beyond the pectoralis muscle limits is marked for selective extraction by pull-through technique if it cannot be removed completely by suction [1].

Procedure

Patients are divided into four groups according to the body type, leading to a different choice of procedure: slim, athletic, fat, and gynecomastic patients (Fig. 9.8) [5].

In thin patients, enhanced definition with superficial liposuction is performed as an adjunct to fat grafting in the muscular and submuscular layers. In athletic patients, definition is created using deep and superficial liposuction alone. Although fat grafting in these patients is seldom required, some of them benefit from limited supramuscular fat grafting. Fat grafting in this plane is possible in athletic patients because when extensive deep liposuction is not performed, fat migration due to tunneling in the supramuscular layer is less likely. For obese

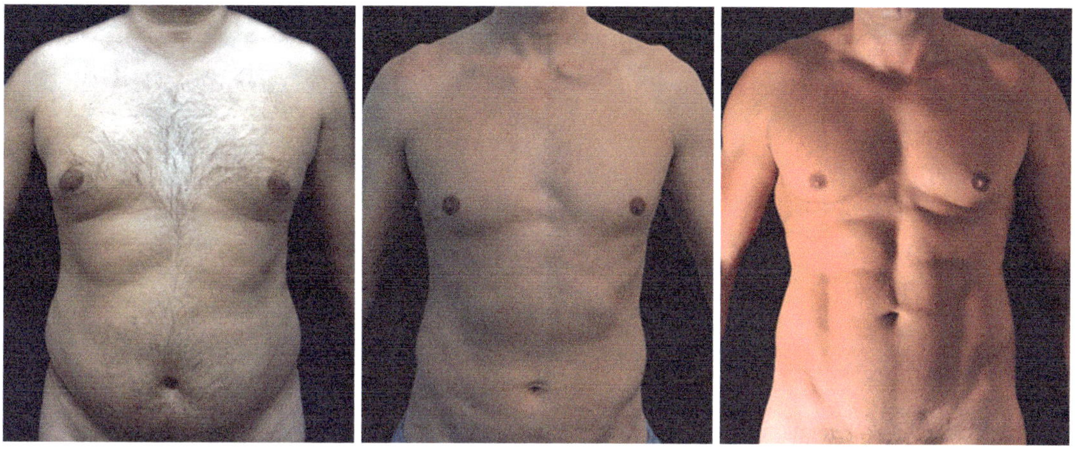

Fig. 9.8 Body types: fat, thin, and athletic

patients or patients with pseudogynecomastia, liposuction is performed to completely remove the deep layer of fat in and around the pectoral area. Superficial fat removal is also required to achieve skin retraction in the area. Fat grafting may also be performed to the upper pole to replace the volume extracted in the lower pole, giving a lifted appearance. Finally, in patients with true gynecomastia, open resection is performed through an omega incision.

Infiltration

Infiltrate the tissues thoroughly using tumescent solution with 1,000 ml of normal saline, 50 ml of 1 % lidocaine, and 1 ml of epinephrine 1:1,000. The ratio of infiltration to volume of fat removed is approximately 2:1. Wait 12–15 min after the deep and superficial planes have been infiltrated for adequate vasoconstriction. Emulsification with third-generation ultrasound can then commence.

Emulsification

Begin by treating the superficial tissues with VASER pulsed mode using a 2.9 mm probe, with 70–80 % power. Use VASER in continuous mode for deep fat fragmentation with a 2.9 mm or a 3.7 mm 2-ring probe at 90 % power.

Extraction

Deep Extraction

Fat is extracted in the deep planes from the subpectoral area, the triangular pectoral area, the triangular area lateral to the muscle, and the axillary fat pad over the superior lateral border of the pectoral beneath the clavicle and the deltoid muscle.

Superficial Framing

In the superficial layer, aspiration is used to sculpt the pectoral line inferior and parallel to the inferior border of the pectoralis major. It is important to notice the position of the arm on the operating table while this line is sculpted; the arms must be adducted (in contact with the torso). If they are abducted (in 90°), sculpturing can lead to an angled line instead of a straight one, resulting in a "sad pectoral" (Fig. 9.9). Subdermal liposuction using compression and pinching techniques is performed in "negative space" areas around the convex mass of the pectoralis major. As suction continues, shadows are created in the pectoralis–latissimus triangle and at the junction of the pectoralis major and linea semilunaris, enhancing definition of the surrounding muscles.

Intermediate Layer

The junction between the superficial and the deep zones are blended to produce defined inferior and lateral borders of the pectoralis major.

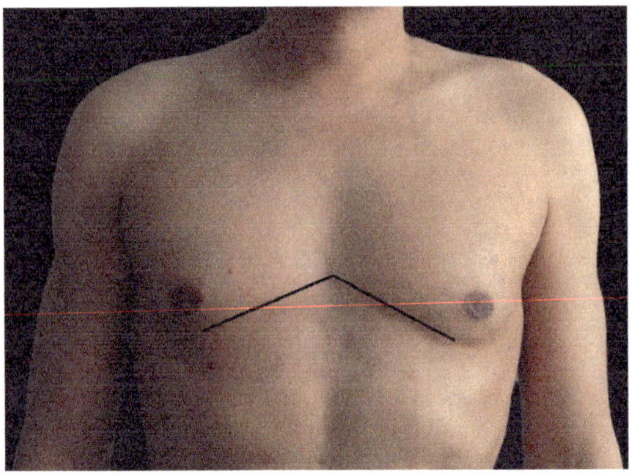

Fig. 9.9 Sad-looking pectorals

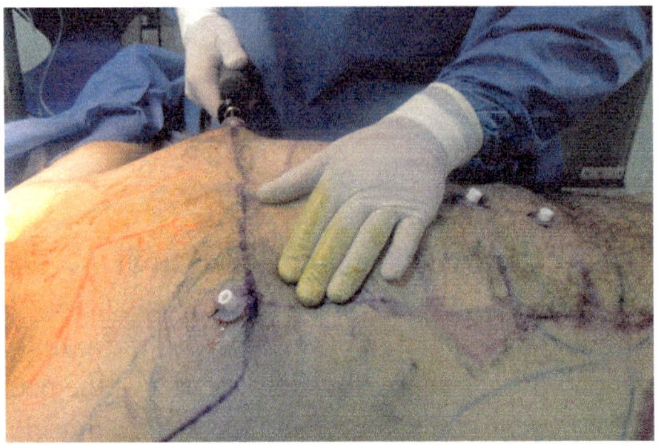

Fig. 9.10 Sculpting of the pectoral negative space

The negative space areas are completed in this step of the surgery (Fig. 9.10).

Fat Grafting

Fat tissue is harvested with a 3 mm blunt cannula from other areas of the body to an empty, sterile bottle trap. An antibiotic, such as cefazolin 1 g, is added to the fat container. The solution is decanted to separate the fat cells from the saline and serosanguinous components. The author also enriches the fat with either platelet-rich plasma (PRP) or stem cells derived from the patient to improve fat cell survival after grafting (see Chap. 7).

First, the pectoralis major is located and grasped between the fingers and thumb. Through the anterior axillary fold incision, a 3.0 mm blunt

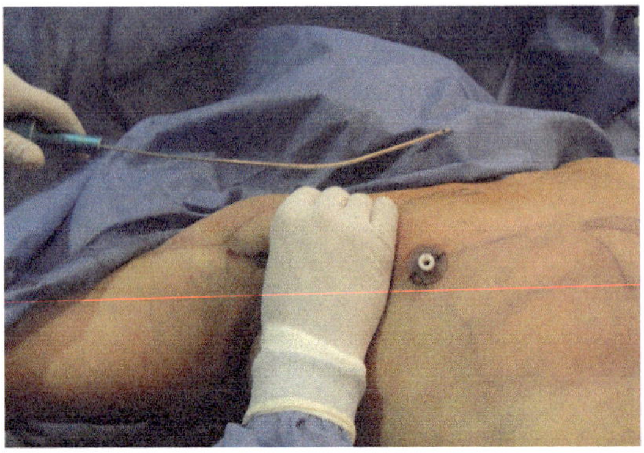

Fig. 9.11 Pectoral fat grafting: pinching technique

30° curved cannula is introduced into the muscle mass and fat is injected retrogradely in a fanning motion (Fig. 9.11). Threads of fat are placed, first, in the intramuscular layer and then in the submuscular plane (Fig. 9.12).

On rare occasions, fat is placed in the supramuscular layer, especially in older men in the medial-superior pectoral area when there is muscle atrophy. In these cases, the author enriches the fat using PRP or stem cells and places the fat with 1.0 mm micro-cannulae using Coleman's technique.

The curvature of the cannula is important because it follows the muscle shape. Avoid injecting the lower pole, because it would accentuate a "glandular appearance." The average of total fat injection is around 150 cc on each side, with a range of 70–300 cc. Closure of all the incisions following fat grafting is mandatory to prevent loss of fat. A continuous subdermal suture is used. Fat grafting to the male chest enhances muscular definition by adding volume in the upper poles. Figures 9.13, 9.14, and 9.15 show results of male chest contouring in heavy and slim individuals.

Postoperative Care

A low-pressure garment is used over the chest area following the procedure. A foam vest over the grafted area is not recommended. The postoperative care regimen should include external ultrasound to all areas except the grafted areas and

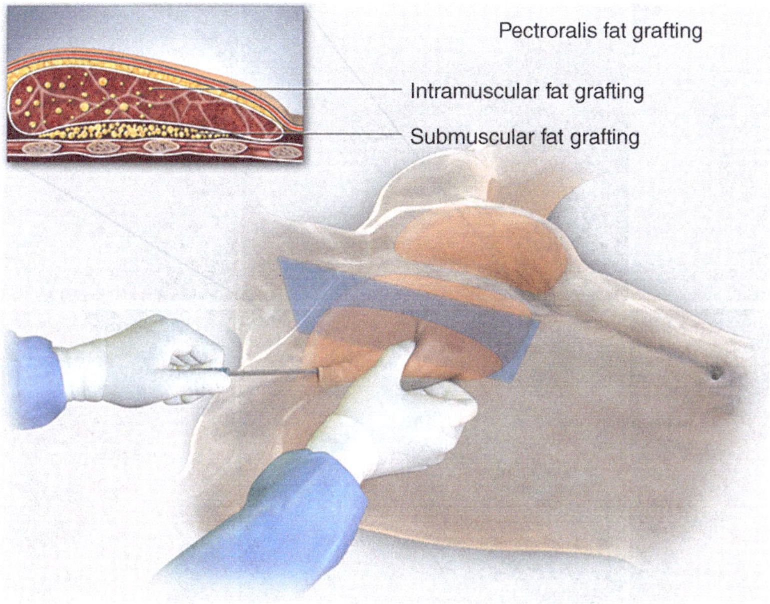

Fig. 9.12 Fat grafting in the male chest. Grafting technique: the pectoralis major is pinched and fat is grafted intramuscularly with a 3.0 mm blunt curved cannula. It is important to keep the cannula curvature facing upward to follow the shape of the muscle and avoid an accidental thoracic penetration. (*Inset*) Fat-grafting scheme. Most of the fat graft is placed in the superior pole to enhance the muscular appearance. Fat is not placed in the lower pole

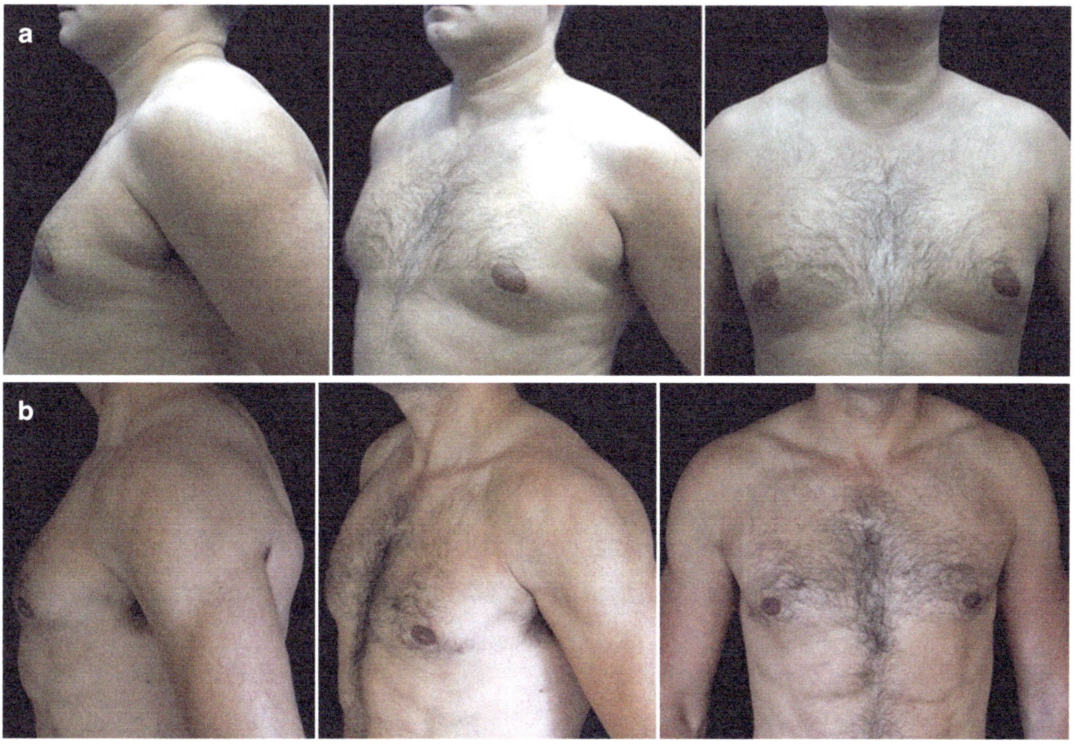

Fig. 9.13 A 42-year-old patient preoperative (**a**) and 6 months postoperative (**b**)

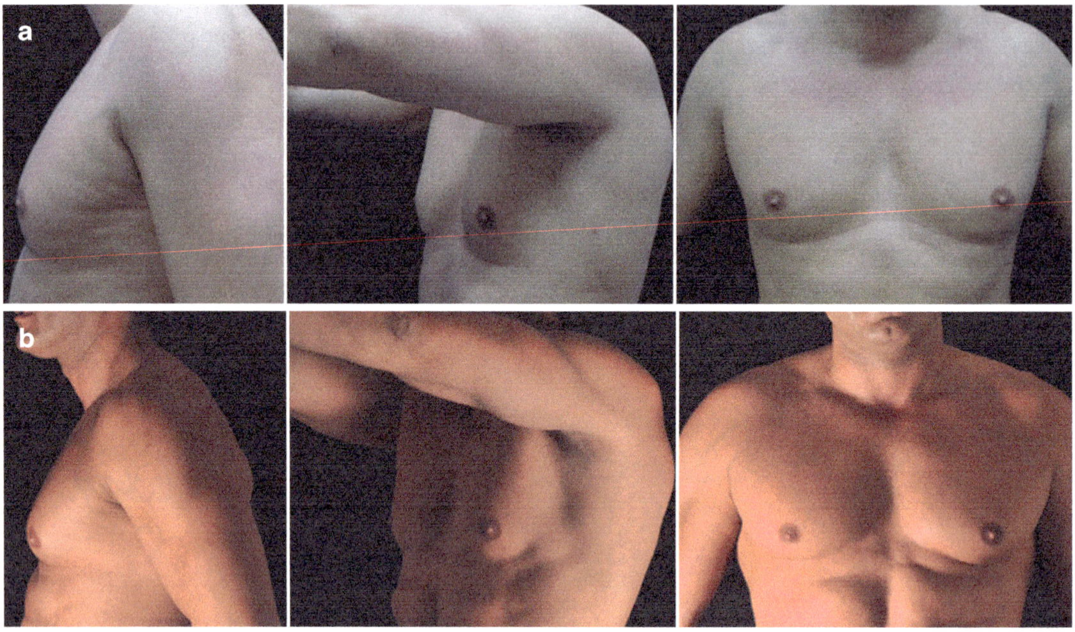

Fig. 9.14 A 42-year-old male patient pre- (**a**) and postoperative (**b**)

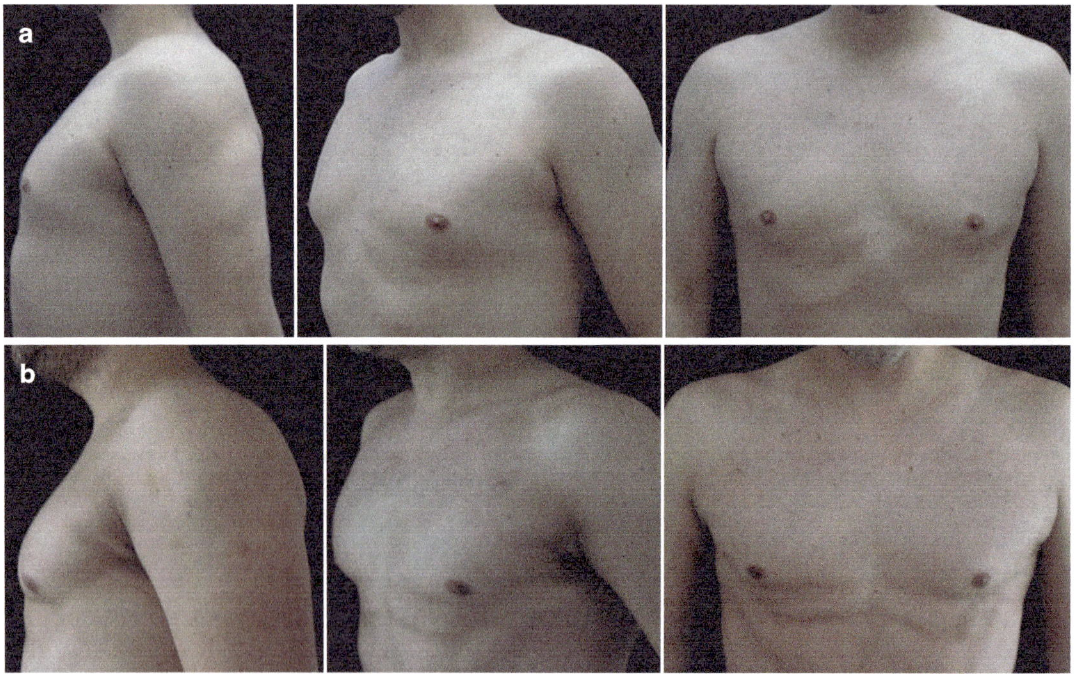

Fig. 9.15 A 26-year-old slim male patient pre- (**a**) and postoperative (**b**)

lymphatic drainage massage. Early stretching exercises are also important to prevent retractions in the lateral border of the pectoralis muscle.

Warning!

Do not use a tight garment, foam vest, or anything that would increase the pressure over the fat-grafted area. Avoid external ultrasound for postoperative therapy over this area as well. This would reduce the viability of the fat and increase its migration to surrounding areas.

References

1. Hammond DC, Arnold JF, Simon AM, Capraro PA (2003) Combined use of liposuction with the pull-through technique for the treatment of gynecomastia. Plast Reconstr Surg 112(3):891–895
2. Horn G (2002) A new concept in male reshaping: anatomical pectoral implants and liposculpture. Aesthetic Plast Surg 26:23–25
3. Mentz HA, Ruiz-Razura A, Newall G, Patronella CK, Miniel LA (2007) Pectoral etching: a method for augmentation, delineation, and contouring the thoracic musculature in men. Plast Reconstr Surg 120(7): 2051–2055
4. Hoyos AE, Millard JA (2007) Vaser-assisted High definition Lipoplasty. Aesthet Surg J 27:594–604
5. Hoyos A, Perez M (2012) Dynamic-definition male pectoral reshaping and enhancement in slim, athletic, obese, and gynecomastic patients through selective fat removal and grafting. Aesthetic Plast Surg 36(5): 1066–1077
6. de Souza Pinto EB, Indaburo PE, Da Costa Muniz A, Martinez YP, Gerent KMM, Iwamoto H, Marão Miziara AC (1996) Superficial liposuction: body contouring. Clin Plast Surg 23(4):529–548
7. Zocchi ML (1996) Ultrasound-assisted lipoplasty. Technical refinements and clinical evaluations. Clin Plast Surg 23:575–598

Male Arms

10

Introduction

No other anatomical region portrays physical strength, power, and masculinity in men than does the arm and shoulder. Ancient Greek and Roman sculptors and artists were aware of this and magnificently displayed these features in their works. In particular, Greek sculptors gloriously showcased the muscularity of the upper arm and deltoids in their sculptures. Their aim was to show the aesthetic ideals in healthy, athletic males, particularly in characters from Greek mythology, warriors, and ancient rulers.

The superficial fat structure, bilateral symmetry, and the skin thickness in this region make the task of contouring the arm one of the most challenging [1–3]. A thorough understanding of the local distribution of fatty tissue and muscular anatomy is essential for successful high-definition sculpting of the arms [4, 5]. The arm is divided into four regions: anterior, external, posterior, and internal. On the anterior, external, and internal regions, the fat is mainly of the superficial (areolar) type. This is usually a thin layer. For contouring, the most important region is the posterior aspect of the arm, where there is also a distinctive deep (lamellar) layer [5]. This layer varies in thickness, depending on the body mass index of the patient. This layer is mainly concentrated in the posterior external and anterior external regions, in the proximal and middle third of the arm. Liposuction in this area can be extensive and this can lead to skin laxity if optimal postoperative skin retraction is not achieved (Fig. 10.1).

The shape and contours of the arm are defined by the muscular disposition and mass [6–8]. In men, increased muscular mass correlates closely with an appearance of health and athleticism. The deltoid, triceps, and biceps muscles are mainly responsible for the shape of the arms and serve as guidelines for the surrounding structures (Fig. 10.2).

The Arm Has Curves

An aesthetically pleasing well-formed arm has defining curves. The shape of the deltoid and biceps muscles defines the anterior arm. The posterior arm, however, is more difficult to define and model due to its unique fat distribution. On profile view with the arm in a 90° position, the athletic posterior arm has curves in the proximal and distal areas. In the ideal arm, the muscle mass of the triceps creates a convex area in the midportion, whereas the triceps tendon flattens the distal posterior arm.

The Youth Angle

The inferior border of the arm, with the shoulder in 90° abduction, defines an angle with a vertical parallel to the midline called the "youth angle." The more acute the angle is, the more pronounced

A.E. Hoyos, P.M. Prendergast, *High Definition Body Sculpting*,
DOI 10.1007/978-3-642-54891-8_10, © Springer-Verlag Berlin Heidelberg 2014

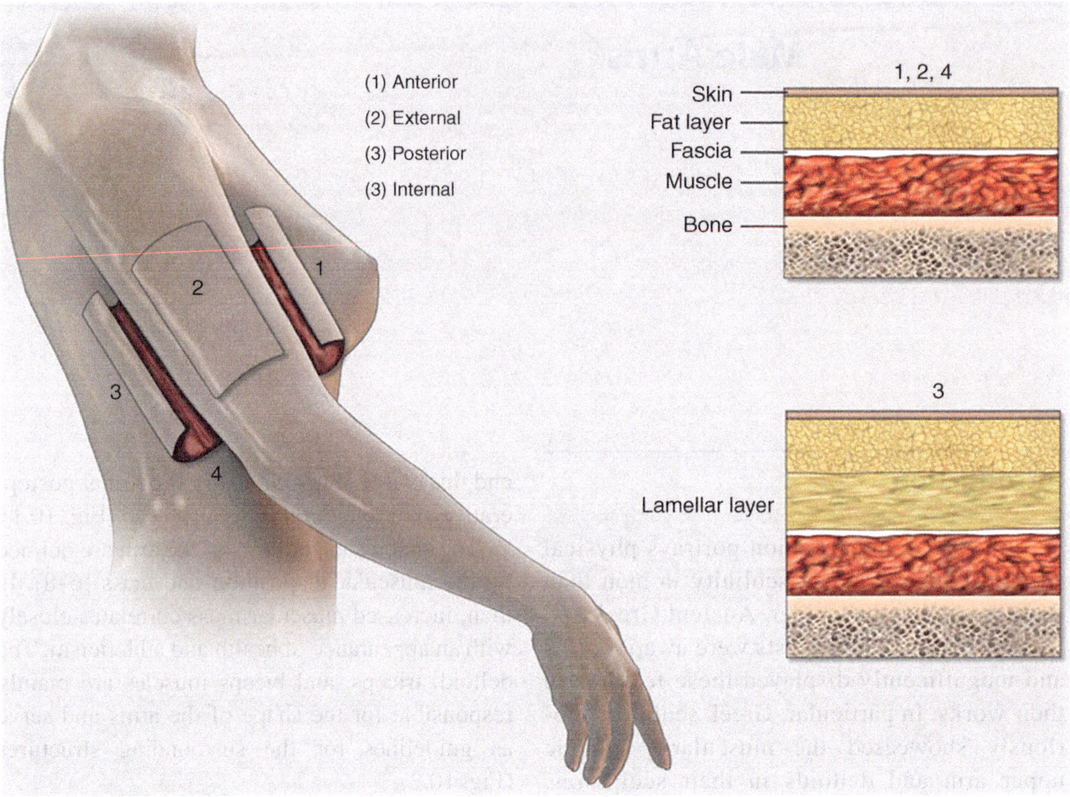

Fig. 10.1 Anatomical basis of fat distribution in the arm according to Avelar [1]. Anterior (*1*), external (*2*), posterior (*3*), and internal (*4*) zones of the arm. Zone 3 is prone to store a larger amount of lamellar (deep) fat, which is the area of focused debulking during liposuction

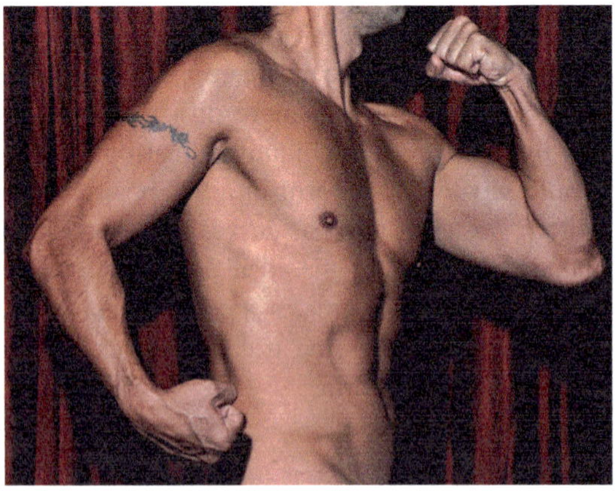

Fig. 10.2 Athletic male arms

the triceps muscle mass. In obese and older patients, the angle tends to be obtuse due to the presence of extra fat and/or laxity of the skin (Fig. 10.3).

High-definition liposculpture helps attain an athletic appearance by shaping the body fat in multiple layers and over the entire arm contour by creating concave and convex zones [5]. This differs considerably from simply flattening the convex areas using conventional liposuction.

Stealth Incisions

The ideal incision points should be placed with the patient in the prone position, with 90° arm abduction, 90° elbow flexion, and complete external rotation. Usually three 5 mm incisions are made: in the posterior axillary crease, in the anterior axillary fold, and the last one at the elbow near the olecranon tip. Silicone ports and discs are placed into the incisions and sutured in place (Fig. 10.4).

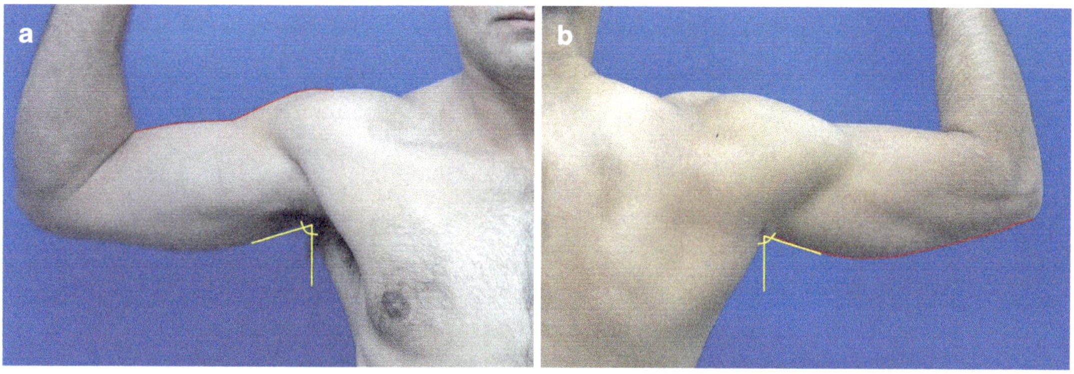

Fig. 10.3 A 42-year-old male. (**a**) The anterior portion of the arm is defined by the curvature of the deltoid and the biceps. Fat deposition in this portion is minimal even with moderate weight fluctuations and normal aging. (**b**) The posterior arm is prone to fat deposition due to the presence of deep (lamellar) fat and thin skin that increases in volume with weight changes (**b**). The posterior arm is not straight in its ideal aesthetic form; areas of curvature (negative spaces) are present in the proximal and distal arm due to the triceps tendon (distal) and the insertion of the proximal triceps. The angle between a vertical line and the proximal posterior arm is defined as the "youth angle" (*yellow lines*). This angle should be less than 90°

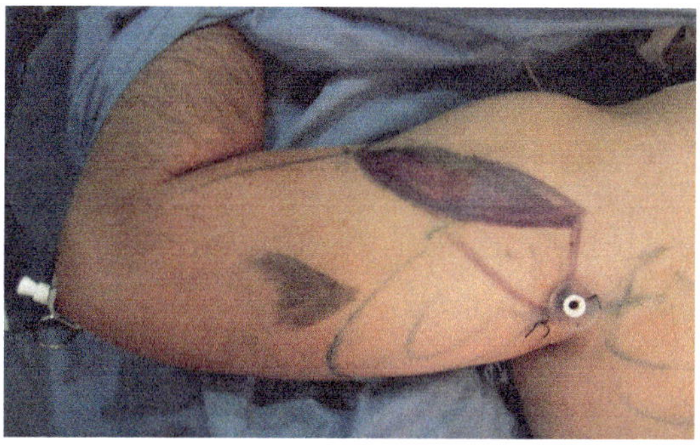

Fig. 10.4 Incision sites with ports at the posterior axillary crease and the elbow

There is a difference in the negative spaces by gender because of the triceps curvature in men (Fig. 10.5).

Deep Markings

The posterior area is divided into thirds. The distal and proximal arm is where most of the fat for extraction is located (Fig. 10.6).

Framing

Three muscles are marked: deltoids, biceps, and triceps. To begin, ask the patient to perform 90° arm abduction with 90° elbow flexion and neutral internal rotation of the shoulder in order to mark the posterior sulcus of the deltoid (Fig. 10.7). Next, with the shoulder externally rotated, mark the anterior sulcus. Then, in complete adduction of the upper limb, ask him to perform a voluntary contraction of the triceps muscle. This creates a new groove at the posterior sulcus. The zone between the initial posterior sulcus groove and this new groove created during muscular contraction is the "dynamic zone." In active contraction of the triceps, another mark is made at the interfascicular zone. The intermuscular creases

The Use of Drains

In general, drains are not required in this area. The incision near the elbow is left open to facilitate permissive drainage postoperatively. Prompt postoperative management, including massage, is important in order to achieve adequate drainage, reduce swelling, and accelerate healing.

Markings

Preoperative marking is performed with the patient in the standing position. The fat is better visualized with the arm relaxed in adduction.

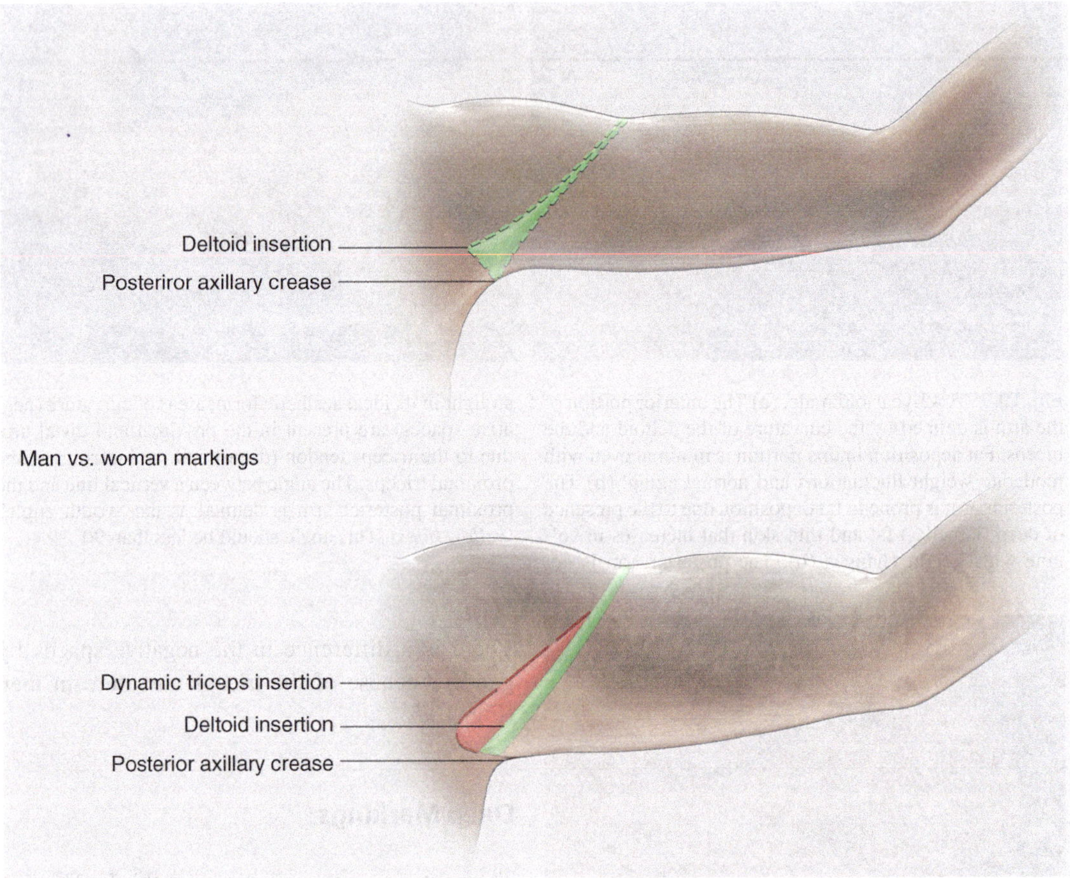

Fig. 10.5 Illustration showing the definition zones for the male and female patient (*in green*). The higher muscular volume of the triceps muscle in male displaces the deltoid m. when in contraction: the dynamic zone (*in red*)

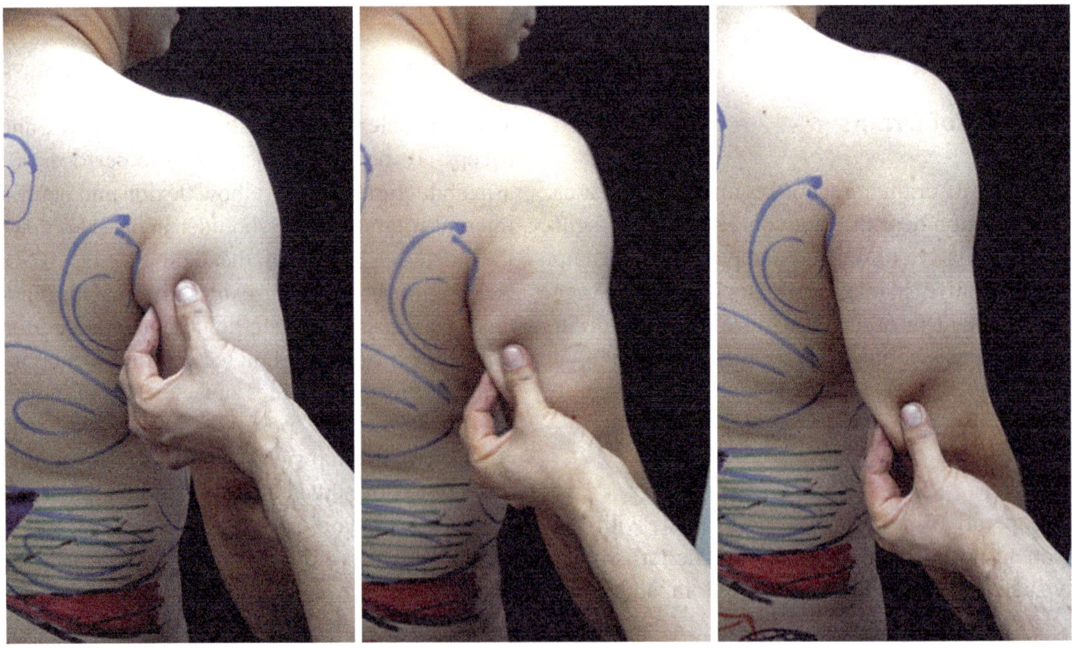

Fig. 10.6 Assessing fat thickness on the posterior arm: proximal, middle and distal portions of the posterior zone

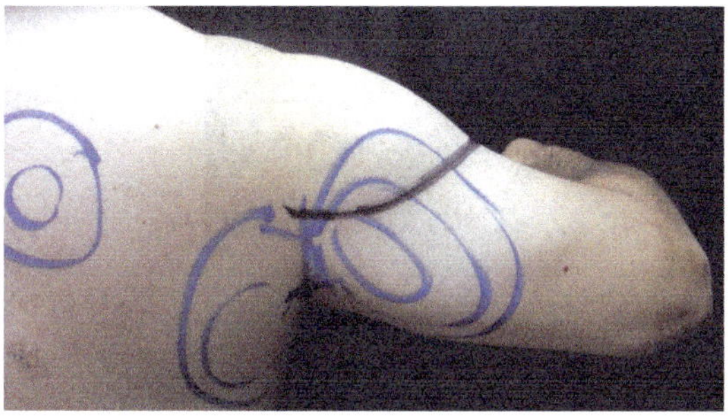

Fig. 10.7 Arm position for the deltoid posterior sulcus marking

between the biceps and triceps are also marked for fat extraction (Fig. 10.8).

Negative Spaces

The bicipital groove is marked internally and externally. Marking the biceps in 90° flexion of the elbow, we sketch a semilunar zone from the distal muscle tendon to the crease of the elbow. A transition area is marked from the posterior border of the deltoid toward the muscle belly. This is used to guide the blending during lipoplasty to avoid unsightly steps (Fig. 10.9).

Procedure

Infiltration

The tumescent solution consists of 1,000 ml of normal saline plus 1 ml of 1:1,000 epinephrine and 100 ml of 1 % lidocaine. Begin by infiltrating the deep layers of fat followed by the superficial layers. The infiltrate/aspirate ratio should be 2:1.

Emulsification

Emulsification begins in the superficial layer. The average timing for emulsification is approximately 2 min per 100 ml of tumescent solution infiltrated. However, the clinical endpoint is the loss of tissue resistance to the probe. The superficial layers are treated in pulsed (VASER) mode to reduce the total amount of energy delivered to the tissues by half, therefore reducing the heat delivered to the skin. The deeper layers can be treated in continuous mode to efficiently and quickly emulsify adipose tissue.

Extraction

Deep Extraction

Deep liposuction is performed using a 3 mm cannula over the marked areas. The majority of the debulking is performed over the proximal posterior aspect of the upper arm (Fig. 10.10).

Warning!
Liposuction in the deep layer of the posterior arm has to be concentrated in the proximal and distal zones. In the middle third caution should be taken to avoid overresection. This creates a "telephone" deformity.

Superficial Framing

The initial goal of superficial liposuction in the arm is to frame the contours in the posterior proximal and distal arm. Superficial liposuction also allows the skin to redrape and enhances skin retraction. We use a curved 45° 3 mm cannula to contour the deltoid sulcus (Fig. 10.11). Similarly, the intermuscular grooves are suctioned to highlight the separation between the triceps and biceps anteriorly and posteriorly.

Warning!
The lipoplasty in the arms must be performed using small (3 mm) cannulae to avoid contour irregularities. For the contouring of the deltoid and triceps, a special curved cannula must be used.

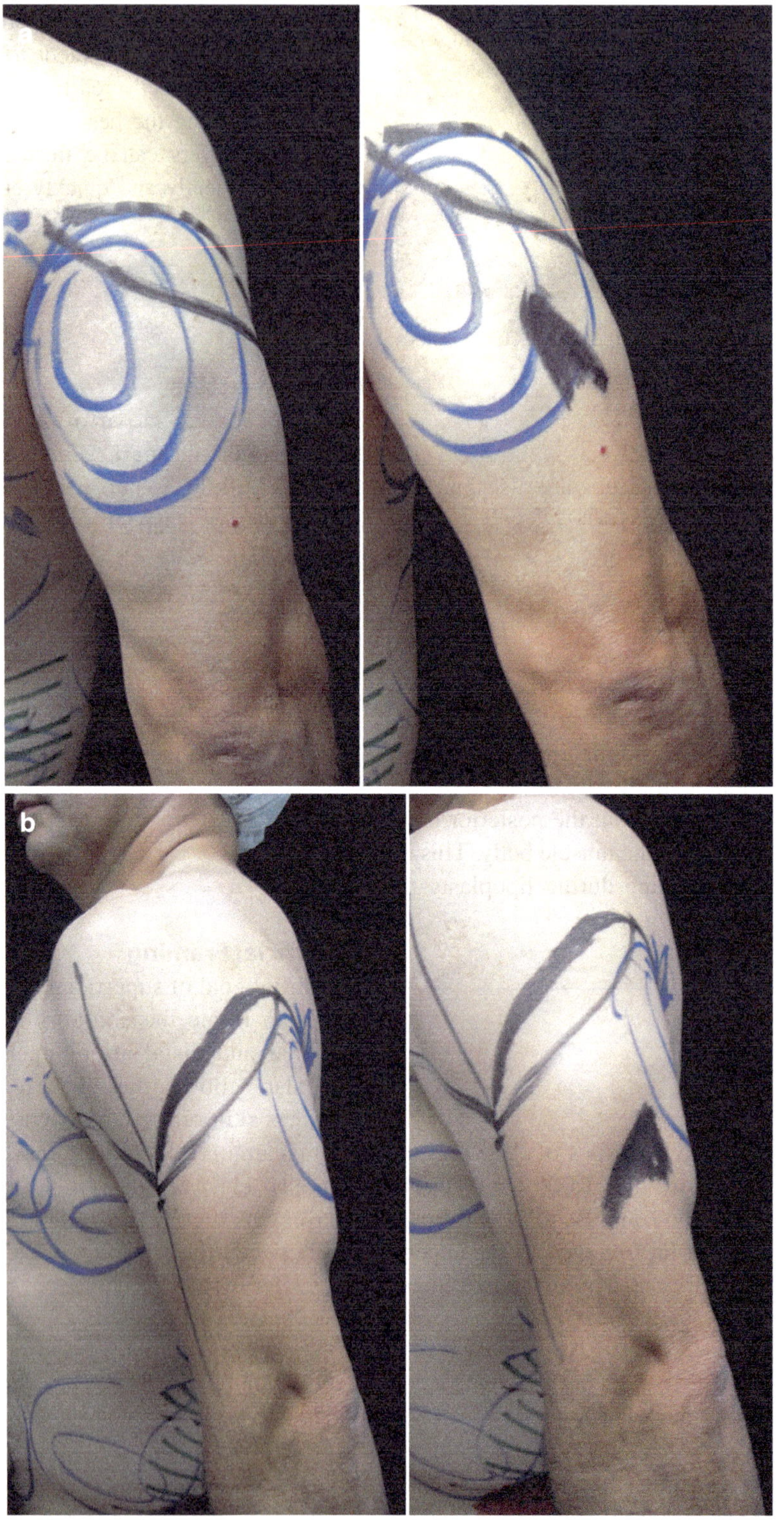

Fig. 10.8 Triceps and dynamic zone markings. Marking of the deltoid dynamic zone and the triceps interfascicular zone: (**a**) posterior and (**b**) lateral view

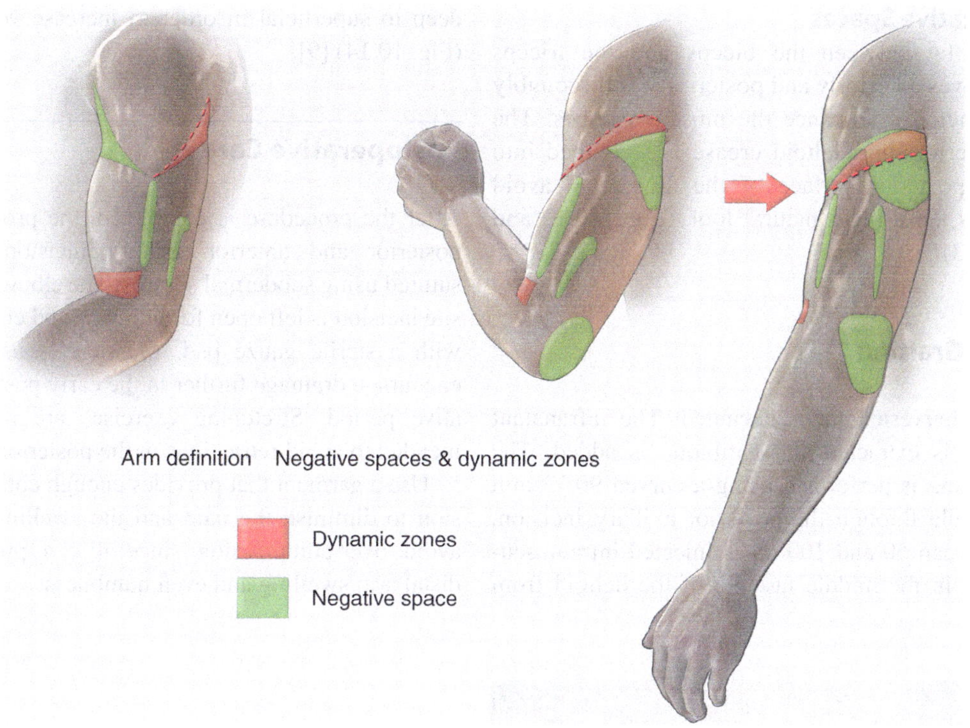

Fig. 10.9 Areas to be marked for arm definition in men. Negative spaces include the bicipital groove (internal and external), the tricipital tendon, and the posterior border of the triceps in the proximal and distal portion. Notice that the zones of dynamic movement are treated as zones of negative space in the area of the posterior deltoid sulcus and the distal bicipital tendon. These markings move as different muscles contract, so for accuracy, a transition zone is outlined in these areas

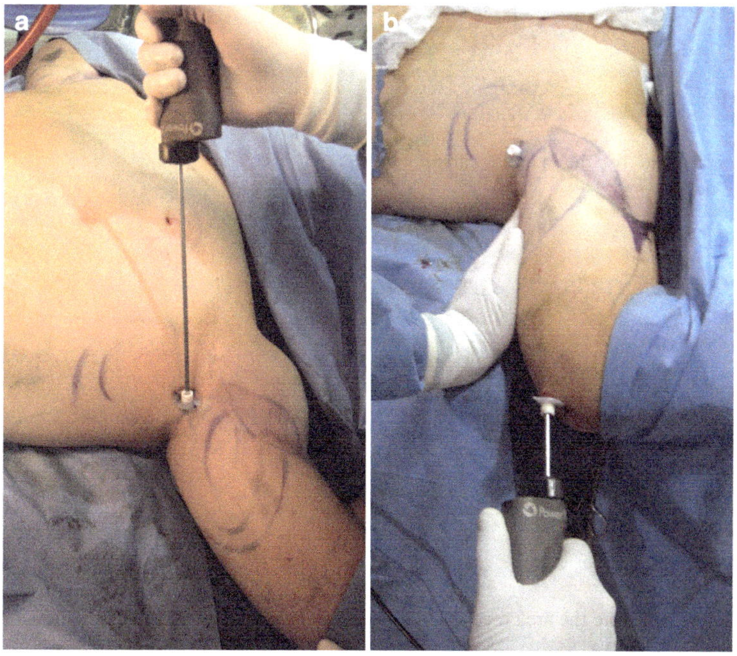

Fig. 10.10 Deep extraction through the posterior axillary port (**a**) and the elbow port (**b**)

Negative Spaces

The fat between the biceps and the triceps grooves anteriorly and posteriorly is thoroughly extracted to enhance the muscular edges. The posterior supradeltoid crease is smoothed into the posterior surface of the muscle to avoid steps, ensuring a natural look (Figs. 10.12 and 10.13).

Fat Grafting

The harvested fat is decanted. The infranatant fluid is extracted and antibiotic is added. The grafting is performed using a curved 90° 3 mm cannula through the posterior axillary incision. Between 50 and 100 ml is injected intramuscularly in the middle fascicle of the deltoid from deep to superficial in order to increase volume (Fig. 10.14) [9].

Postoperative Care

After the procedure is completed, the proximal posterior and anterior axillary incisions are sutured using subdermal sutures. The elbow port-site incision is left open for drainage and covered with a sterile gauze pad. Massage is used to encourage drainage further in the early postoperative period. Stretching exercises are recommended to avoid retractions in the posterior arm.

Use a garment that provides enough compression to diminish the pain and the swelling, but avoid over-compression since it can produce distal arm swelling and even numbness.

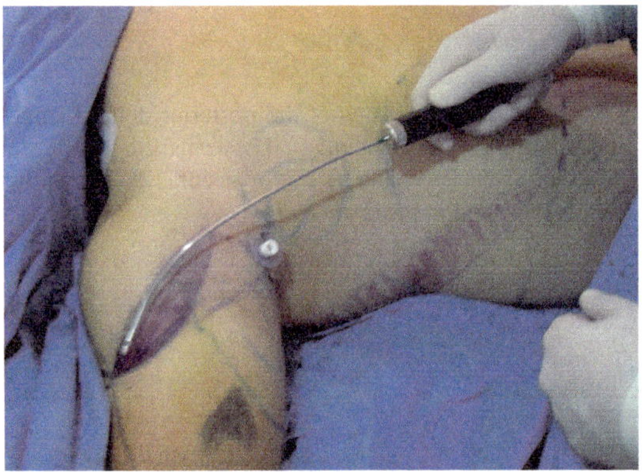

Fig. 10.11 Approach used by the curved cannula to access the posterior deltoid

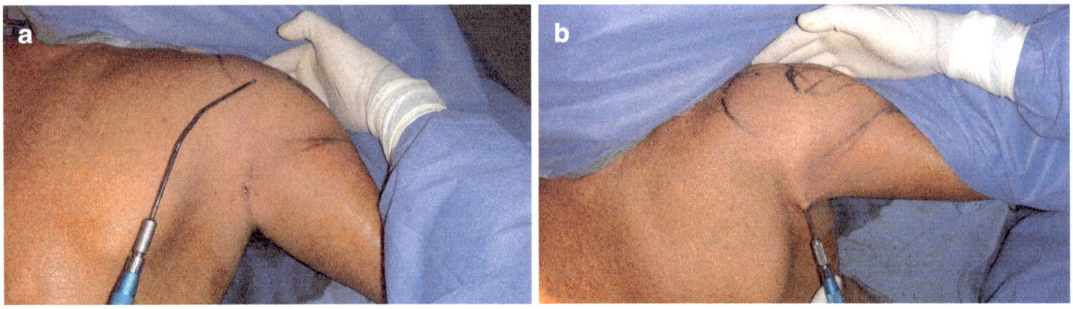

Fig. 10.12 Fat grafting. (**a**) Note the area reached by the curved cannula. (**b**) Fat injection procedure

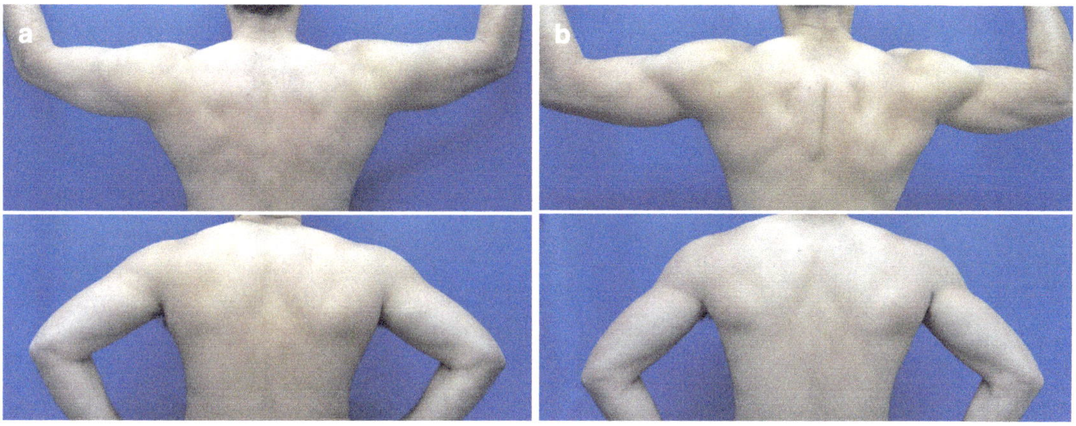

Fig. 10.13 A 45-year-old overweight male patient, preoperative (**a**) and 1 year postoperative (**b**) anterior and posterior view

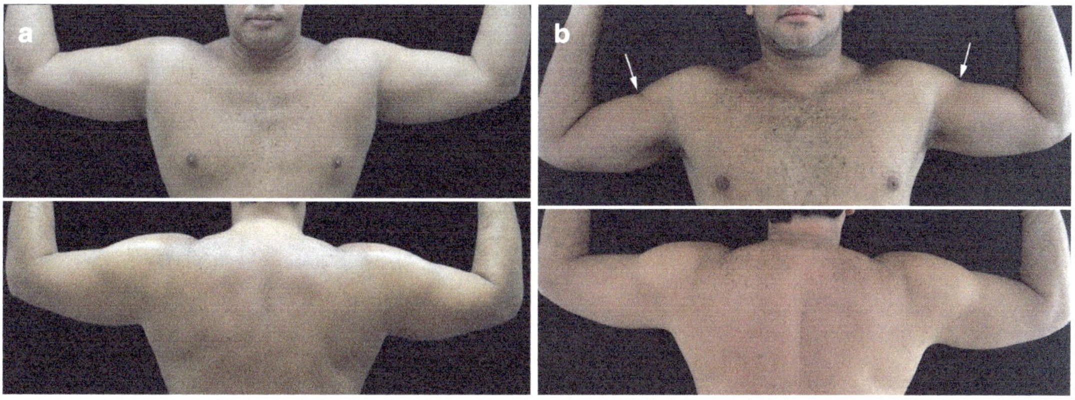

Fig. 10.14 A 42 year-old patient, preoperative views (**a**) anterior (*up*) and posterior (*below*); and six months postoperative (**b**) anterior (*up*) and posterior (*below*). Liposuction with definition and fat grafting of 60 ml was performed. The *arrow* shows the definition of the deltoid sulcus giving the sensation of higher muscularity

References

1. Avelar J (1989) Regional distribution and behavior of the subcutaneous tissue concerning selection and indication for liposuction. Aesthet Surg J 13: 155–165
2. de Souza Pinto EB, Indaburo PE, Da Costa Muniz A, Martinez YP, Gerent KMM, Iwamoto H, Marão Miziara AC (1996) Superficial liposuction: body contouring. Clin Plast Surg 23(4):529–548
3. Rochrich RJ, Beran SJ, Di Spaltro F et al. (1998) Extending the role of liposuction in body contouring with ultrasound assisted liposuction. Plast Reconstr Surg 101:1090–1102
4. Duncan DI (2012) Improving outcomes in upper arm liposuction: adding radiofrequency-assisted liposuction to induce skin contraction. Aesthet Surg J 32(1):84–95
5. Hoyos A, Perez M (2012) Arm dynamic definition by liposculpture and fat grafting. Aesthet Surg J 32(8): 974–987
6. Appelt EA, Janis JE, Rohrich RJ (2006) An algorithmic approach to upper arm contouring. Plast Reconstr Surg 118:237–246
7. Chamosa M, Murillo J, Vázquez T (2005) Lipectomy of arms and lipograft of shoulders balance the upper body contour. Aesthetic Plast Surg 29(6): 567–570
8. Gilliland MD, Lyos AT (1997) CAST liposuction of the arm improves aesthetic results. Aesthetic Plast Surg 21(4):225–229
9. Toledo L, Mauad R (2006) Fat injection: a 20-year revision. Clin Plast Surg 33:47–53

11 Male Torso and Back

Introduction

The shape, size, and definition of the back play an important role in the aesthetics of the male human anatomy [1, 2]. Ideally, the posterior torso should be "V" shaped, broader superiorly, and tapering inferiorly. The deltoid volume should be pronounced and there should be visible separation between these muscles and the rest of the back [3]. With underdeveloped musculature and excess fatty deposits around the flanks and waist, definition is poor and the ideal shape becomes an inverted "V" or pear shape. In men, fat deposits around the posterior and lateral waist, the so-called love handles, are particularly problematic because they often do not respond to exercise and dieting [4]. The main objective of body sculpting in the back is to obtain the "V"-shaped posterior torso. This is achieved by thorough liposculpture to extract most of the fat and highlight the dominant muscles, particularly the latissimus dorsi and paraspinal muscles (Fig. 11.1) [5–7].

Stealth Incisions

Extensive lipoplasty of the posterior aspect of the torso requires incision sites that allow access to most of the surface area of the back and flanks. Placing incisions on almost any point over the surface of the back poses the risk of visibility, so we use stealth incisions to hide them. Incisions are placed in the posterior axillary folds and in the intergluteal crease.

For accessing the entire treatment area from these limited incisions, specially designed long and curved cannulae are used. These allow access to the flanks and upper and lower back and follow the curvature of the torso and lower back as the sculpting progresses laterally (Fig. 11.2).

The Use of Drains

A single drain is used in the posterior torso in the intergluteal incision. Open drainage is useful for very mobile patients who prefer not to be restricted, although it is messier and requires the concomitant use of diapers or highly absorbent dressings or pads (Fig. 11.3).

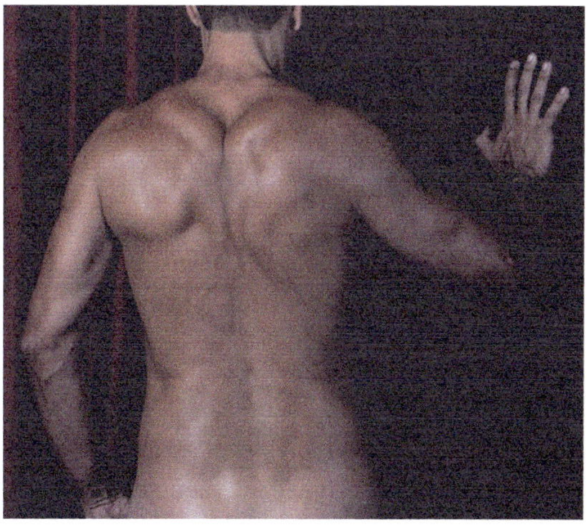

Fig. 11.1 Athletic male torso showing the ideal "V" shape

A.E. Hoyos, P.M. Prendergast, *High Definition Body Sculpting*,
DOI 10.1007/978-3-642-54891-8_11, © Springer-Verlag Berlin Heidelberg 2014

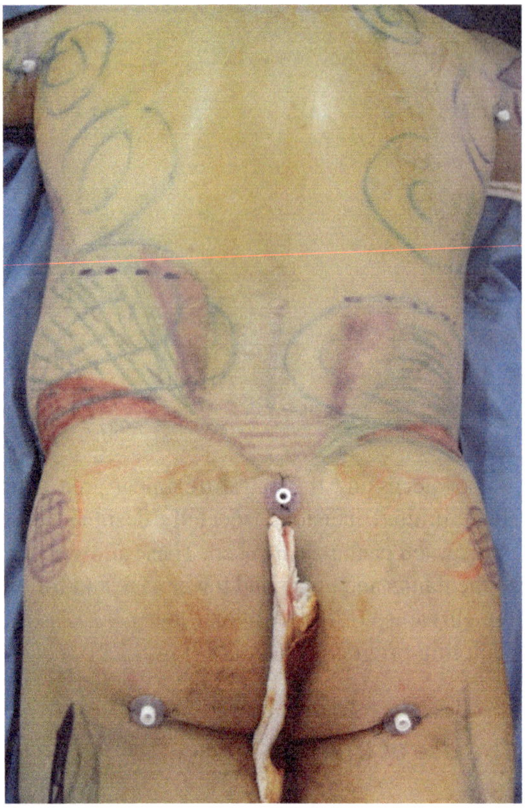

Fig. 11.2 Intraoperative image showing the preferred incision and port sites

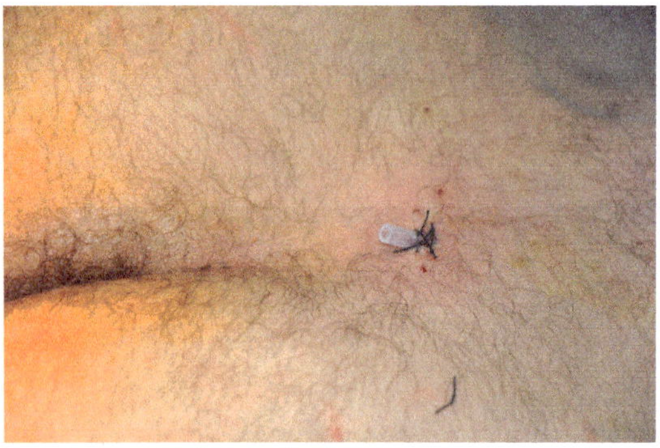

Fig. 11.3 Open drain in sacral incision

Closed drains are more bulky and difficult to conceal. Although they tend to be more cumbersome with the foam vest and garment, their potential benefits should be discussed with the patient preoperatively. The vacuum generated may improve skin redraping. Naturally, they also contain much of the blood-stained drainage fluid.

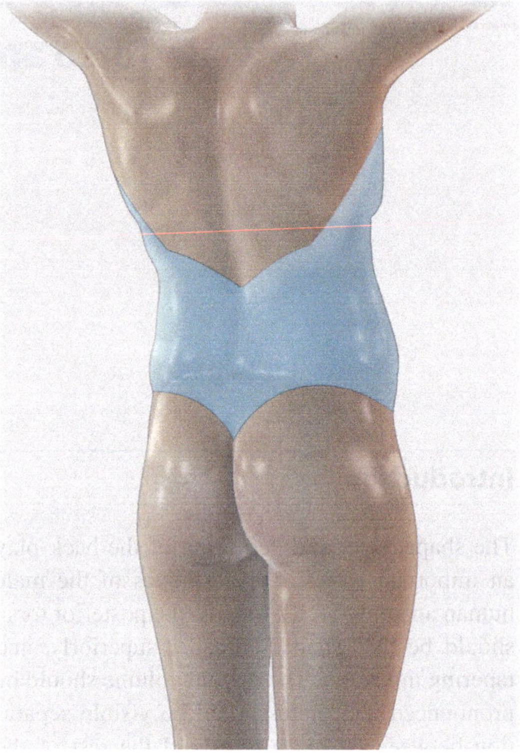

Fig. 11.4 Illustration showing the areas requiring debulking of extra fat (*in light blue*)

Markings

Deep Markings

The initial liposuction markings are made in the areas where extra fat is located (Fig. 11.4): the axillary fat pad, the mid back where the fat rolls are located in some patients, and the lower back over the hips (love handles). The latter area is often under-resected, leading to a suboptimal result, particularly if the patient gains any weight subsequently (Fig. 11.5). The key in this important area is to thoroughly remove the fat in order to achieve the desired shape and provide a long-lasting result.

Framing

Framing delineates the position of the muscles and other superficial anatomy landmarks. In the

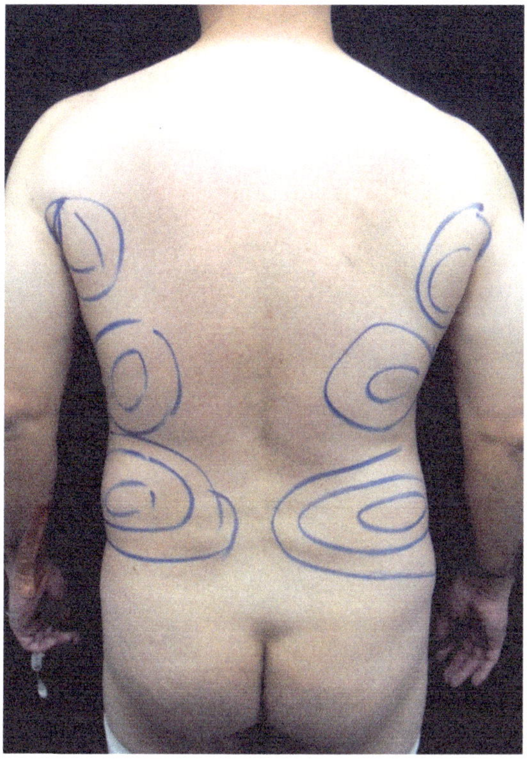

Fig. 11.5 Marking of the axillary fat pad, mid back, and love handles

upper back, the lateral border of the latissimus dorsi is outlined, although most of the definition of this muscle is achieved with the patient in the supine position. In practice, some definition of the upper back muscles is achieved simply by removing superfluous fat. It is not necessary to mark and sculpt the smaller muscles like trapezius and rhomboids. Attempting to define these muscles individually tends to produce an unnatural result.

The lower back is different. The important muscles to reveal are the paralumbar muscles, paired columns of muscle adjacent to the lower spine [3]. The lines formed by these create a hollow area lateral to them when the love handles are empty. These continue inferiorly with the sacral dimples (Fig. 11.6). In some men the sacral dimples are visible, but they are not key features that determine an athletic shape, since men do not tend to have an appreciable sacral fat pad.

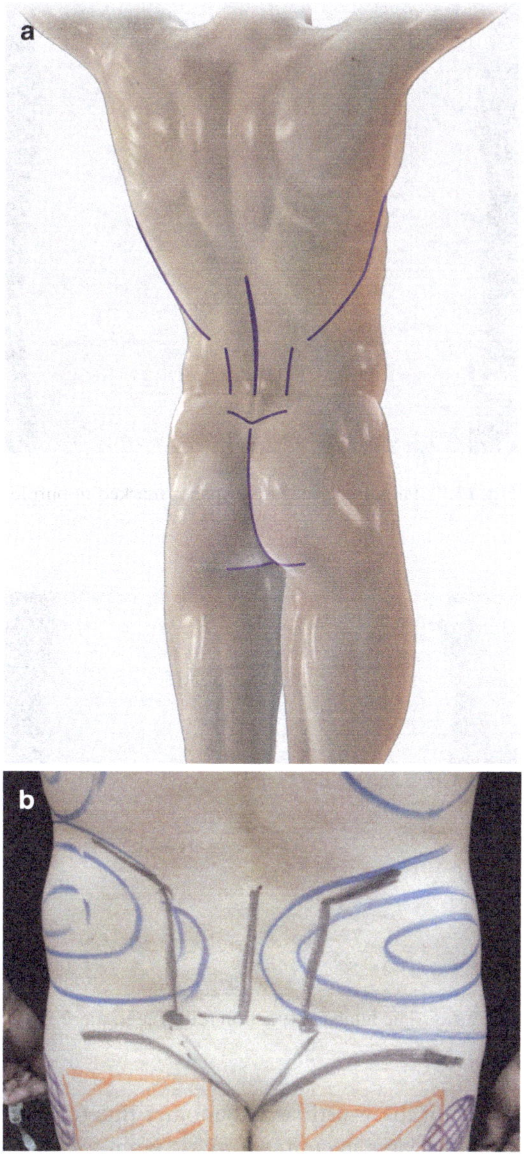

Fig. 11.6 (a) Framing the latissimus dorsi and paralumbar muscles (b) preoperative markings to define the paralumbar muscles

Negative Spaces

There are three key areas for negative spaces in men: one is a triangular-shaped area lateral to the paralumbar muscles, with an upper limit along the lower costal margin (Fig. 11.7).

The second negative space in this region is delineated by a line from the upper intergluteal crease to the point of maximum indentation

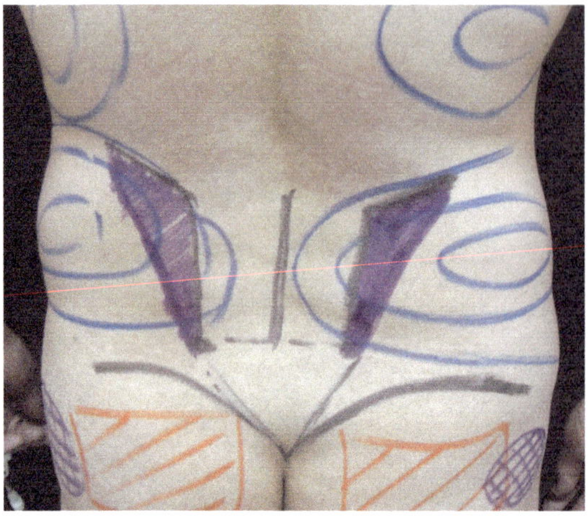

Fig. 11.7 Paralumbar negative spaces marked in purple

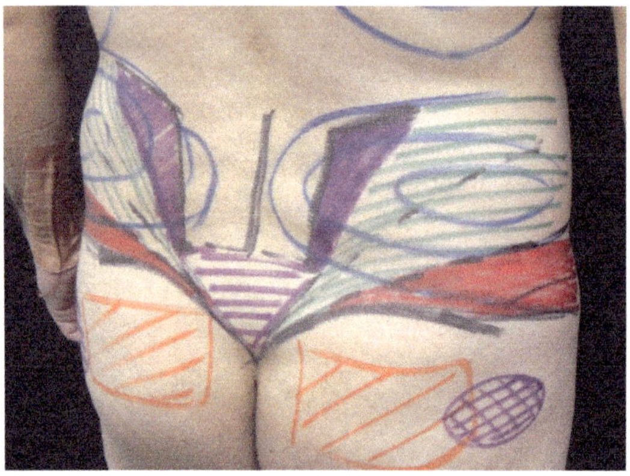

Fig. 11.8 The lumbar extraction red zone in men

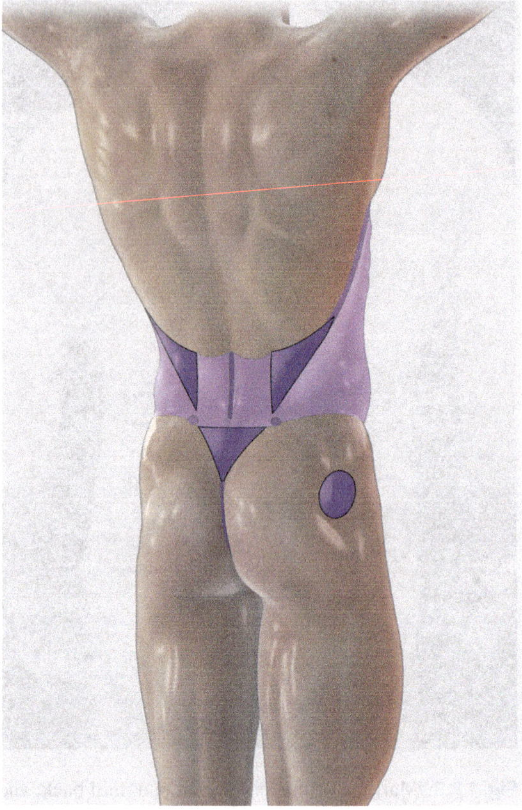

Fig. 11.9 Illustration showing the dorsal extraction areas for the male patient: the areas of preferred deep extraction (*light purple*) and the negative spaces (*in dark violet*)

(PMI) of the waistline and another line (curved) from the same intergluteal crease point following the superior limit of the gluteus maximus muscle, ending in the upper limit of the trochanteric depression. In females this area produces a slightly smooth contour, whereas in men this area is a complete depletion zone that creates a lower waistline and improved muscular definition (Fig. 11.8).

The third negative space is the sacral triangle, marked by connecting the sacral dimples and these dimples to the intergluteal crease point (Fig. 11.8). The dorsal areas for fat extraction in the male patient are shown in Fig. 11.9.

Procedure

Infiltration

The procedure initiates with infiltration. When we use general anesthesia, the solution consists of 1,000 cc Ringer's lactate and 1:100,000 epinephrine and lidocaine 20 cc 1 % solution.

Following a 2:1 ratio of infiltrate to aspirate, aim to infiltrate half of the volume in the superficial layer and half in the deep layer. The infiltration begins in the deep layer and is completed in the superficial layers. This order is important, since tumescence is a transient state. If infiltration began in the superficial layer, much of the wetting fluid could migrate more deeply by the time the ultrasound delivery commenced. Delivery of ultrasound energy to dry tissues is ineffective and potentially dangerous. Once the deeper layers are thoroughly infiltrated, the superficial layer is filled, trying to make it as even as possible, until a state of turgid tumescence is achieved (Fig. 11.10).

Emulsification

In this step, emulsification begins in the superficial layer and moves later to the deeper layers. This is the opposite order to infiltration. Emulsification should begin in the subdermal plane once optimal vasoconstriction following the infusion of tumescent fluid has been reached and before the wetting solution has migrated deeply away from this plane. Slow, deliberate strokes are used so that the VASER probes emulsify evenly and smoothly. For the superficial plane, the system is tuned to pulsed (VASER) mode to prevent excessive heat generation.

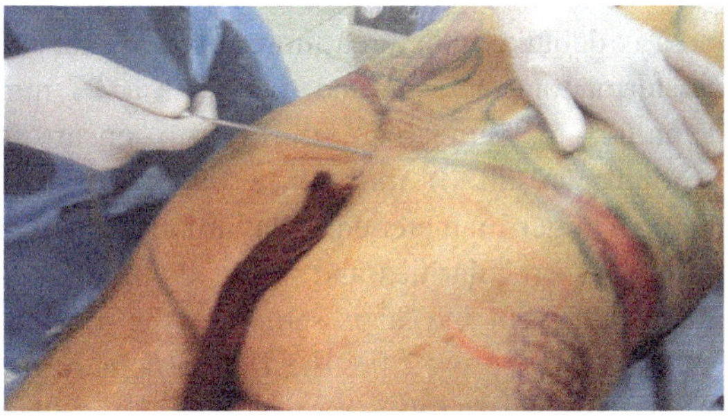

Fig. 11.10 Tumescent solution infiltration through the intergluteal incision

Additional VASER time is utilized along the areas of framing to prepare for more aggressive extraction in these areas.

Later, proceed to the deep layer. Begin with the deepest areas to ensure complete emulsification, gently rubbing the probe against the muscular layer. Do this with very slow, controlled strokes. Once there is little or no resistance in the deep subcutaneous fat, return again superficially to blend with the previously treated area in the subdermal plane (Fig. 11.11).

Extraction

Deep Extraction

From the intergluteal crease access incision, the deep love handle region is approached first from medial to lateral. From deep to superficial, the aim is to almost completely empty the fat here in order to ensure a good contour and minimize the likelihood of an undercorrection. From the same incision, any fat in the sacral triangle is also removed. Although this region requires aggressive liposuction, it should be performed using a safe technique, always aware of the location of the tip of the cannula. The guiding hand feels for the tip of the cannula and protects the posterior costal margin.

One of the key points to treat the waistline is to start with a small cannula (3.7 mm) in the deep layer and later advance to a 4.6 mm cannula to sculpt the negative space of the supragluteal area. In order to achieve lateral extraction, a specially designed curved 4.6 mm cannula is used to reach

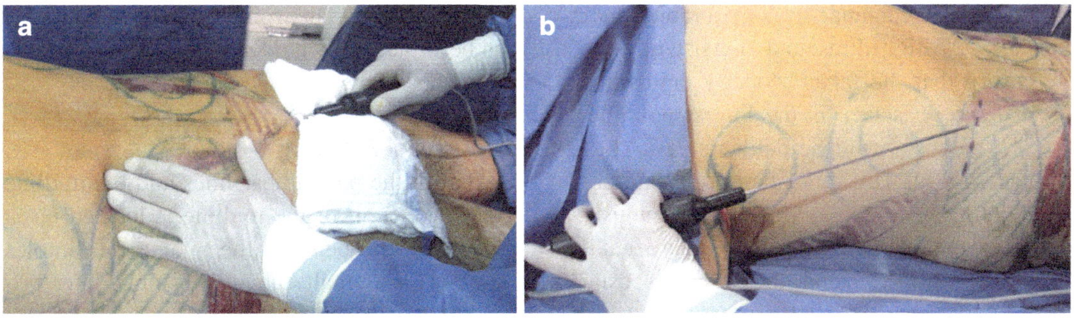

Fig. 11.11 VASER emulsification through the intergluteal port (**a**); notice the reach of the cannula when inserted through the posterior axillary port (**b**)

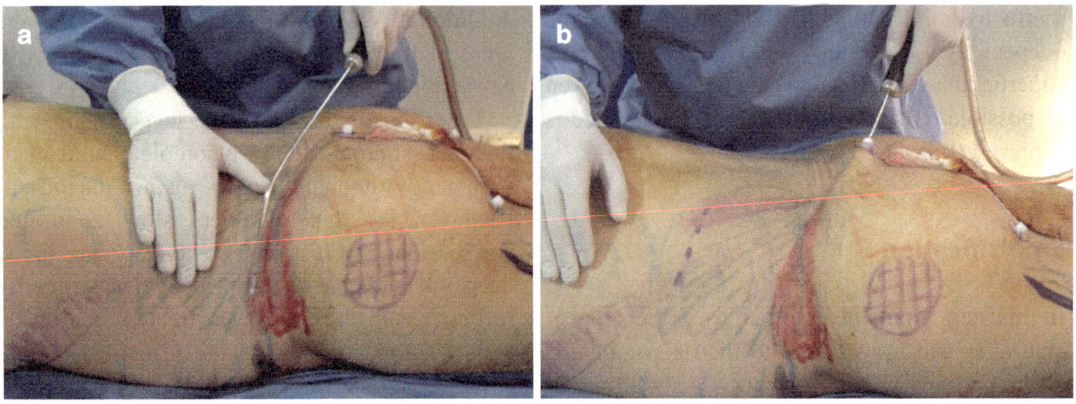

Fig. 11.12 Deep fat extraction over the red zone using a curve cannula. (**a**) Area reached by the cannula, (**b**) extraction procedure

distally around the waist. Remember that the stroke motion with this cannula has to follow the curvature of the cannula. The arm movement of the surgeon is not to and fro in a linear pattern, but adopts a slightly semicircular pattern (Fig. 11.12).

Warning
The lower back is one of the most dangerous areas to work on, especially during infiltration and deep extraction from the upper intergluteal crease incision. The access is difficult and the angle is awkward. The costal margin is very low and sometimes difficult to identify. In addition, the fat is dense in the deep layer simulating superficial fat. Adjust the surgical table so that the torso is flexed and the costal margin moves away from the trajectory of the probes and cannulae. It is important to use the VASER ultrasound persistently to ensure that the fat is properly emulsified and the resistance is the lowest possible. The passes should be deliberate but slow and careful. The smart hand (the one not holding the cannula) should continuously locate the tip of the cannula to ensure that it never passes beyond the inferior costal margin. The authors advise that only experienced surgeons should contour this area.

Once the dorsal lumbar area is contoured, proceed to the upper back. The area of fat close to the posterior axillary fold is treated initially using a short, large-diameter cannula (4.6 mm × 12 cm cannula "4.6 baby") since this is a difficult area for extraction due to the angulation. Once this area is debulked, the area more distally over the posterior torso is aspirated, first with a 3.7 mm cannula, to "tunnelize" the fat to ensure a smoother result. If this dense fat is extracted using a larger-diameter cannula initially, the likelihood of irregularities and ridges is high. Once the majority of the fat is removed, the 4.6 mm cannula can be used for the final touch. In the presence of back rolls, treat superficially with a 3.7 mm cannula in order to release the dense fibrous tissue in this area until there is loss of resistance. An additional incision may be used that can provide better longitudinal access to the rolls for release. In women, this extra incision can be strategically hidden in the bra line; in men it may be visible.

Superficial Framing

Start with the paralumbar lines and the midline. The lower limit of the midline is located on an imaginary line between the two sacral dimples. Begin with a small cannula (3 mm), later proceeding to deepen the groove using a 3.7 mm cannula. The paralumbar lines are sculpted in the same way.

The Negative Spaces

Since there are only two areas, start with the paralumbar negative space, using a 3.7 mm cannula. For a thorough extraction, the same area should be approached from the axillary incision using a long 3.7 or 4.6 mm cannula (Fig. 11.13).

Later, complete the second negative space (lateral supragluteal) with a 4.6 mm curved cannula for the deeper areas and a 3.0 mm semi-curved cannula for the superficial plane, using an arm movement that correlates with the degree of curvature of the cannula.

If gluteal fat grafting is planned, the final touch in the lumbar area is completed *after* performing fat grafting [8, 9]. This is important to prevent a staircase appearance of the gluteal region, from the augmented buttock to the concave lower back. As with all sculpting, a tonal progression from convexities to concavities is important to achieve a natural aesthetic appearance. Results following liposculpture of the male torso and back are shown in Figs. 11.14 and 11.15.

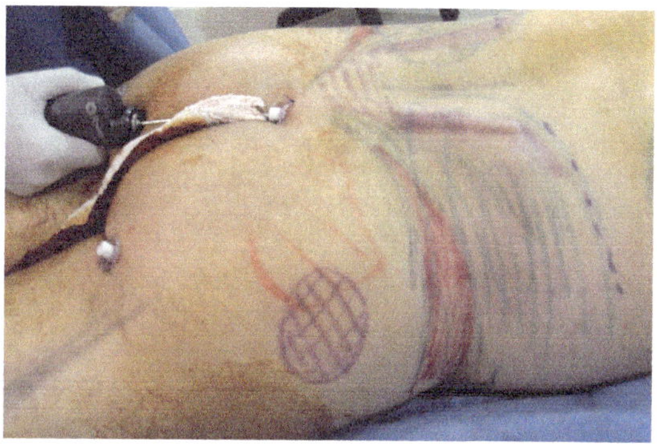

Fig. 11.13 Extraction of the negative paralumbar zone

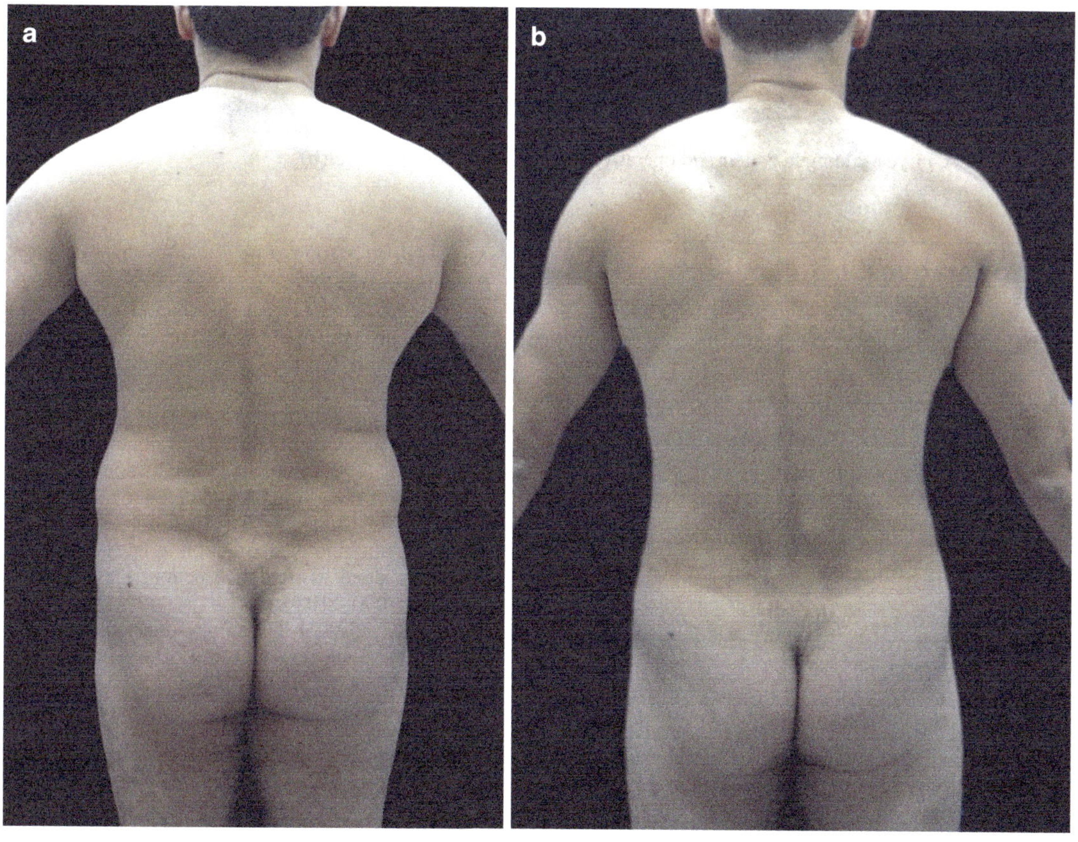

Fig. 11.14 A 42-year-old male patient, preoperative (**a**) and 6 months postoperative (**b**)

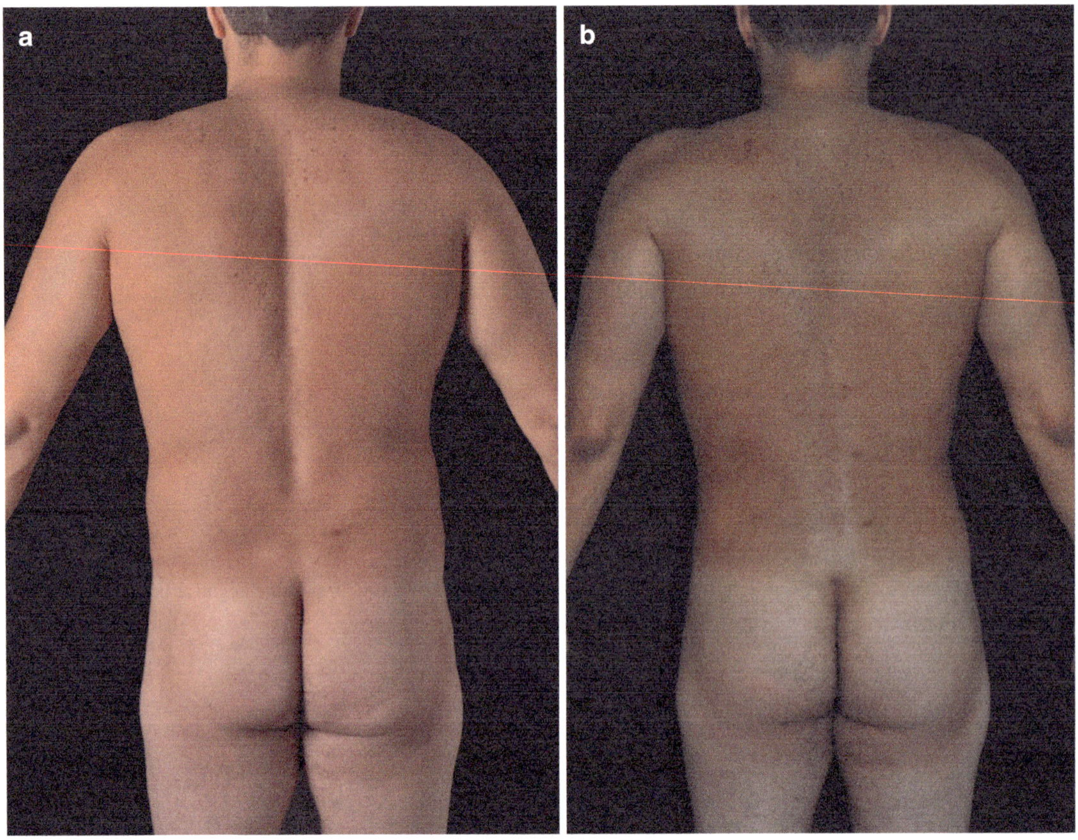

Fig. 11.15 A 46-year-old male patient, preoperative (**a**) and 1 year postoperative (**b**)

Postoperative Care

The posterior axillary fold incision is closed with subdermal sutures. Usually a drain is placed in the intergluteal crease incision, although in certain cases permissive drainage is achieved simply by leaving the incision open.

Padding is placed over the sacral triangle for extra compression. A high-definition foam vest and overlying compression garment are applied.

References

1. Hoyos AE, Millard JA (2007) Vaser-assisted high definition lipoplasty. Aesthet Surg J 27:594–604
2. Hoyos A, Perez M (2012) Arm dynamic definition by liposculpture and fat grafting. Aesthet Surg J 32(8): 974–987
3. Matarasso SL (1999) Liposuction of the chest and back. Dermatol Clin 17(4):799–804
4. Avelar J (1989) Regional distribution and behavior of the subcutaneous tissue concerning selection and indication for liposuction. Aesthet Surg J 13: 155–165
5. de Souza Pinto EB, Indaburo PE, Da Costa Muniz A, Martinez YP, Gerent KMM, Iwamoto H, Marão Miziara AC (1996) Superficial liposuction: body contouring. Clin Plast Surg 23(4):529–548
6. Rochrich RJ, Beran SJ, Di Spaltro F et al (1998) Extending the role of liposuction in body contouring with ultrasound assisted liposuction. Plast Reconstr Surg 101:1090–1102
7. Zocchi ML (1996) Ultrasound-assisted lipoplasty. Technical refinements and clinical evaluations. Clin Plast Surg 23:575–598
8. Chajchir A (1996) Fat injection: long-term follow-up. Aesthetic Plast Surg 20:291
9. Toledo L, Mauad R (2006) Fat injection: a 20-year revision. Clin Plast Surg 33:47–53

Male Buttocks and Thighs

12

Introduction

The gluteal area in men is defined by the shape and volume of the gluteus maximus muscle. A well-developed and aesthetically pleasing gluteal region is a trait unique to primates, which is an evolutionary adaptation to erect posture and bipedal locomotion. The gluteus maximus muscle and fat deposits in the superficial fascia largely form the buttock projection. In addition, our erect posture contributes to the lumbosacral curve, which is also unique to primates (Fig. 12.1).

In terms of evolutionary instincts, a developed gluteal region and muscular lower limbs denote power and strength. These are traits that make for a good hunter and thus a good provider. Well-defined, muscular buttocks, therefore, correlate closely with physical attractiveness [1]. It is the muscularity, shape, and definition of the male buttocks that are cues for sexual attraction, and not merely the size. Large, rounded, buttocks in obese patients are not cues for attractiveness. Intramuscular fat grafting combined with high-definition liposculpture improves the gluteal region and the overall body shape by uniting the torso with the muscular lower limbs [2–4].

The male buttock shape is different than the female counterpart. While in females the silhouette forms a smooth curve from the waistline onto the hips and the leg without sharp edges, in men it is sharp edged by definition. The form of the female buttocks is almost hemispherical, whereas in men it tends to be square. One of the key surface anatomical features in men is the presence of the trochanteric depression. This concavity on the lateral surface of the buttocks highlights the definition of the gluteus muscles along its perimeter. In the female buttocks, an obvious trochanteric depression is not preferred (Fig. 12.2).

There is an important relationship between the buttocks and thighs in males. The male fat anatomy shows a fusion between the superficial fascia and the deep tissues in the lateral thigh. This usually necessitates treating the gluteal and thigh regions together as one aesthetic unit. The high density of deep fat in the buttocks makes it behave like superficial fat. Hence, there is little room for

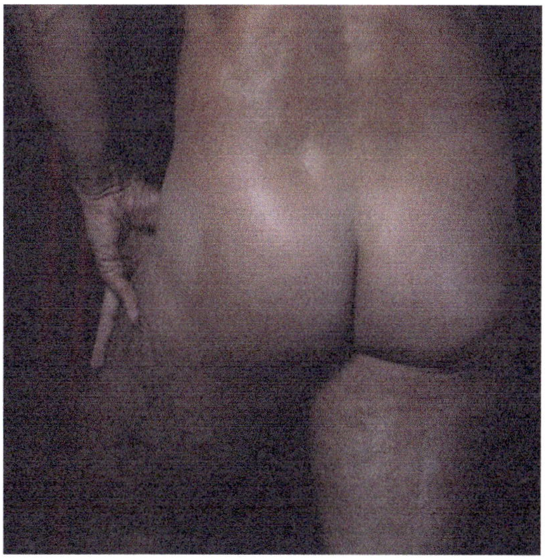

Fig. 12.1 Athletic male buttocks

A.E. Hoyos, P.M. Prendergast, *High Definition Body Sculpting*,
DOI 10.1007/978-3-642-54891-8_12, © Springer-Verlag Berlin Heidelberg 2014

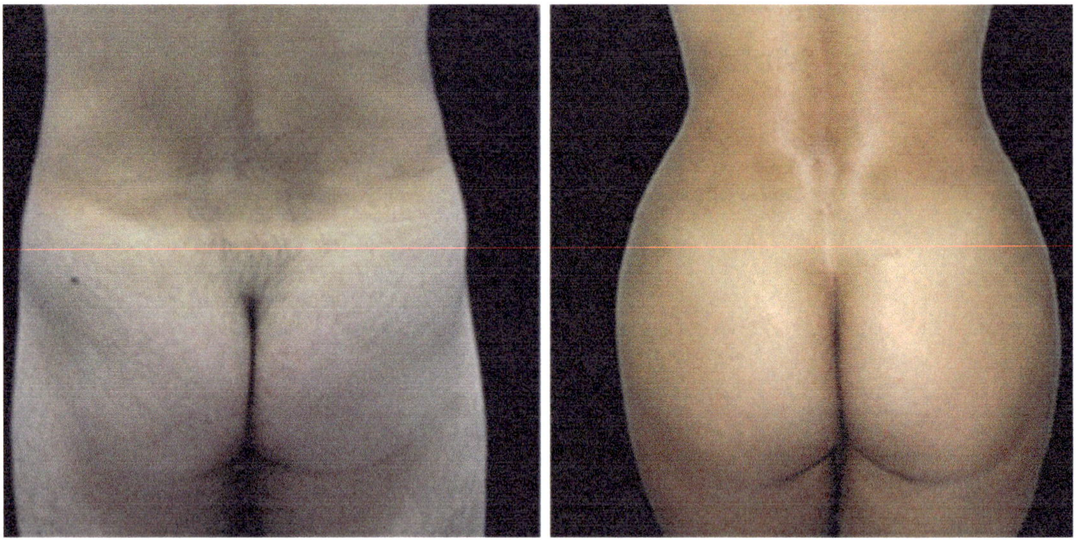

Fig. 12.2 Comparison between male and female buttocks: female contour is more rounded with a smooth transition in the trochanteric depression, which should not be noticeable. In men, a more squared shape is desirable, also a visible trochanteric depression gives an idea of high muscular development

fat storage in the lateral thigh and in the gluteal area in men. The majority of male patients who seek contouring of the buttock area request augmentation rather than reduction. There are exceptions. Male patients with gynecoid features require liposculpture of the buttocks and thighs to define the muscles and produce a convincing picture of athleticism and strength [5, 6].

Stealth Incisions

Three main incisions are used: the first is in the intergluteal crease. This allows the surgeon to reach the superior gluteus, the lower back, and part of the midgluteal area. The second incision is made in the midpart of the infragluteal crease (see below), allowing easy access to the lower gluteal area. The inner thigh can be reached by the lower pubic incisions with the patient supine and by the infragluteal crease incisions for posterior access with the patient prone. In cases when full leg definition is wanted, two additional incisions can be placed in the posterior fold of the knee area: one medial and one lateral (Fig. 12.3).

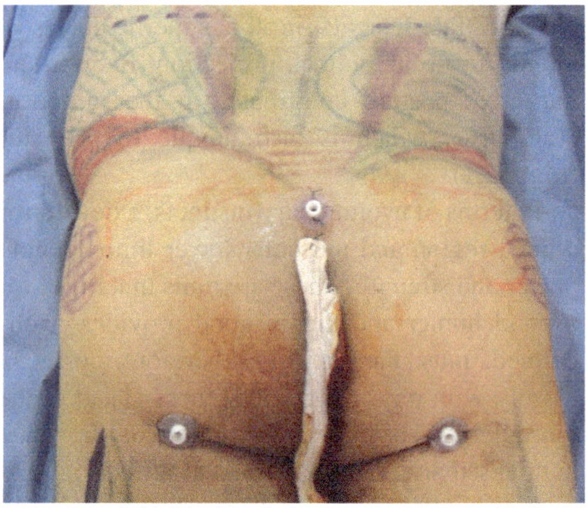

Fig. 12.3 Incision and ports sutured in place

The Use of Drains

As we stated in the previous chapter, the intergluteal incision is either left open for permissive drainage or a closed drain is placed in it. The infragluteal fold incisions should always be closed by subdermal sutures, since these are the ports of entry of fat grafting, to prevent protrusion of fat or migration. The posterior knee-fold incisions can be closed or left open for drainage.

Markings

Deep Markings

The ideal buttock shape in males resembles the shape of the underlying gluteus maximus muscle. The absence of fat is the standard, so there is little space for transition areas in this specific region. Later in the female chapters, we will observe that the gluteal area has specific zones for smooth contour, while in men sharp edges are often desired to produce a sculpted, muscular appearance. Usually the perigluteal area in males does not have a lot of excess fat, but the inner thigh can store some fat. This is marked for resection.

Framing

The superior portion of the gluteal area is discussed on the previous chapter. However, it is important to remember the definition zones:

With the patient in the upright position, begin by identifying the superior gluteal edge. Pressing over the superior aspect of the buttocks while the patient contracts the muscle helps define the superior gluteal edge.

Proceed to identify the maximum point of indentation (PMI) in the waistline and trace a line to the top of the intergluteal crease and then a line from this point to the superior iliac crest; this forms a triangle area we called the green zone where the fat can be freely removed.

Next, identify the trochanteric depression on the lateral side and trace a line from the upper limit of it to the top of the intergluteal crease. By doing this, a new triangle is formed; we called this area the red zone. In females it is a transition zone, whereas in men it is an area of complete deep and superficial fat removal, with a lower limit defined by the upper gluteal crease (Fig. 12.4).

The inferior gluteal area is divided into four zones by placing a vertical line through the center of the gluteus maximus and a horizontal line through the inferior gluteal crease. The lines intersect at the infragluteal midpoint (IGM).

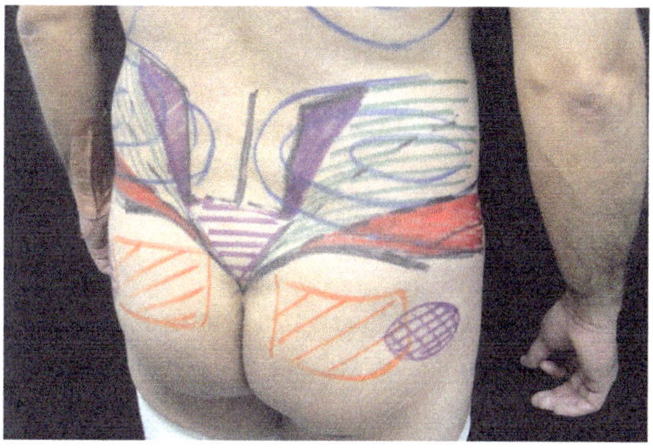

Fig. 12.4 Framing marking in the male patient: green and red zones

Negative Spaces

There are three main areas for negatives spaces in the male buttocks: the proximal portion of the inner thigh, the red zone until the upper intergluteal crease, and the trochanteric depression. In the thigh, there is a negative space over the posterior portion of the lateral intermuscular sulcus, between the quadriceps and the biceps femoris.

The middle third of the inner thigh contains an adhesion zone composed only of superficial fat. A line is drawn from the superior border of the zone of adherence to the infragluteal midpoint. The lower gluteal edge should normally end at the IGM. Lateral to the IGM, the border of the gluteus can be identified by grasping the posterior thigh muscles and rotating them externally. This maneuver helps in identifying extra fat on the lateral buttocks (Fig. 12.5).

The trochanteric depression is desirable in men. If it is not present, it is created by performing superficial liposuction over the lateral buttocks (Fig. 12.6).

The gluteal area itself is now divided into horizontal thirds. The major projection zone must be located over the middle third. So it is important to identify the characteristics of each area to know where and how much fat to remove.

In the lower limb, the differentiation between muscular groups is important, especially in the lateral thigh. With the patient flexing at the hips and knees in a partial squat position, the depression

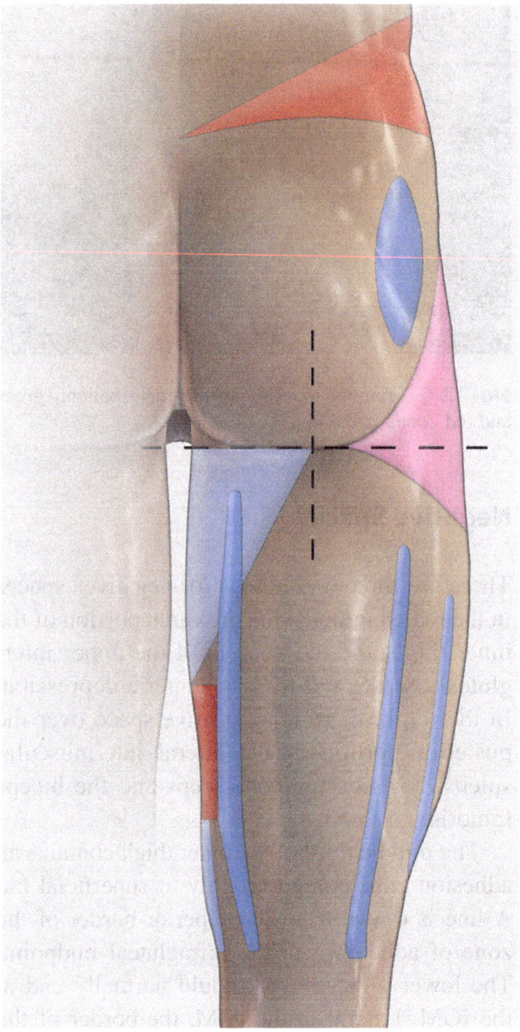

Fig. 12.5 Illustration of the negative spaces markings on male: The inferior gluteus and thigh. Notice the trochanteric depression as a negative space (*blue*), also the intermuscular areas between the biceps femoris and the surrounding muscles (also in *blue*). The transition zone (*pink*) must be carefully identified as muscular and fat deposits do blend. There are some negative spaces (*red* and *light blue*) that define the contour of the buttock

between quadriceps and biceps femoris can be visualized and marked. The lateral and medial borders of biceps femoris in the posterior view can be marked in the same position.

The distal insertion of quadriceps can be marked if the patient wishes to have more definition in the area. However, additional incisions in the anterior knee might be required.

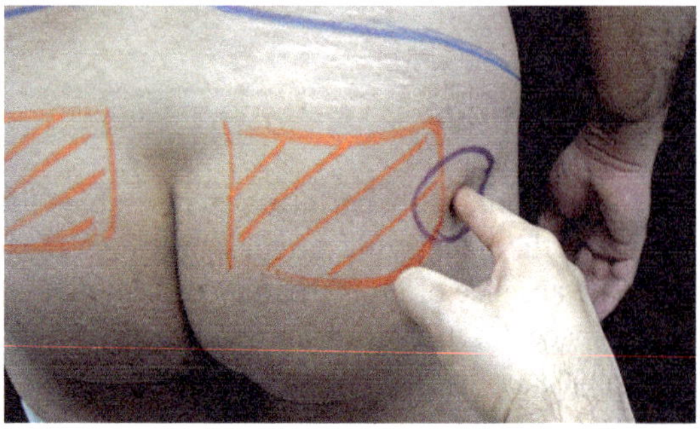

Fig. 12.6 The trochanteric depression. The orange area (gluteal middle third) indicates the major projection zone

Procedure

Infiltration

Tumescent solution is infiltrated uniformly in the fat layers, starting in the deep layer and later in the superficial layer. The solution consists of 1,000 mL of normal saline and a vial of 1:1,000 epinephrine together with sodium bicarbonate. The ratio of infiltration to suction should be 2:1.

Emulsification

Emulsification is performed using third-generation ultrasound. The maximum time of emulsification is 2 min per 100 mL of tumescent solution infiltrated, but remember that the clinical endpoint is the loss of the tissue resistance [6]. For the gluteal area a 3.7 mm 2-ring probe is the probe of choice, while in the distal thigh a 2.9 mm 3-ring probe is a better choice (Fig. 12.7).

Extraction

Deep Extraction

Deep liposuction is performed using a 3.7 mm cannula over the lower back and upper gluteal area through the intergluteal crease incision (Fig. 12.8).

Accessing from the infragluteal midpoint (IGM), begin the extraction of the lower and the lateral gluteal area and especially the inner thigh

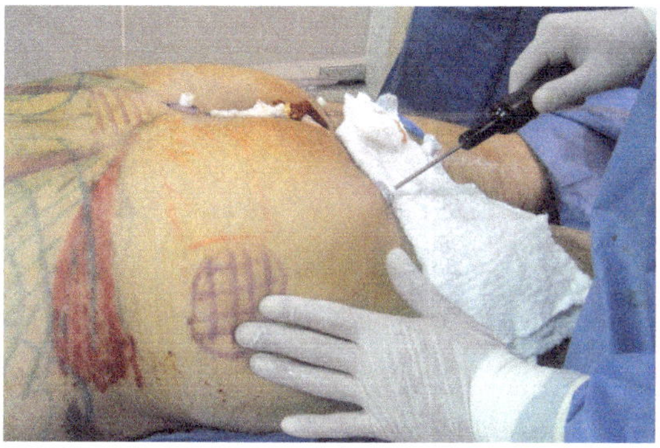

Fig. 12.7 Fat emulsification over the trochanteric area

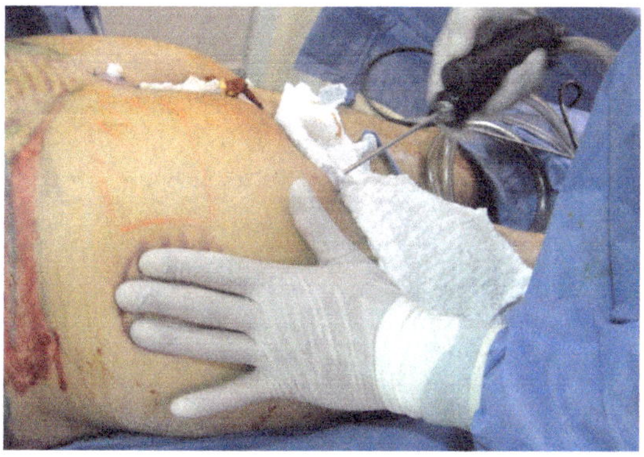

Fig. 12.8 Superficial extraction over the trochanteric area

area. The extraction starts from distal to proximal; in men a more aggressive extraction is permitted. The inner thigh is completed later when the patient is in supine position.

Warning
Remember to start from distal to proximal in the inner thigh extraction to avoid over-resection over the mid-thigh adhesion zone.

Superficial Framing

The upper gluteus maximus line is defined, as well as the lower internal area. Through the posterior knee-fold incision, definition of thigh between the quadriceps and the biceps femoris is achieved. An inter-quadriceps line can be done as well. Definition of the lateral and medial borders of the biceps femoris is performed through the posterior knee-fold incisions.

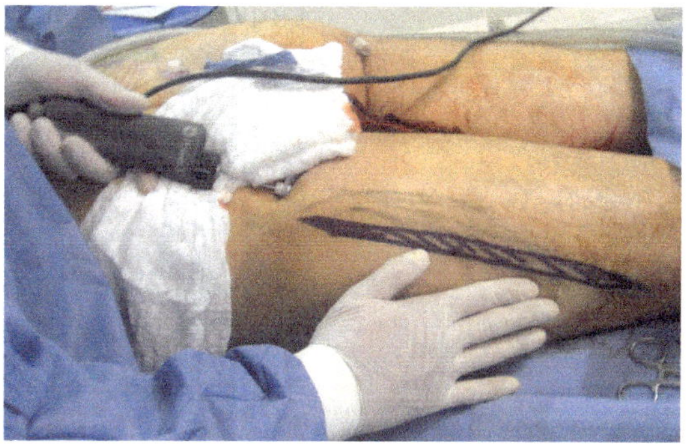

Fig. 12.9 Lateral thigh negative space

Negative Spaces

Negatives spaces are located over the red zone bordered by the upper border of the gluteus maximus, the trochanteric depression if there is extra fat located there, and over the medial infragluteal crease. A small transition zone is made over the lateral leg between the iliotibial tract and biceps femoris, a sharp edge is done anterior, but while moving to posterior, a transition zone is done to smooth the area (Fig. 12.9).

Fat Grafting

Fat tissue is harvested with a 3 mm blunt cannula to an empty, sterile bottle trap. Add 1 g of cefazolin. Use decantation to separate the fat cells from the saline and serosanguinous components. Through the midinferior gluteal point, insert the cannula and start placing the grafting with a slow movement injecting only when the cannula is moving out. The graft will be mostly placed on the middle third of the gluteus. No injection over the trochanteric depression is necessary. On the contrary, when the intragluteal grafting is done, this concavity should appear more pronounced [4, 7].

Postoperative Care

Mild compression is recommended in the buttock area to prevent reabsorption of the fat grafted. In the thighs a normal compression garment is required to prevent swelling. Therapeutic lymphatic drainage

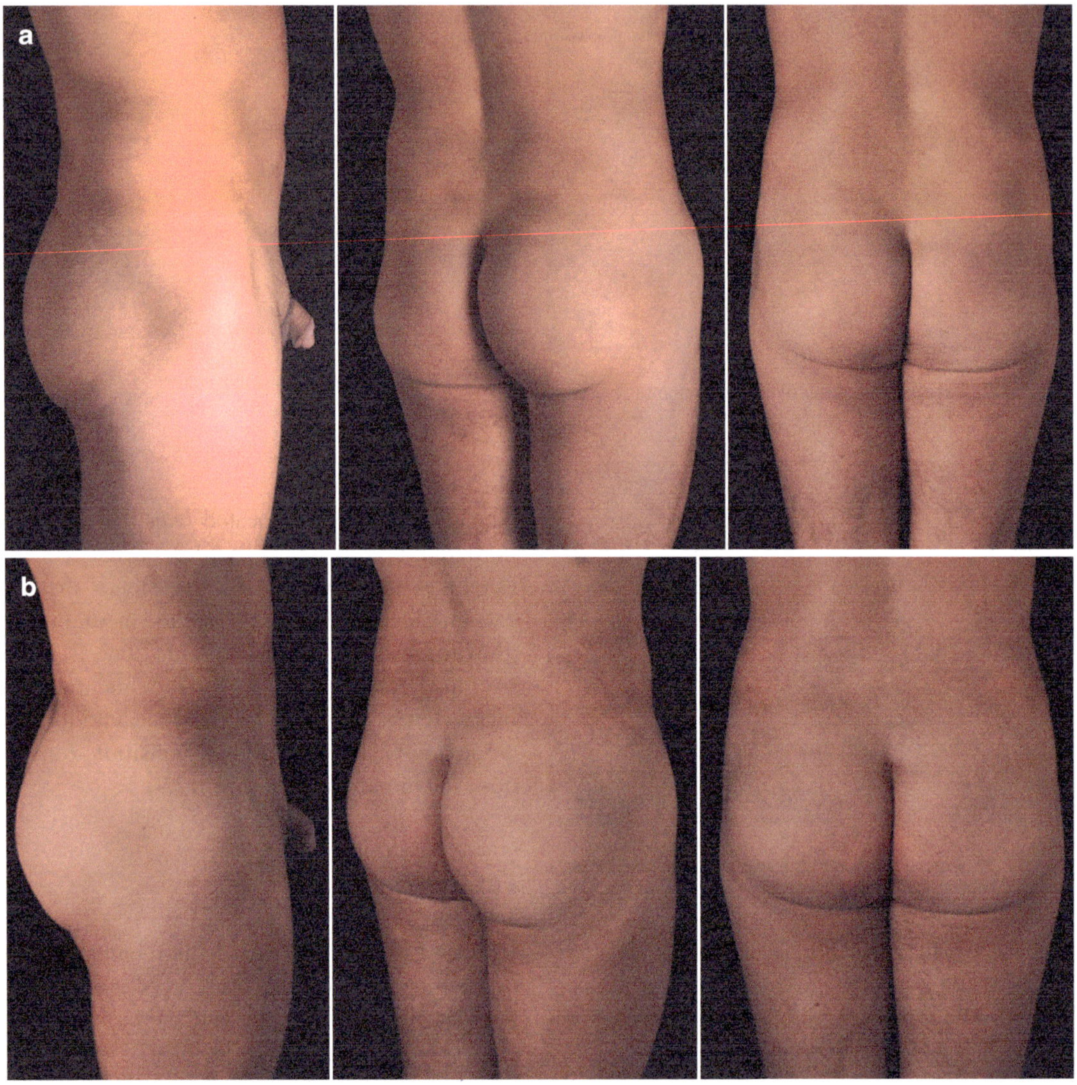

Fig. 12.10 A 34-year-old male patient preoperative (**a**) and 6 months postoperative (**b**). Note the change in the contour and the convexity

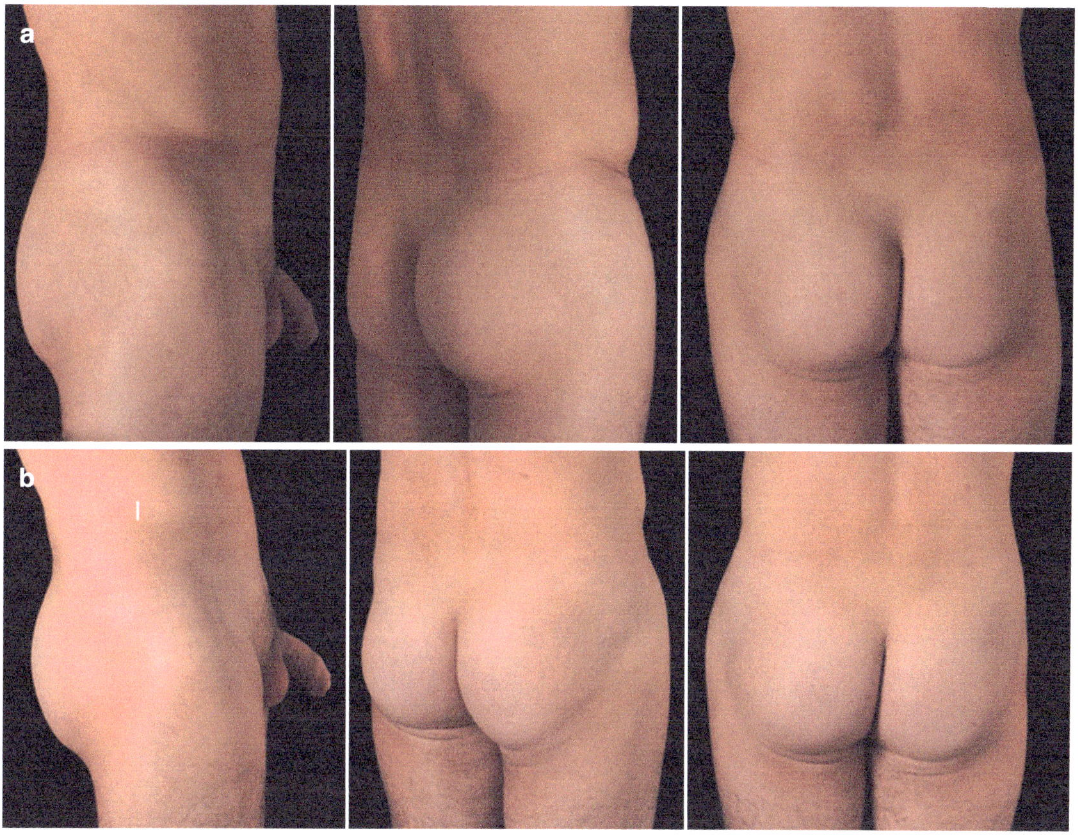

Fig. 12.11 A 42-year-old male patient preoperative (**a**) and 6 months postoperative (**b**)

is used over the thigh areas, directed to the inguinal lymph nodes on the inner thigh, and to the posterior knee-fold incisions for the lateral and medial thighs. Postoperative results are shown in Figs. 12.10 and 12.11.

References

1. Singh D (2006) Universal allure of the hourglass figure: an evolutionary theory of female physical attractiveness. Clin Plast Surg 33(3):359–370
2. De Pedroza LV (2000) Fat transplantation to the buttocks and legs for aesthetic enhancement or correction of deformities: long-term results of large volumes of fat transplant. Dermatol Surg 26(12):1145–1149
3. Hoyos AE, Millard JA (2007) Vaser-assisted high definition lipoplasty. Aesthet Surg J 27:594–604
4. Mendieta CG (2006) Intramuscular gluteal augmentation technique. Clin Plast Surg 33(3):423–434
5. de Souza Pinto EB, Indaburo PE, Da Costa Muniz A, Martinez YP, Gerent KMM, Iwamoto H, Marão Miziara AC (1996) Superficial liposuction: body contouring. Clin Plast Surg 23(4):529–548
6. Rochrich RJ, Beran SJ, Di Spaltro F et al (1998) Extending the role of liposuction in body contouring with ultrasound assisted liposuction. Plast Reconstr Surg 101:1090–1102
7. Toledo L, Mauad R (2006) Fat injection: a 20-year revision. Clin Plast Surg 33:47–53

Part III

The Female Patient: Technique

13 Female Abdomen and Torso

Introduction

The abdomen is one of the most important regions in aesthetic body contouring. It is also one of the most challenging. Since the early days of aesthetic surgery, various surgical approaches have been used to improve the appearance of the abdomen, including liposuction, abdominoplasty, and various combinations or variations of these procedures [1, 2]. The difficulty in achieving a beautiful, convincing result lies in the complex and elegant arrangement of the anatomical structures beneath the skin. If the surgeon does not have a good knowledge of the anatomy of the fat, musculature, and bony landmarks, the results of surgery become unpredictable. In the early days of aesthetic surgery, complications after abdominal contouring such as asymmetries, unsightly irregularities, and an unnatural appearance explained womens' reluctance and reservations about undergoing such procedures. Today, liposuction of the abdomen is the most frequently performed procedure for women in aesthetic plastic surgery. Lessons have been learned over the years, allowing us to achieve beautiful results with few complications [3–6].

The ideal abdomen is not just flat; it is a combination of convexities and concavities that follow the anatomy of the bones and muscles underneath [7]. Although variations are multiple and complex, the more defined we want the abdomen to appear, the more thorough and aggressive the treatment should be.

The female torso is characterized by a perfect combination of curves and projections that influence the well-known waist-to-hip ratio. Achieving an ideal waist-to-hip ratio and seamless smooth contours in this zone are important objectives in order to achieve female attractiveness. Achieving the correct degree of definition is a challenge. In women, definition must be appropriate to obtain athletic, slim, and feminine results, while in men, a harder, more muscular appearance is preferred (Fig. 13.1).

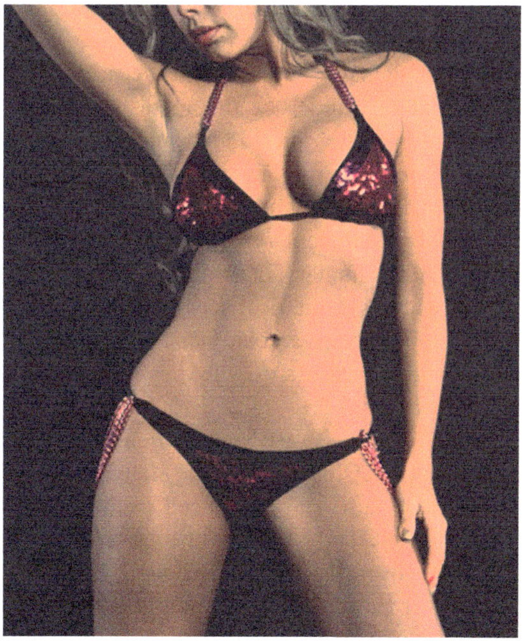

Fig. 13.1 Athletic female abdomen

A.E. Hoyos, P.M. Prendergast, *High Definition Body Sculpting*,
DOI 10.1007/978-3-642-54891-8_13, © Springer-Verlag Berlin Heidelberg 2014

Stealth Incisions

High-definition body sculpting in the female patient involves defining rectus abdominis by revealing its lateral borders and midline, but not the horizontal tendinous intersections. Women almost never request a "six-pack" appearance, but prefer the more feminine "two pack." Rarely, very athletic patients may want some definition of the rectus bellies horizontally. Once the rectus is defined, the surrounding areas must be carefully sculpted to obtain a natural appearance. Incision placement is important in the female abdomen because the incisions should be hidden yet the entire abdomen must be reached. The ideal incision points should be:

1. Pubis: In line vertically with the lateral border of the rectus abdominis, 5 mm incisions are placed in the inguinal region within the hair-bearing area. These incisions allow access to almost the entire abdominal region. From these sites, we can define the waist, the rectus abdominis, and the midline.
2. Umbilicus: For the superior midline and the inferior abdomen definition, an incision is hidden in the navel.
3. Inframammary Crease: For both sides of the abdomen, an incision must be made in the inframammary crease in line vertically with the lateral border of the rectus abdominis. These incisions are hidden and allow us to access the superior abdomen and flanks. If the breast is not big enough to create an appreciable inframammary fold, we should avoid the inframammary incision so that there are no visible symmetrical scars. In women with small breasts, an areolar incision is preferable to provide access to the upper abdominal region.

Additional Incisions: Some patients may need additional incisions when the fatty tissue is excessive. These may be placed in the anterior axillary fold and the midline at the pubis. Incisions over the abdominal area should be avoided if possible. If one additional incision over the abdomen is essential for access, it should be over the horizontal tendinous intersections of the rectus abdominis. If more than one additional incision is needed, they should be placed asymmetrically to avoid the stigmata of aesthetic surgery (Fig. 13.2).

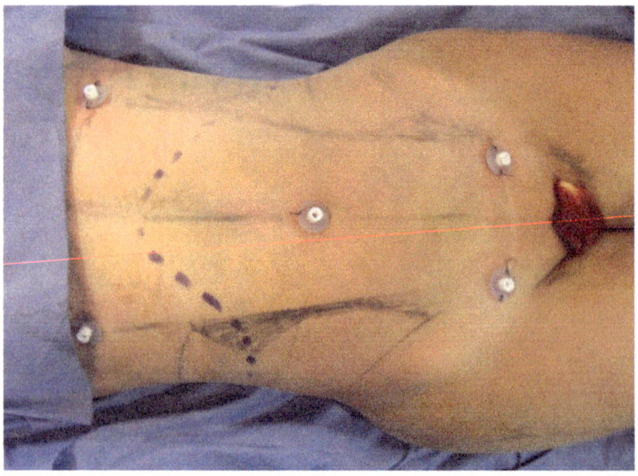

Fig. 13.2 Incision points with ports in place

The Use of Drains

Drains for women are seldom used in the abdomen. We prefer to leave the distal wounds open for drainage with massage and gravity. The upper incisions are closed with continuous subdermal sutures. When large fat volumes are extracted, we sometimes leave a drain in each pubic incision in order to avoid fluid collections in the flanks and the inguinal regions. A drain is left in the sacral incision.

Markings

Deep Markings

First, mark the most protuberant areas on the abdomen and flanks. There is a central area that has less fat, where the belt creates chronic compression. Mark it in red as an adhesion zone for careful extraction (Fig. 13.3).

Framing

The linea alba and the linea semilunaris are the key framing lines in females. The midline is

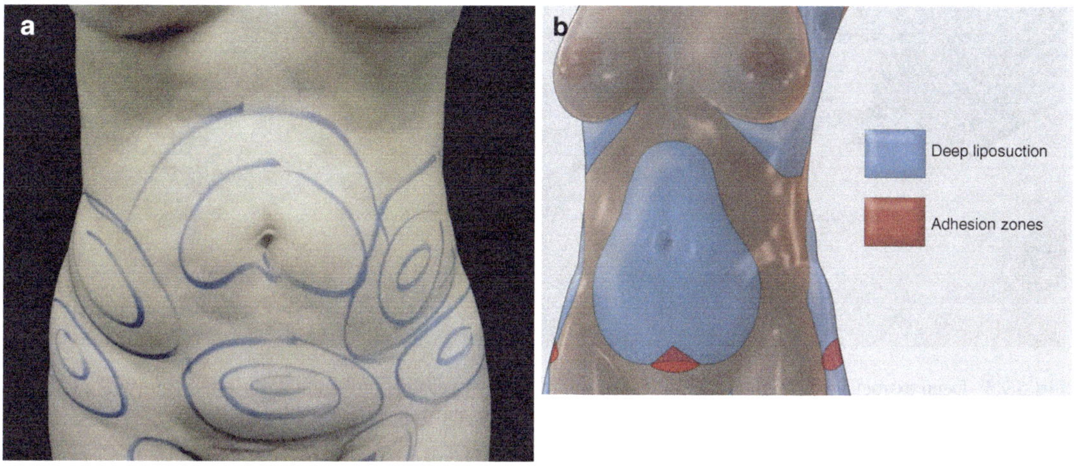

Fig. 13.3 Markings for deep extraction: (**a**) preoperative in vivo markings. (**b**) General (*blue*) zones for deep liposuction

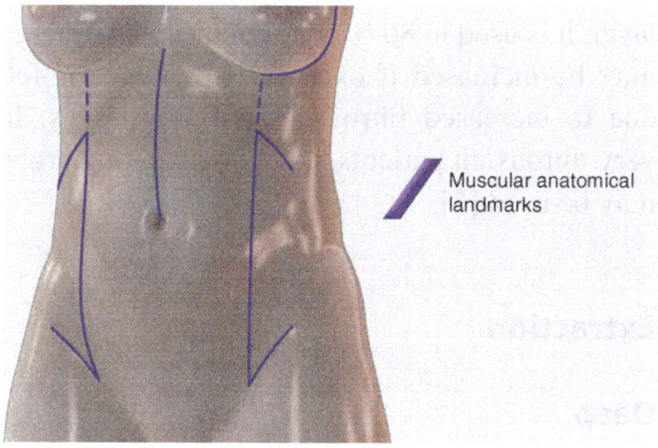

Fig. 13.4 Marking of the underlying anatomy

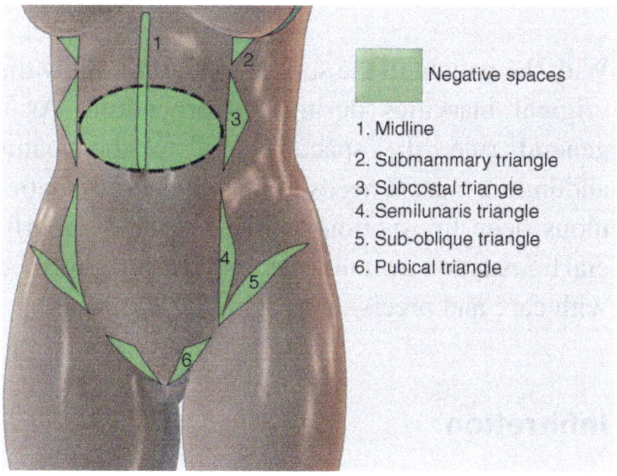

Fig. 13.5 Abdominal negative spaces (*green*) in the female patient

marked by palpation of the linea alba from the umbilicus to the xiphoid process (Fig. 13.4). The lateral border of the rectus is marked as continuous lines in the resting position. If the patient specifically requests a "six-pack," a light shadow is drawn over the horizontal tendinous intersection above the umbilicus.

Negative Spaces

In order to highlight the muscles, the surrounding areas must be sculpted thoroughly to create negative spaces. By removing more fat, more shadow is cast and the definition improves. There should always be a tonal progression from the highlight to the shadow to ensure the contours appear smooth and natural. The negative spaces that are key to abdominal sculpting are as follows:

1. Midline negative space.
2. Subcostal negative space.
3. Subcostal triangle.
4. Semilunaris triangle, between the semilunaris and the inguinal ligament.
5. Suboblique triangle, just below the external oblique muscle. Mark it only in the athletic female.
6. Pubic triangle, a wedge area to decrease the pubic angle (Fig. 13.5).

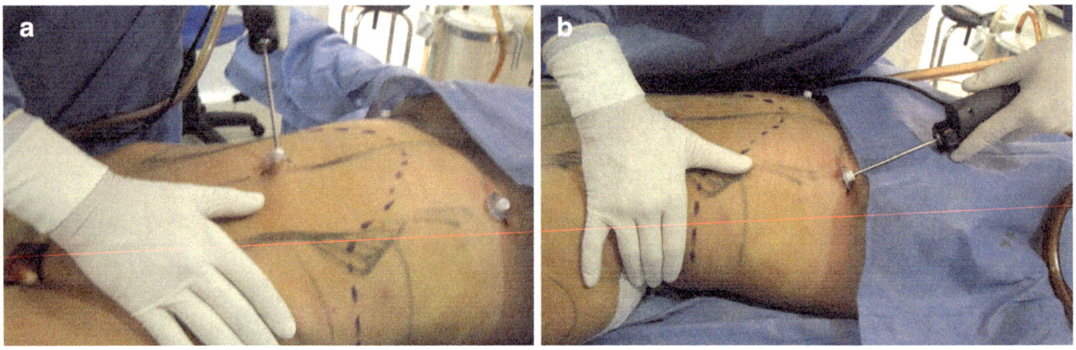

Fig. 13.6 Deep extraction through the umbilical incision (**a**). Extraction through the inframammary incision (**b**): the dotted line marks the landmark of the ribcage. For safety reasons, the cannula inserted from the pubic incisions must never cross this line

Procedure

With the patient in the supine position, follow the original markings during the procedure. As a general rule, the space lateral to the rectus abdominis muscle needs to be treated with meticulous deep liposuction, while deep and superficial liposuction over the rectus sheets is performed with care and precision to achieve definition.

Infiltration

Each area is infiltrated with standard tumescent solution (1,000 cc of normal saline, 10 cc 1 % lidocaine, and 1 ml of epinephrine 1:1,000), in the deep and superficial fat layers. Always begin with the deep layer, and later advance to the superficial layer to avoid migration from the superficial into the deep layers prior to emulsification with ultrasound.

Emulsification

Fat emulsification is performed with third-generation ultrasound, blending between the superficial, intermediate, and deep fat layers with a 3.7 mm 3-ring probe for the lower abdomen and a 3.7 mm 2-ring probe for the upper abdomen. In the superficial and intermediate layer, VASER is used in 80 % pulsed mode, while in the deep layer, it is used in 80 % continuous mode. Energy may be increased if excessive resistance is felt due to increased fibrousness of the tissues. In very fibrous, fit patients, the 3.7 mm 1-ring probe may be used [5].

Extraction

Deep

Deep liposuction is performed in the lateral and midregion of the abdomen using initially a 3.7 mm and later a 4.6 mm long cannula supply [4]. In slim patients, only the 3.7 mm cannula is used to avoid contour irregularities. The waistline area is suctioned using the 3.7 mm long and 4.6 mm curved VentX cannulas. By using small-diameter, atraumatic cannulas (SST-6, Valeant Pharmaceuticals North America LLC), injury to the subdermal vascular plexus is minimized, preserving the skin's blood supply [3]. The waistline is contoured by taking advantage of the three main incisions, where the approaches converge into the point of maximum indentation (PMI) (Fig. 13.6).

Superficial Framing

Superficial lipoplasty is performed for definition along the linea alba, linea semilunaris, and external oblique abdominal muscles. Small cannulas (3.0, 3.7 mm) are used for a smooth contour. The

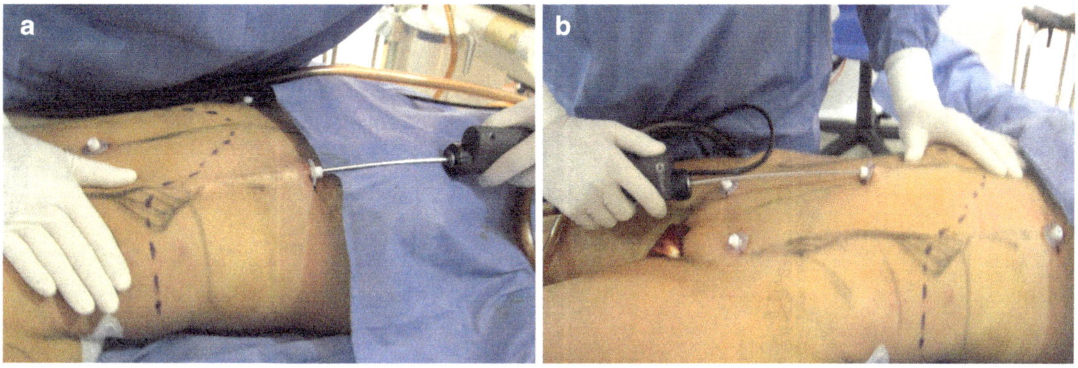

Fig. 13.7 Superficial framing along the linea semilunaris (**a**) and the linea alba (**b**)

finer the cannula is, the more predictable the skin retraction will be (Fig. 13.7).

Negative Spaces

The secret to success in high-definition lipoplasty belongs in this step of the surgery. The artistry of transforming carved fat into a shape that looks and feels natural takes its origins in how the light is going to affect the shape. Follow two simple rules and your results will be better than expected.

1. Turn lines into curves.
2. Create shadows along the natural concavities of the anatomy.

Start with the lower negative space, between the external oblique muscle and the inferior extent of the semilunar line. Start every negative space with a full extraction just next to the line, and make it smoother as you sculpt further away from the line.

Proceed with the semilunar lines from the inframammary incisions, defining the lines from superiorly to inferiorly along the line. Remember that these lines are slightly curved and not straight. Using curved cannulas, these slightly convex lateral curved lines are defined first, followed by the shadows lateral to them.

Later, the subcostal negative space is defined, keeping in mind that the space changes position from standing to supine. The original marking made on standing should be followed during sculpting.

Fat Grafting

In this area we do not perform fat grafting, as we do not need to augment any abdominal muscles. The feminine appearance is achieved only using liposculpture.

Postoperative Care

Close the upper and lower incisions with subdermal sutures. The lower pubic sites can be left open for permissive drainage in patients with large-volume liposuction to avoid seromas.

Lymphatic drainage massage is indicated for at least ten sessions to reduce postoperative swelling and bruising. The massage also speeds up the results and prevents fibrosis in the central abdomen, an area very prone to produce it.

A foam vest is used in the trunk. This provides better skin retraction, reduces the pain, and increases the pressure over the central abdomen, where most garments do not provide adequate compression. Over the foam vest, a compression garment is indicated to evenly compress the foam vest over the abdominal contours. This garment should be used for a period of up to 2 months.

With meticulous attention to detail in planning, marking, technique, and postoperative care, high definition can be achieved in patients of varying body types (Figs. 13.8, 13.9, 13.10, and 13.11).

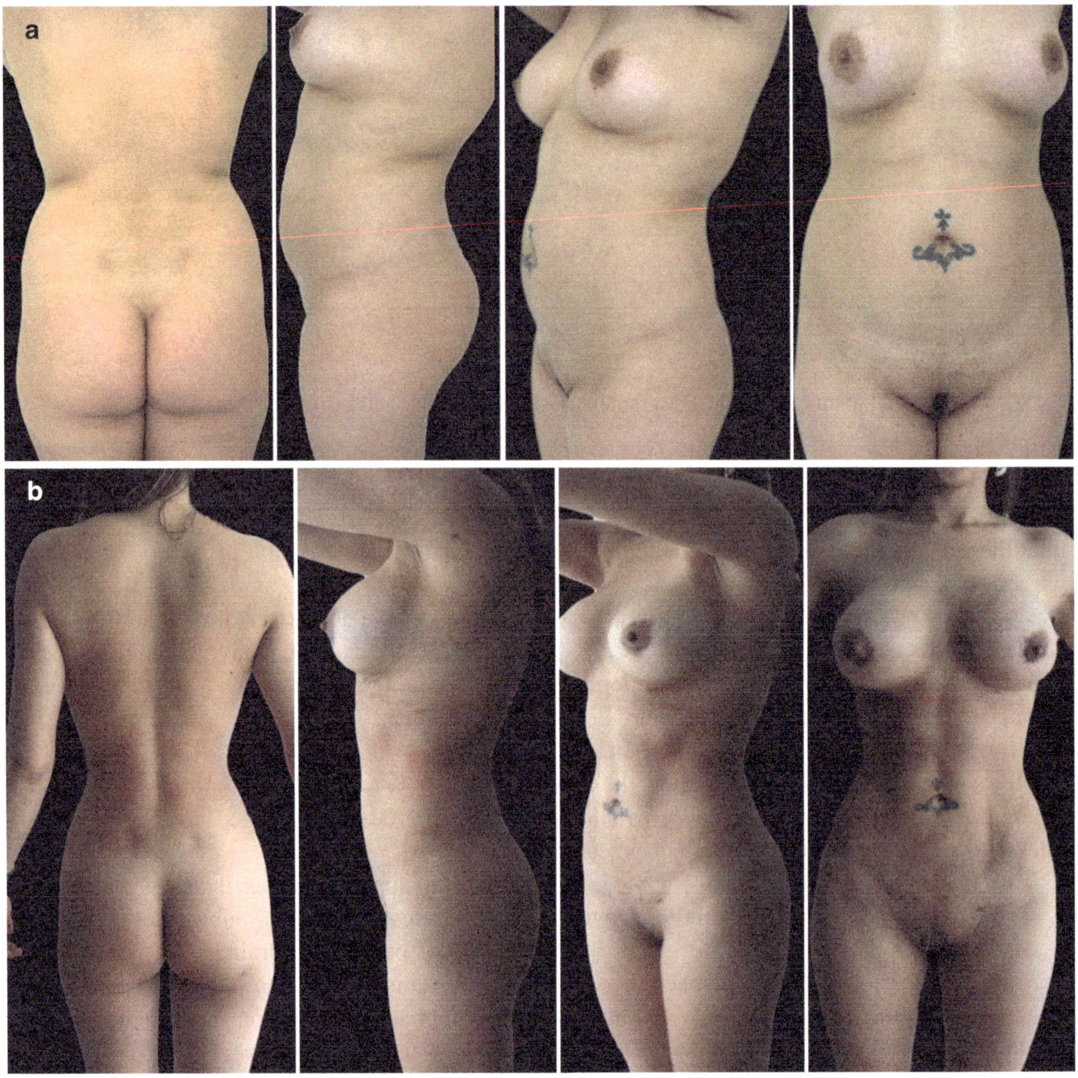

Fig. 13.8 A 24-year-old fat female patient preoperative (**a**) and 5 years postoperative (**b**)

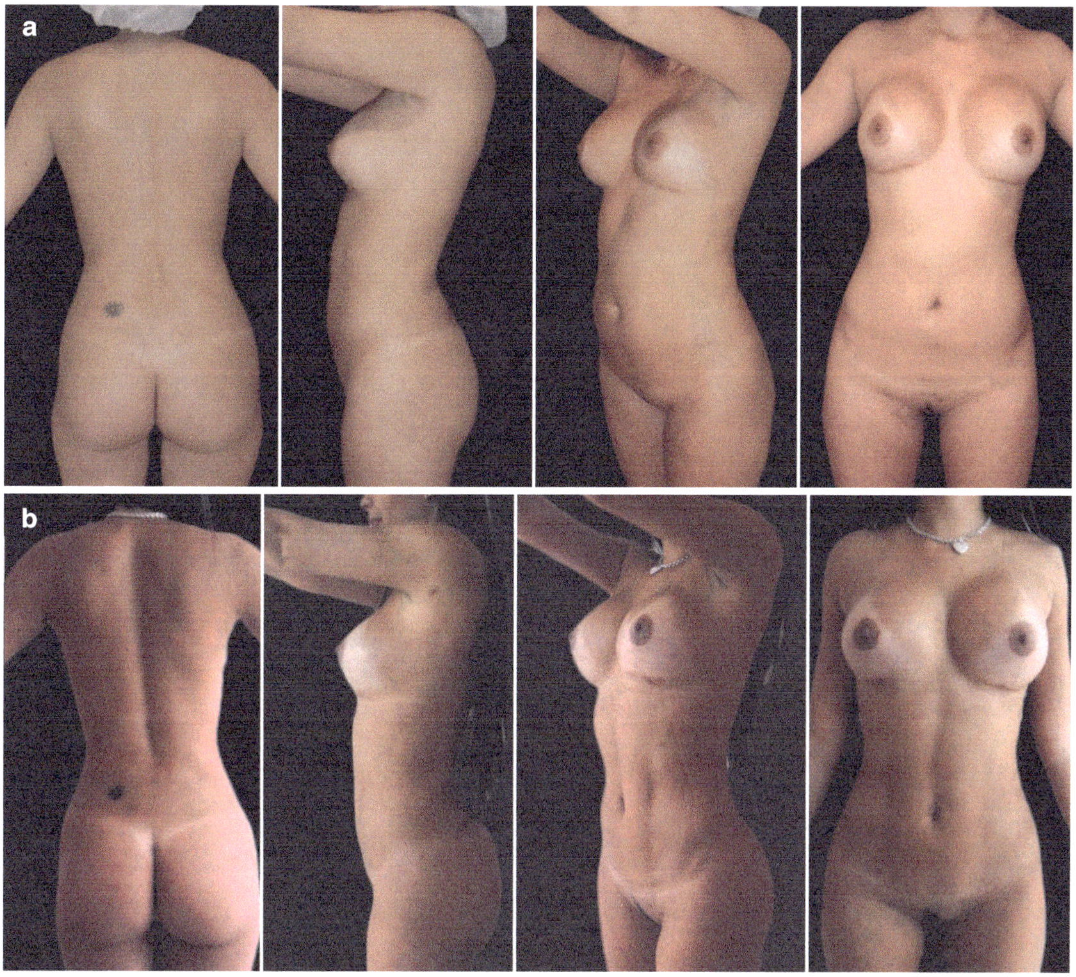

Fig. 13.9 A 29-year-old slim female patient preoperative (**a**) and 1 year postoperative (**b**)

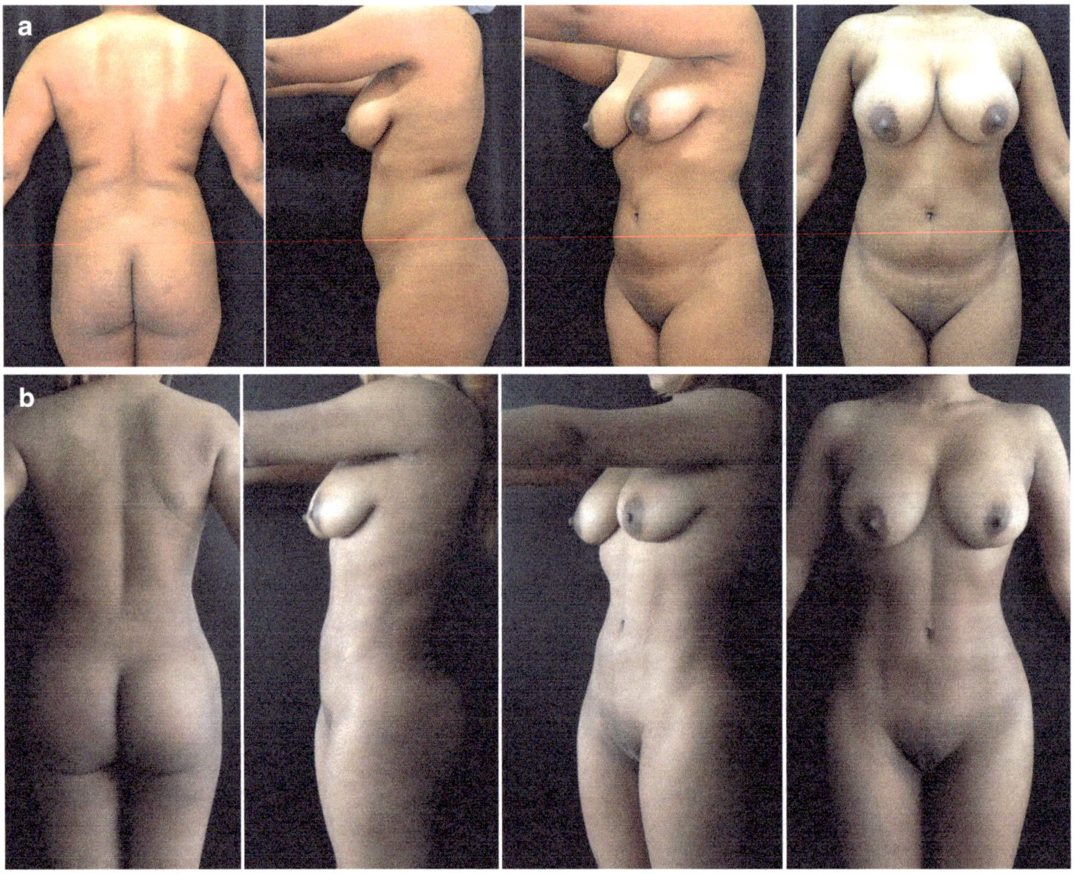

Fig. 13.10 A 27-year-old fat female patient, preoperative (**a**) and 1 year postoperative (**b**)

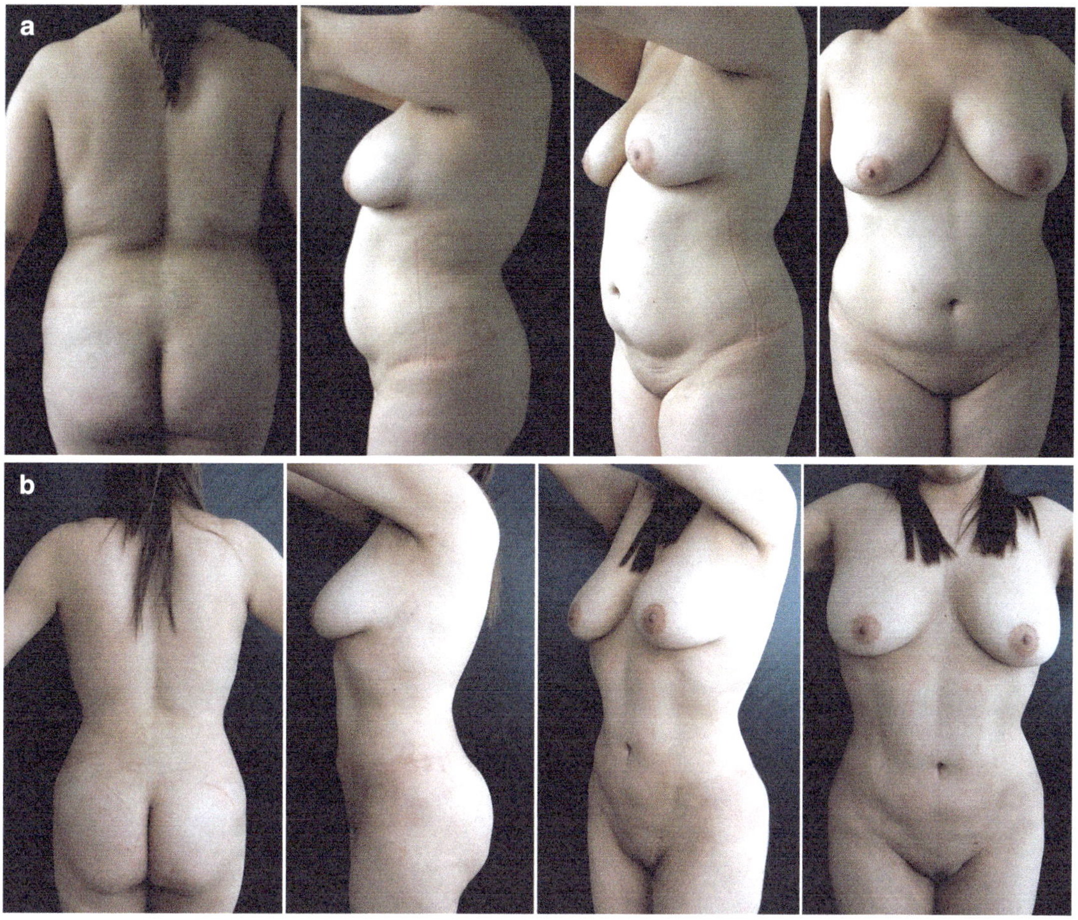

Fig 13.11 A 37-year-old overweight female patient, preoperative (**a**) and 1 year postoperative (**b**)

References

1. Hoyos AE, Millard JA (2007) Vaser-assisted high definition lipoplasty. Aesthet Surg J 27:594–604
2. Shiffman MA, Mirrafati S (eds) (2005) Aesthetic surgery of the abdominal wall. Springer, Berlin/Heidelberg
3. de Souza Pinto EB, Indaburo PE, Da Costa Muniz A, Martinez YP, Gerent KMM, Iwamoto H, Marão Miziara AC (1996) Superficial liposuction: body contouring. Clin Plast Surg 23(4):529–548
4. Fodor PB, Cimino WW, Watson JP, Tahernia A (2005) Suction-assisted lipoplasty: physics, optimization, and clinical verification. Aesthet Surg J 25(3): 234–246
5. Rochrich RJ, Beran SJ, Di Spaltro F et al. (1998) Extending the role of liposuction in body contouring with ultrasound assisted liposuction. Plast Reconstr Surg 101:1090–1102
6. Zocchi ML (1996) Ultrasound-assisted lipoplasty. Technical refinements and clinical evaluations. Clin Plast Surg 23:575–598
7. Avelar J (1989) Regional distribution and behavior of the subcutaneous tissue concerning selection and indication for liposuction. Aesthet Surg J 13:155–165

Female Dorsum, Flanks, and Hips

14

Introduction

The curves, slimness, and proportions of the female back play a key role in physical attractiveness. A slim waist, lumbar lordotic curve, and curvaceous hips define beauty and femininity and increase sex appeal (Fig. 14.1). With advanced lipoplasty, the idea is to create smooth, seamless contours, some definition of important anatomical landmarks, and a deep waist above the buttocks [1–6]. The hips should be contoured to improve curvaceousness and proportions, adding fat where necessary [7, 8]. Pay attention to the patient's desires and expectations, since the results that are desirable often vary between patients, ethnicities, and age groups. For instance, a curvaceous hip is often requested in Latin or African-American patients, whereas Caucasians might prefer slimmer hips. As we mentioned in previous chapters, the aesthetic ideal and goal is to provide a waist-hip ratio of 0.7.

In most books on body contouring, liposuction over the back is mentioned as an aside and has not been given the importance or attention it deserves [9]. As in all forms of sculpture, treating the surrounding areas is fundamental to achieving good definition and smooth transitions between each aesthetic unit. We use a systematic approach to achieve ideal female form, carefully addressing the flanks, dorsum, and hips so that the final result appears not simply better, but beautiful (Fig. 14.2).

Stealth Incisions

The back is an area of high exposure and scars in this area are difficult to conceal. For this reason, we need to place incisions in the natural folds where they are not likely to be seen when the patient wears a bathing suit. The use of special long cannulae allows us to reach the whole back without the need for extra back incisions. Additional incisions should be avoided as much as possible.

The ideal points for incisions should be (Fig. 14.3):

1. Axillary fold: One incision in the posterior axillary fold on both sides, strategically placed in the natural wrinkle of the fold at the posterior axillary line.

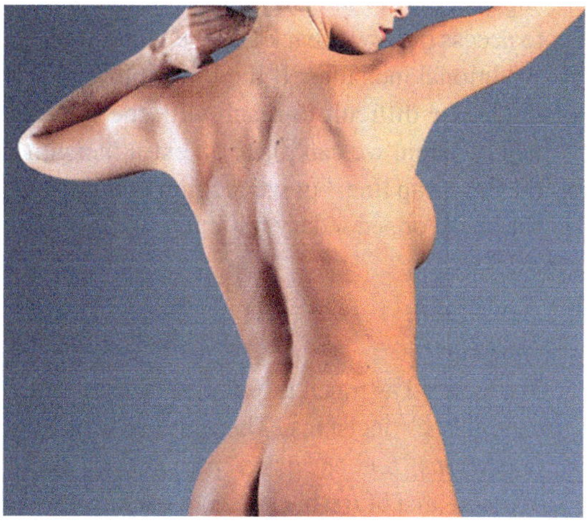

Fig. 14.1 Beautiful female form

A.E. Hoyos, P.M. Prendergast, *High Definition Body Sculpting*,
DOI 10.1007/978-3-642-54891-8_14, © Springer-Verlag Berlin Heidelberg 2014

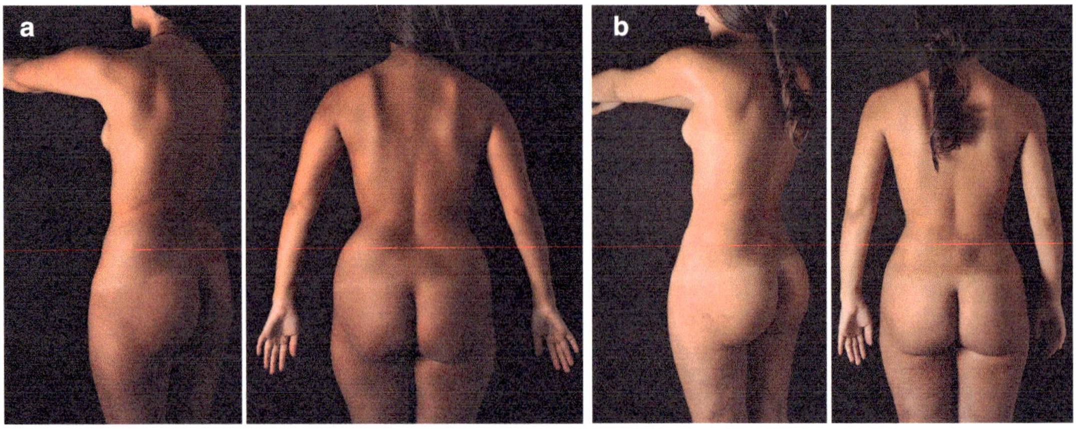

Fig. 14.2 A 22-year-old female patient preoperative (**a**) and 15 days postoperative (**b**)

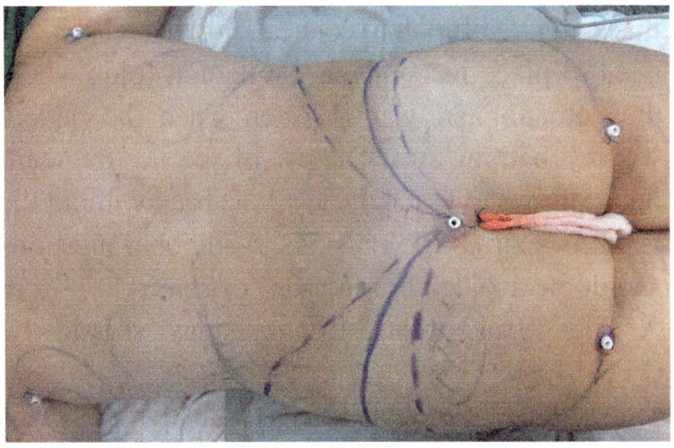

Fig. 14.3 Female dorsum incisions

2. Intergluteal crease: One incision is made in the superior part of the intergluteal crease in order to access the lower back and the gluteal spaces.
3. Additional incisions: If the lower back and the flanks are difficult to reach with the intergluteal incision, we can place an extra incision at the bra-strap line, but we recommend this only for obese or secondary patients.

Warning!
Try to avoid as much as possible placing the central back incisions. There are two main indications for an extra incision in the exposed area of the back: heavy patients that have back rolls due to significant fatty deposits in the central back and secondary patients that have fat below the costal margin.

The Use of Drains

A drain, open or closed, is left in the sacral, intergluteal incision (Fig. 14.4).

Markings

Deep Markings

Fat deposits are marked from the center to the periphery, extending superiorly and inferiorly from the point of maximum indentation (PMI). Back rolls are marked for aggressive liposuction (Fig. 14.5).

Framing

Special markings are made in the flanks to enhance the waistline. The only framing point is the paired sacral dimples and the midline above the line between them. These markings define the posterior inferior iliac spines and paralumbar muscles, respectively. The lateral borders of the paralumbar muscles are palpated and marked with the patient standing and hyperextending the hips (Fig. 14.6).

Negative Spaces

First, we locate the point of maximum indentation (PMI) of the waist. This is found by palpating the inferior costal margin and the anterior supe-

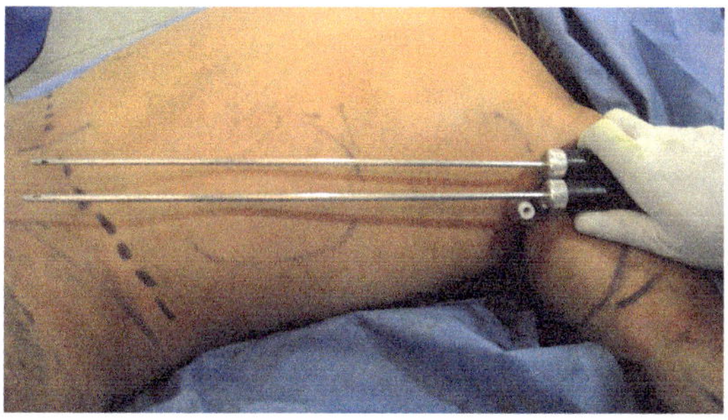

Fig. 14.4 Areas reached using long cannulae in the back

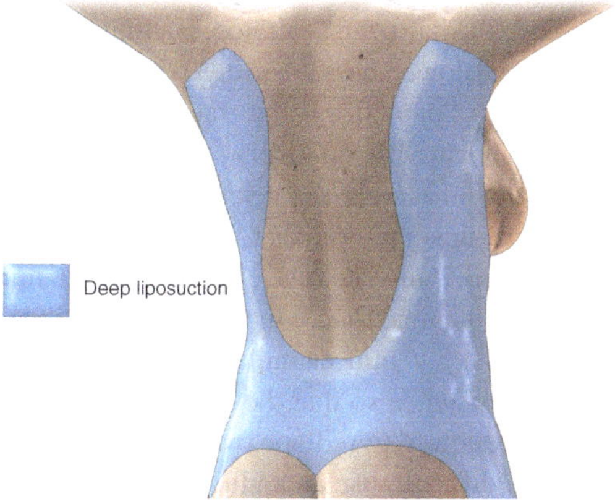

Fig. 14.5 Markings for deep extraction

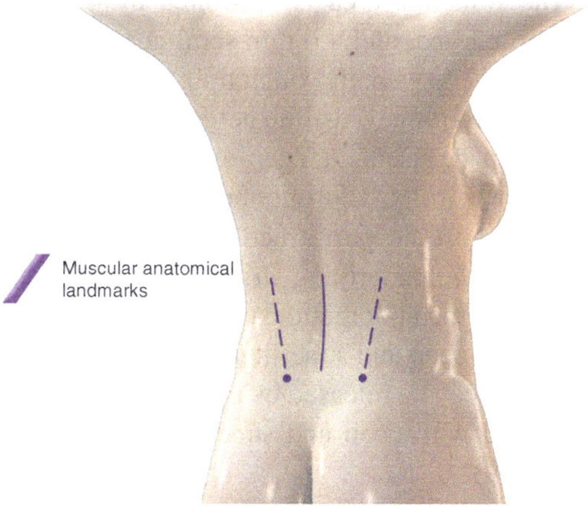

Fig. 14.6 Markings of the sacral dimples, muscular anatomical landmarks, and the midline for framing

rior iliac crest and following the lateral muscular structure between these until the point of maximum concavity is reached. Later, we divide the dorsum into two: upper back and lower back. The

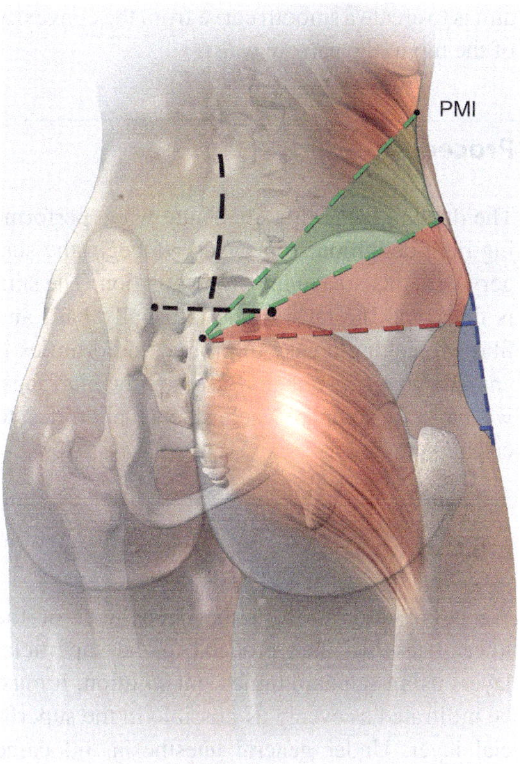

Fig. 14.7 Illustration showing the point of maximal indentation (*PMI*) and the negative spaces: *green* and *red* zones

upper back is located from the arm to the PMI and the lower from this point to the trochanteric depression.

The Green and Red Zones

First, draw a line from the PMI to the superior point of the intergluteal crease and then a line from this point to the superior iliac crest laterally. This forms a triangular area we call the green zone where fat should be removed thoroughly (Fig. 14.7).

Identify the trochanteric depression on the lateral side of the gluteus maximus muscle and trace a line from the top of the trochanteric depression to the upper limit of the intergluteal crease. By doing this, a new triangle is formed; we call this area the red zone. This zone requires special management because it is a transition zone between the green zone and the trochanteric depression. The red zone area should be treated with caution in order to avoid overresection. The aim is to create a smooth curve from the convexity of the hip to the narrow waist.

Procedure

The dorsum is the first challenge when performing high-definition surgery, as we begin the surgery with this area in the prone position. The skin is thick and the fatty tissue is usually hard and fibrous, making it easy to produce deformities if enough care is not taken. Based on the markings, we have to compare each side at all times to ensure symmetry.

Infiltration

We begin infiltration in the deep layer of the lower back and then proceed to the superficial layers using standard tumescent solution. It must be infiltrated as evenly as possible in the superficial layer. Under general anesthesia, lidocaine may or may not be used for infiltration. We add lidocaine in secondary patients to reduce pain in the postoperative period.

Emulsification

In the fibrous fat of the back and flanks, VASER is going to be used for up to 2 min for every 100 cc of infiltrated solution. We begin by emulsifying the superficial layer and then the deep layer with a 3.7 mm 2-ring or 1-ring probe. In the superficial and intermediate layer, VASER is used in 90 % pulsed mode, while in the deep layer, it is used in 90 % continuous mode [5].

Extraction

Deep Extraction

Proceed to the upper back. This area is approached using a short, large-diameter cannula (4.6 × 12 cm VentX cannula or "4.6 baby"). Without such a cannula, this area proves to be awkward and difficult due to the angulation (Fig. 14.8). Once this area near the axilla has been aspirated, continue toward the mid and lower back, starting with a 3.7 mm cannula, to "tunnelize" the fat to achieve a smoother result. If you begin aspiration in this fibrous fat with a larger-diameter cannula, you will create some unsightly ridges for sure. After finishing with the 3.7 mm cannula, change to the 4.6 mm cannula for the final touch. In the presence of back rolls, use the 3.7 mm cannula superficially until you lose resistance so that the fat is removed and the skin is allowed to redrape over the back. If this is proving difficult, use an additional incision that provides better longitudinal access to the rolls for release. In women, this incision should be placed in the location of the bra straps.

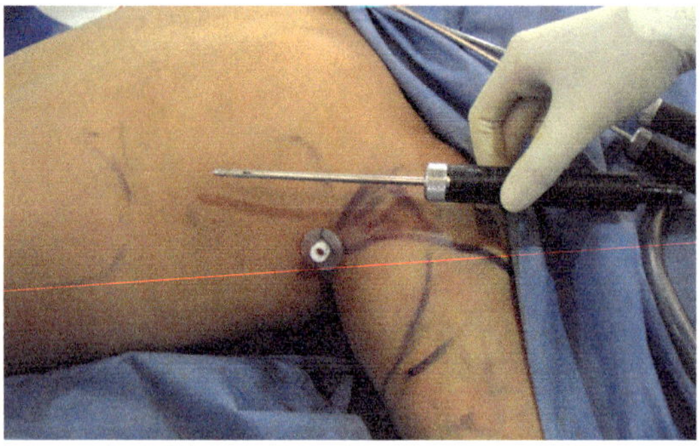

Fig. 14.8 4.6 × 12 mm "baby" cannula

The waistline area is suctioned by 4.6 mm, 4.6 mm curved, and 4.6 mm semi-curved VentX cannulae [2]. Deep, thorough liposuction must be performed for the waistline definition. Short cannulae can be used for deep extraction over the upper back rolls. Liposuction over the lumbar triangle must be performed carefully to avoid trauma to the underlying structures or even penetration of the abdominal cavity. The green zone also needs deep and superficial lipoplasty. Tough back rolls can be released using a basket cannula, combined with deep and superficial liposuction (Fig. 14.9).

Superficial Framing

Superficial lipoplasty must be performed over the lumbar triangle in order to achieve definition of the underlying muscles and the sacral dimples, as they are considered aesthetically pleasant and youthful (Fig. 14.10). The red zone requires gentle

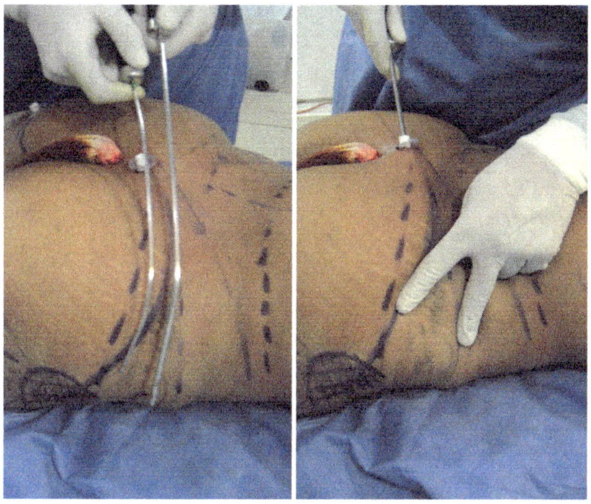

Fig. 14.9 Curved cannula extracting fat from the green zone

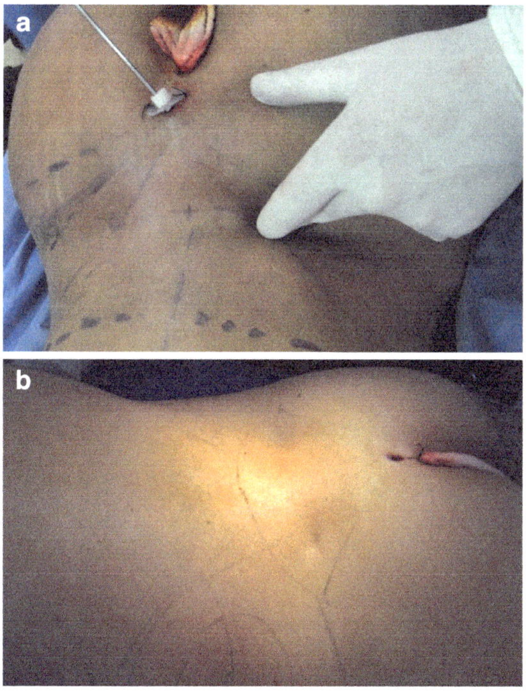

Fig. 14.10 Superficial framing: (**a**) marking of the sacral dimples, (**b**) final result

superficial and intermediate lipoplasty, creating a smooth transition between the PMI and the trochanteric depression and a natural tonal progression between the superior aspect of the buttock below and the deep waist above. Remember, a narrower cannula is more forgiving and more precise when blending two adjacent zones.

Negative Spaces

In order to achieve a natural appearance, a smooth transition with intermediate and superficial lipoplasty needs to be done between the lumbar triangle, the buttocks, and the red zone. Also, the intermediate layer lipoplasty allows us to define the lumbar and dorsal muscles in women to sculpt a more muscular appearance in selected cases.

Fat Grafting

Fat grafting is only necessary in the trochanteric depression when a patient with small hips has a boy-like appearance. The technique of buttock enhancement is described in Chap. 15. Liposuction alone without fat grafting is often enough to accomplish the enhancement of waist-hip ratio [7, 8]. Results of the procedure are shown in Figs. 14.11, 14.12, and 14.13.

> **Warning!**
> Liposuction between the red zone and the upper gluteus muscle needs to be performed gently. Overresection of this area is detrimental because it can masculinize the dorsum. The gluteal area must project sufficiently and extend appropriately to give a natural and beautiful result. If the upper pole of the buttock is inadvertently resected, it is very difficult to correct since it will need repeated fat grafting. There is a long learning curve and proper training is essential in order to avoid overcorrections.

Postoperative Care

The posterior axillary fold site is closed with subdermal sutures. A draitis placed in the intergluteal crease incision to avoid seromas.

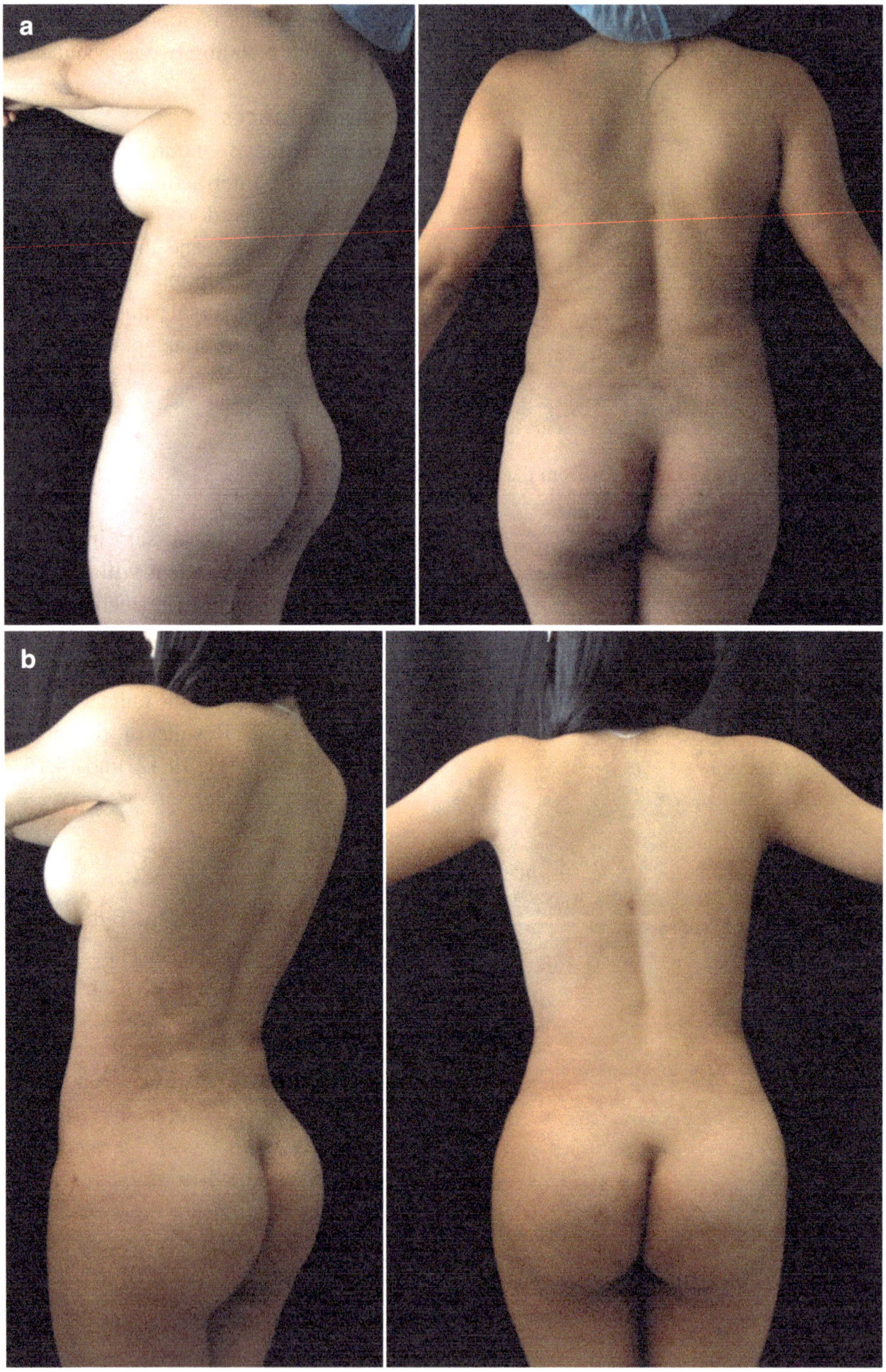

Fig. 14.11 A 27-year-old female patient preoperative (**a**) and 3 months postoperative (**b**). The patient had a previous procedure on the back. Asymmetrical liposuction was performed due to scoliosis

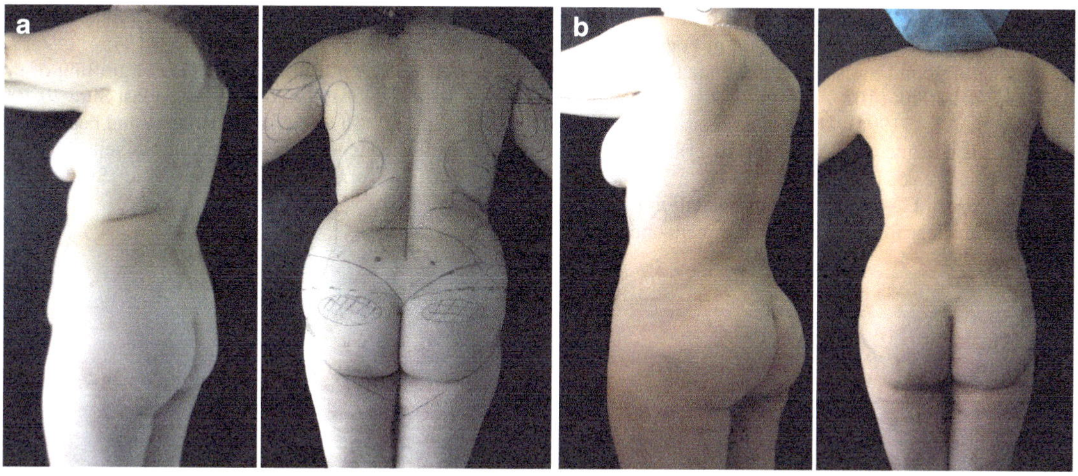

Fig. 14.12 A 42-year-old fat female patient preoperative (**a**) and 1 year postoperative (**b**)

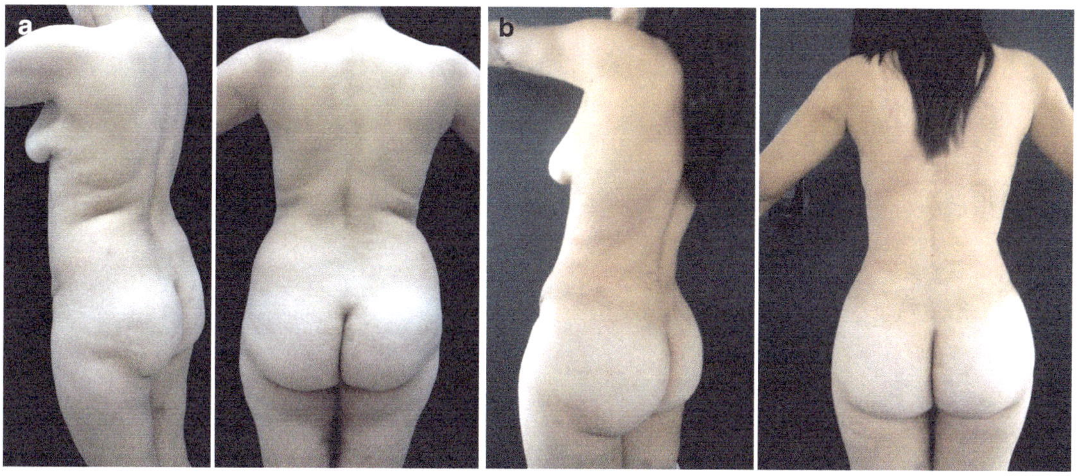

Fig. 14.13 A 36-year-old fat female patient preoperative (**a**) and 1 year postoperative (**b**)

Alternatively, the incisions can simply be left open here for permissive postoperative drainage.

Padding is left on the sacral area for extra compression. A foam vest and compression garment over the waist and torso are important for smooth, even skin retraction.

Postoperative massage and lymphatic drainage are important in this area since the lower back tends to retain fluid. This should commence within 1–2 days following surgery.

References

1. De Souza Pinto EB, Indaburo PE, Da Costa Muniz A, Martinez YP, Gerent KMM, Iwamoto H, Marão Miziara AC (1996) Superficial liposuction: body contouring. Clin Plast Surg 23(4):529–548
2. Fodor PB, Cimino WW, Watson JP, Tahernia A (2005) Suction-assisted lipoplasty: physics, optimization, and clinical verification. Aesthetic Surg J 25(3):234–246
3. Hoyos AE, Millard JA (2007) Vaser-assisted high definition lipoplasty. Aesthetic Surg J 27:594–604
4. Matarasso SL (1999) Liposuction of the chest and back. Dermatol Clin 17(4):799–804, vi

5. Rochrich RJ, Beran SJ, Di Spaltro F et al (1998) Extending the role of liposuction in body contouring with ultrasound assisted liposuction. Plast Reconstr Surg 101:1090–1102
6. Zocchi ML (1996) Ultrasound-assisted lipoplasty. Technical refinements and clinical evaluations. Clin Plast Surg 23:575–598
7. De Pedroza LV (2000) Fat transplantation to the buttocks and legs for aesthetic enhancement or correction of deformities: long-term results of large volumes of fat transplant. Dermatol Surg 26(12):1145–1149
8. Pereira LH, Radwansky H (1996) Fat grafting of the buttock and lower limbs. Aesthetic Plast Surg 20:409
9. Avelar J (1989) Regional distribution and behavior of the subcutaneous tissue concerning selection and indication for liposuction. Aesthetic Surg J 13: 155–165

15 Female Buttocks

Introduction

Evolutionary biology suggests that an hourglass figure, with a narrow waist and full buttocks, is associated with female reproductive potential and physical health across cultures, generations, and ethnicities. Rounded, well-projected buttocks indicate youth and provide an indirect index of the pelvis size and thus fertility.

Our close primate ancestors had in the buttocks a sexual presentation and primary arousal site. Some anthropologists have even proposed that breast fetishism is a derivative of the buttocks' similarity with the breasts.

Early human civilizations artwork clearly portrays the importance of this anatomical area. The Venus de Willendorf (Museum of Natural History of Vienna) is a Paleolithic sculpture dated between 24,000 and 22,000 BCE, which clearly shows a female body with notable buttocks and breasts. In ancient China the buttocks were compared to the full moon. Ancient Greek and Roman sculpture also recreates magnificently the buttock's ideal anatomy as can be seen in the Venus Callipyge (Naples National Archaeological Museum). Nowadays, the buttocks still play a prominent role in eroticism, sexuality, and physical attraction. There is no universally accepted ideal buttock shape, and differences in preference exist across cultures and ethnicities, both in size and shape [1]. However, most have a preference for buttocks that are pert, with smooth round contours (Fig. 15.1).

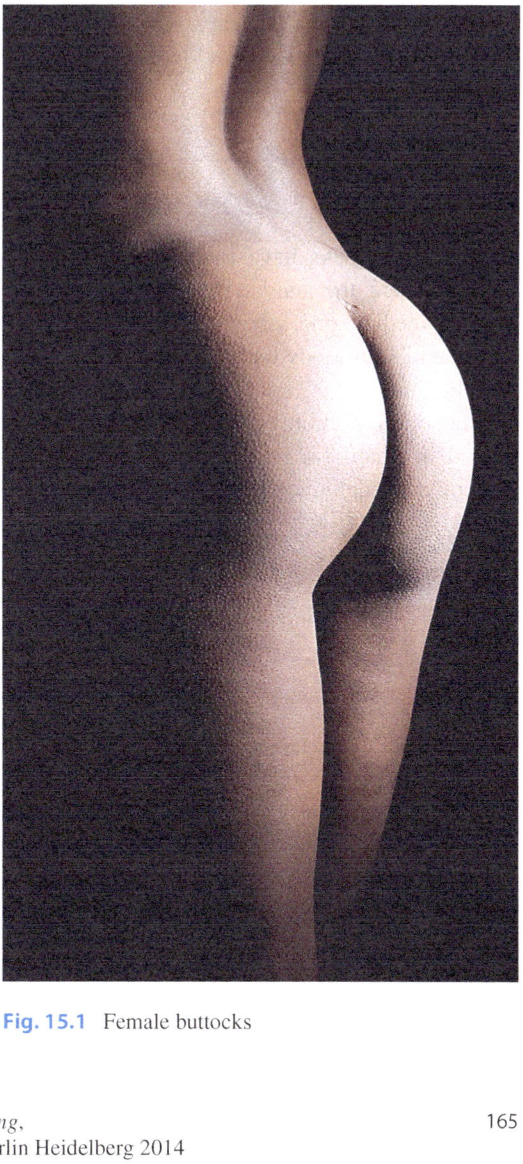

Fig. 15.1 Female buttocks

A.E. Hoyos, P.M. Prendergast, *High Definition Body Sculpting*,
DOI 10.1007/978-3-642-54891-8_15,

Stealth Incisions

Two main 5 mm incisions are used. The first is at the superior limit of the intergluteal crease that allows access to the superior gluteus, the lower back, and part of the mid gluteal area. The second incision is placed at the midpoint of the infragluteal fold. From here we can easily access the lower gluteal area and the internal and external posterior thigh (Fig. 15.2).

The Use of Drains

A drain is used in the intergluteal incision, open or closed. Drains are not needed for the infragluteal incisions; on the contrary, when fat grafting is performed, it must be closed to avoid fat leakage.

Markings

The ideal buttocks have the shape of a hemisphere where the only defined edge is at the inferior-medial zone, whereas the rest of the borders blend seamlessly with the surrounding thigh and the torso.

The upper portion of the gluteal area is discussed in Chap. 14. However, it is important to remember the definition of the red and green zones.

Deep Markings

Mark the fat deposits that are located in the flanks, the sacral fat pad, the hips, and the lateral and medial thighs. These areas are going to be extracted by deep liposuction.

Framing

In females, the only areas for pure framing are the sacral dimples, but we have to establish a guideline for contouring after the deep extraction (Fig. 15.3) [2].

We describe a simple but reliable classification of the zones to provide better contouring. We call them the green and red zones.

Identify the maximum point of indentation (PMI) (Fig. 15.4) in the waistline and trace a line to the upper limit of the intergluteal crease. Then, mark a line from this point to the superior iliac crest; this forms a triangular area we called the green zone where the fat can be freely removed (Fig. 15.5).

Next, identify the trochanteric depression on the lateral side and trace a line from the top of the trochanteric depression to upper limit of the intergluteal crease. By doing this a new triangle is formed, the so-called red zone. The red zone is a transition area between the green zone and the trochanteric depression and requires gentle careful lipoplasty to a avoid overresection (Fig. 15.6).

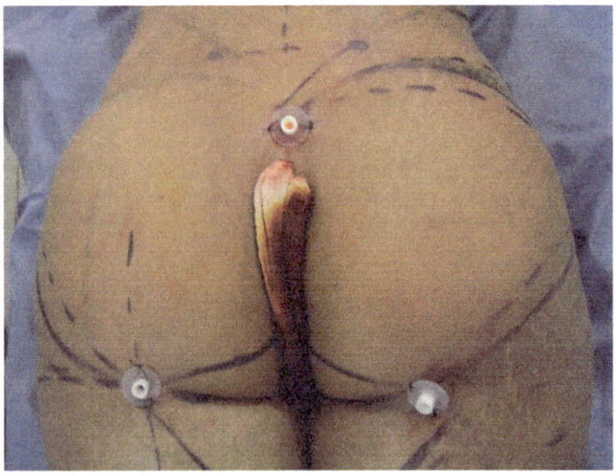

Fig. 15.2 Incisions with ports sutured in place on the superior intergluteal crease and over the mid inferior gluteal point bilaterally

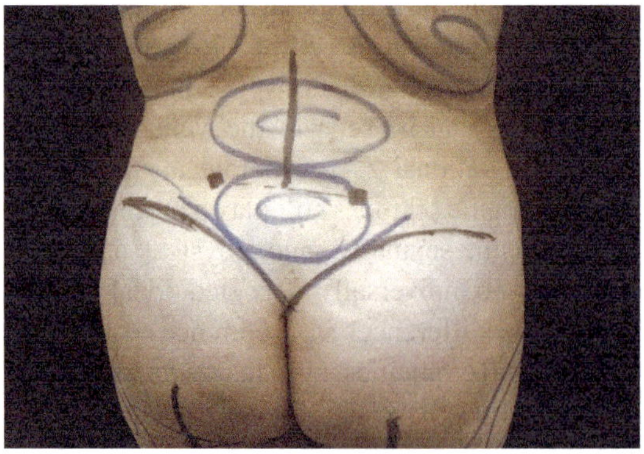

Fig. 15.3 Superior gluteal edge marking

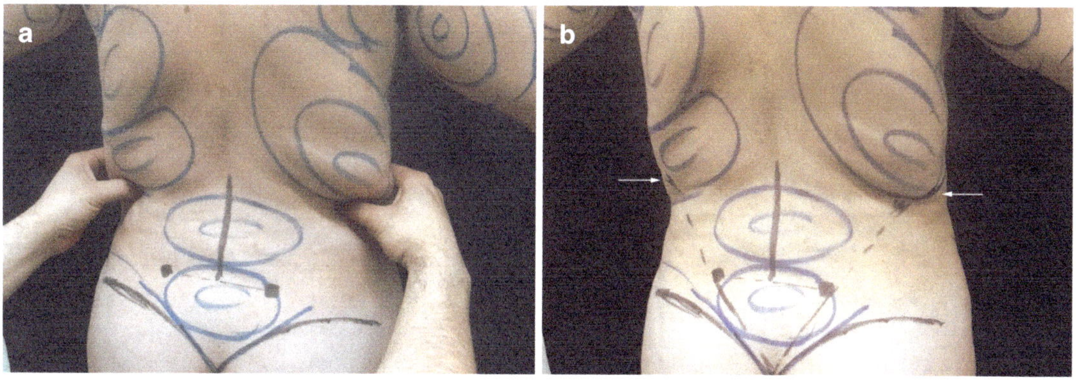

Fig. 15.4 Point of maximum indentation (PMI): (**a**) identification, (**b**) marking. The *white arrows* show that the PMI is asymmetric in this patient

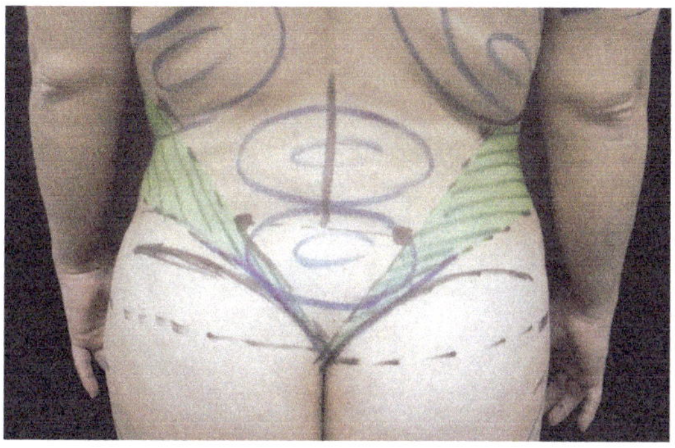

Fig. 15.5 The green zone: free extraction area

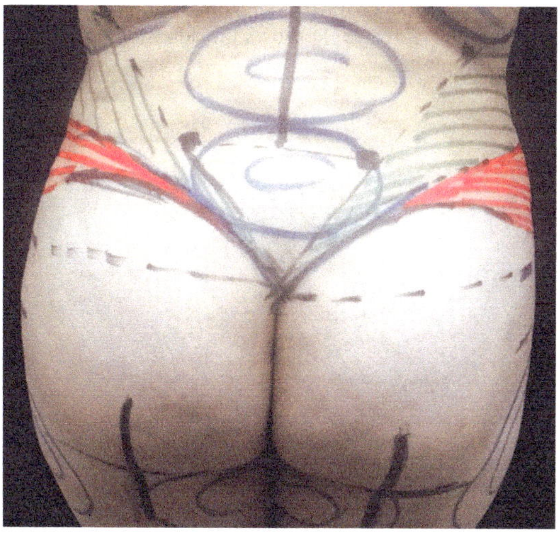

Fig. 15.6 The red zone: extract with caution to avoid overresection

The upper border of gluteus maximus delineates the lower border of the red zone. To find the border, ask the patient to contract the muscle and mark it.

Negative Spaces

Part of the upper aspect of the buttock lies inside the red zone, so the negative space of the red zone in the lower back must blend with the inferior limit of the red zone over the smooth convexity of the buttock. Similarly, the green and red zones must blend seamlessly with one another although liposuction in the green zone is more thorough in order to sculpt the waist near the PMI (Fig. 15.7).

The inferior gluteal area is divided into four zones by tracing a vertical line from the center of the gluteus and a horizontal line that crosses through the infragluteal fold (Fig. 15.8):

Zone 1, the lower internal gluteal area: It forms an acute angle in an aesthetically pleasant buttock, as stated by Mendieta [3] in his classification of female buttocks.

Zone 2, the lower external gluteal area: Producing a smooth contour here is often elusive. It is the transition between the lateral leg and the buttock.

Zone 3, the inner thigh: The markings for fat removal should extend distally into the middle third of the inner thigh where there is an adhesion zone.

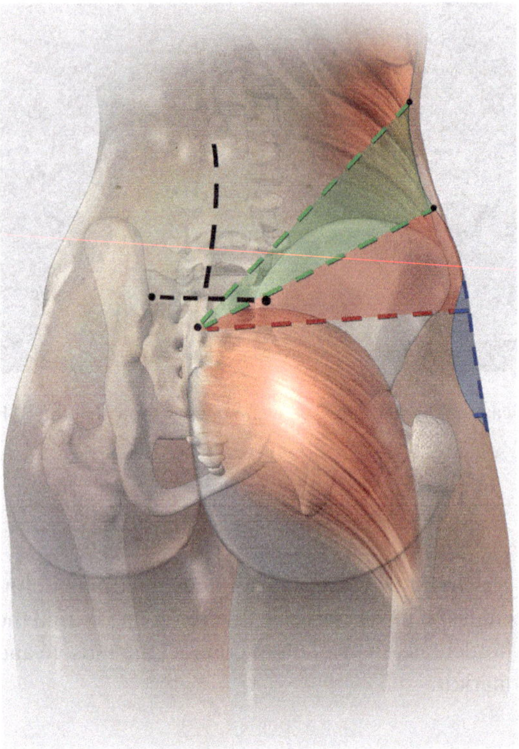

Fig. 15.7 Muscular landmarks and the *green* and *red* zones. The *green* zone is comprehended between the point of maximum indentation (PMI), and the iliac crest. The *red* zone between the lateral and the superior border of the trochanteric depression. The trochanteric depression is an area of fat grafting in female when it is visible (*blue*)

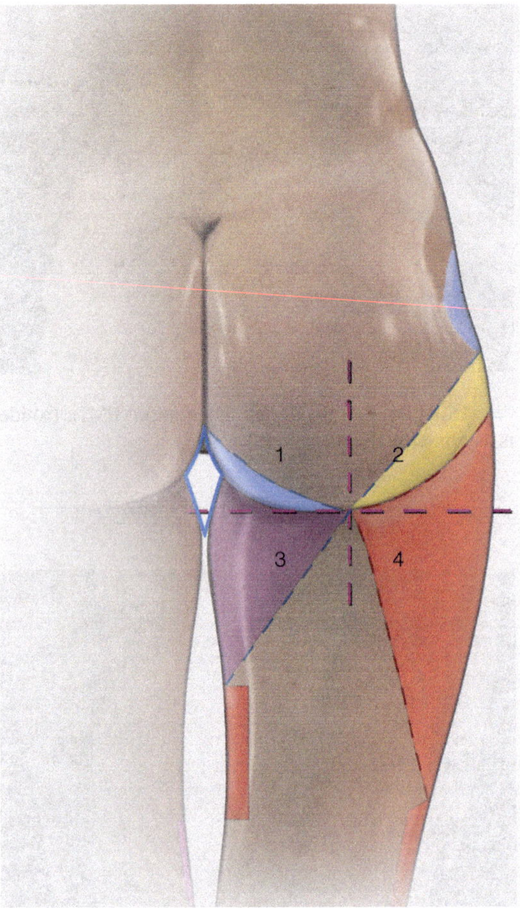

Fig. 15.8 Zones in the inferior gluteal area: *1* lower internal (*light blue*), *2* lower external (*yellow*), *3* inner thigh (*purple*), *4* outer thigh (*red*). Areas with colors do delimitate negative spaces for free and smooth liposuction. The inner thigh *red* rectangle shows the adhesion zone where lipo is prohibited

Zone 4, the outer thigh: It extends from the lateral portion of the buttocks and requires deep liposuction to remove the extra fat that deforms the hips. The markings for fat removal extend from the inferior portion of the trochanteric depression and end at the distal third of the thigh at the adhesion zone.

The inner thigh is divided into thirds; the middle one is an adhesion zone, which contains only superficial fat, so overresection should be avoided in this area. From the upper limit of the adhesion zone, a line is drawn upward to the infragluteal midpoint. The resulting area is safe for extraction and has the advantage of holding a high stem cell concentration (Fig. 15.9).

The lower gluteal edge should normally end at the infragluteal midpoint. However, it is important

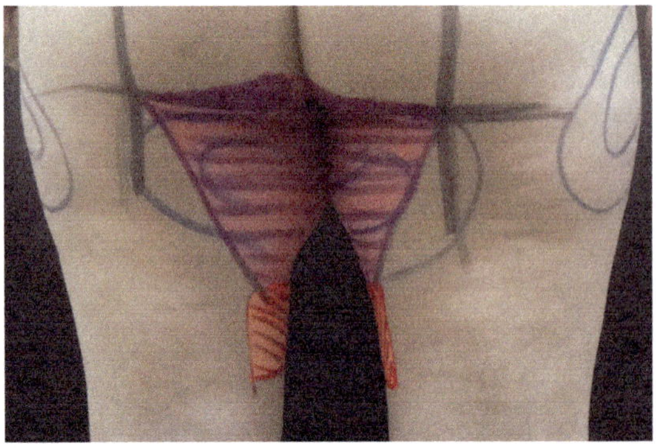

Fig. 15.9 The adhesion zone (in *red*) and the inner thigh safe extraction area (in *pink*)

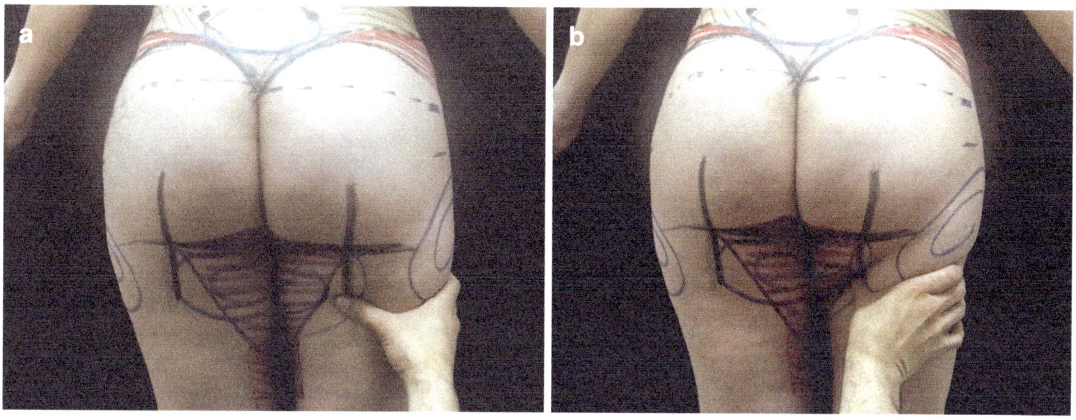

Fig. 15.10 Thigh internal rotation maneuver allows identify the lateral projection of the gluteal fold, following the gluteus maximus. (**a**) Neutral position, (**b**) after rotation

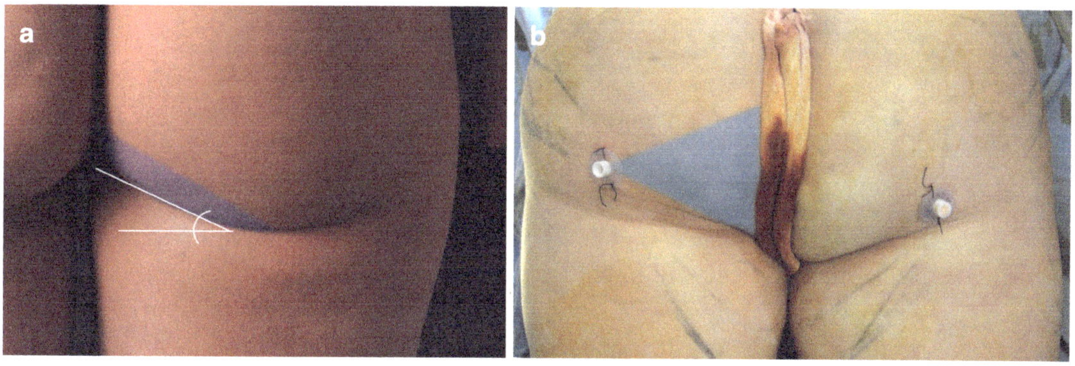

Fig. 15.11 Internal buttock angle. (**a**) The ideal angle must be acute. (**b**) Note results of extraction on the left by liposuction only (in *blue*) vs. the right side (*untouched*). This technique is described by Mendieta [3]

to identify the entire border of gluteus maximus on the lateral side. By making an internal rotation of the thigh, this border can be easily seen and drawn. This maneuver allows identification of the extra fat on the lateral buttocks (Fig. 15.10).

The inferior internal quadrant contributes to the inferior internal border of the buttocks. This border forms an angle that determines the roundness of the gluteus (Fig. 15.11). This angle should be acute in order to provide a youthful look and permit a "rhomboid" of light to be seen between the inferior borders of the buttocks and the upper inner thighs.

A line from the infragluteal midpoint to the inferior edge of the trochanteric depression is drawn. This forms a transition area that also requires a smooth transition (Fig. 15.12).

The gluteal area is divided into horizontal thirds. The middle third should project the most, whereas the upper and lower thirds transition to the red zone and upper thigh, respectively. Usually, the upper and lower thirds undergo varying degrees of liposuction, whereas the middle third receives fat grafting to enhance projection (Fig. 15.13). It is important identify the characteristics of each area to know where and how much to remove (Fig. 15.14).

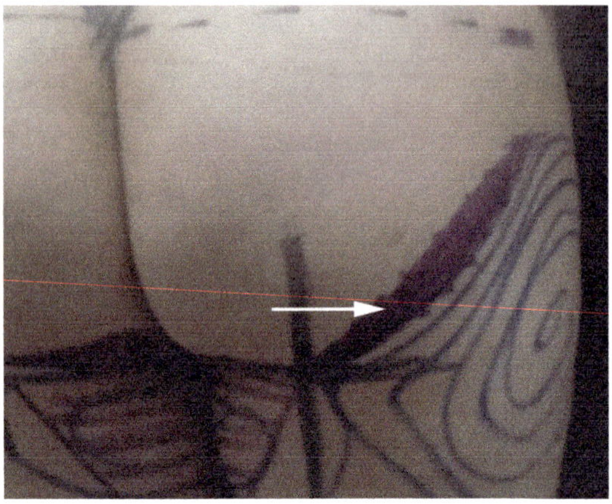

Fig. 15.12 Lower external transition area (*arrow*): comprehended between the lower border of the trochanteric depression and the external projection of the gluteal fold. This is an area of care to shape the ideal spherical shape of the buttock

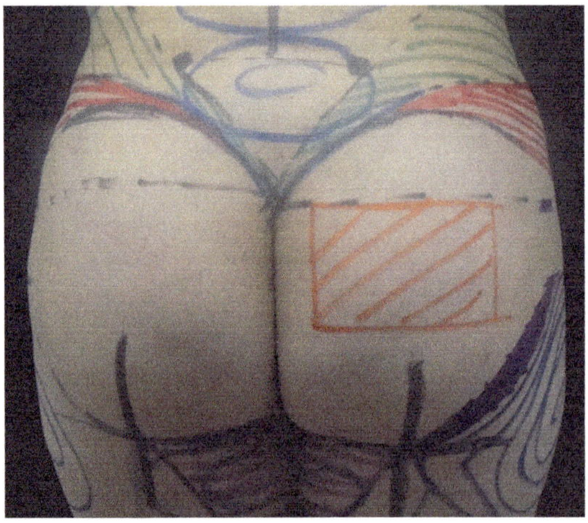

Fig. 15.13 Major gluteal projection zone (*orange*)

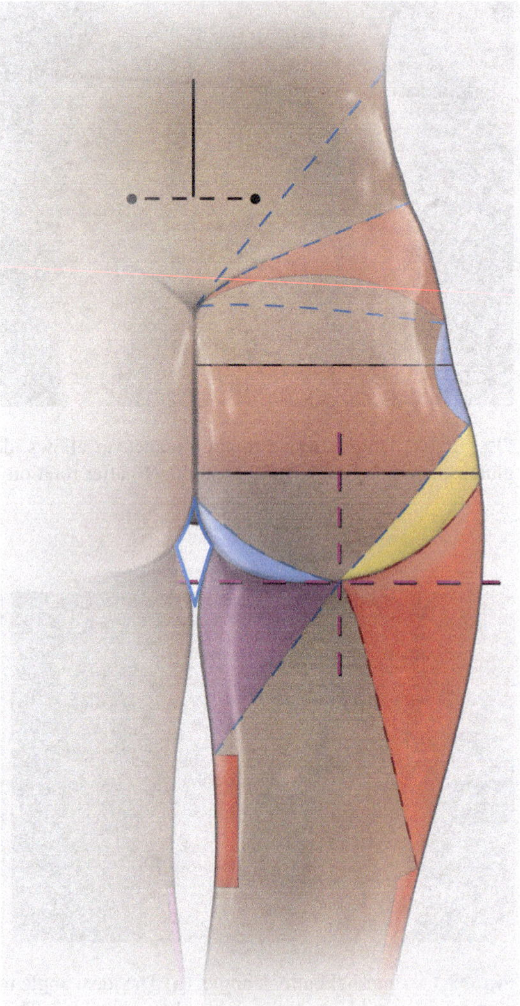

Fig. 15.14 Illustration of all the markings in the gluteal and perigluteal area. Notice the mid gluteal area markings for intramuscular fat grafting (*pink*). The trochanteric area (*blue*) might need extramuscular lipofilling in selected cases. The upper perigluteal red zone (in *pink*) and the lower external transition area are very important: overresection here is very difficult to correct

Procedure

Under general anesthesia the patient is placed in the prone position. The aim of the procedure is to define and enhance the buttocks by revealing the rounded appealing shape. This is performed through selective debulking, fat grafting, and blending of the various zones described above [2–5].

Infiltration

Tumescent solution is infiltrated uniformly in the fat layers, starting in the deep layer and ending in the superficial layer. The solution consists of 1,000 mL of normal saline, sodium bicarbonate, 1 ml of 1:1,000 epinephrine, and varying amounts of lidocaine. The ratio of infiltration to suction should be 2:1.

Emulsification

Emulsification is performed using third-generation ultrasonic probes. The average time of emulsification is 2 min per 100 mL of tumescent

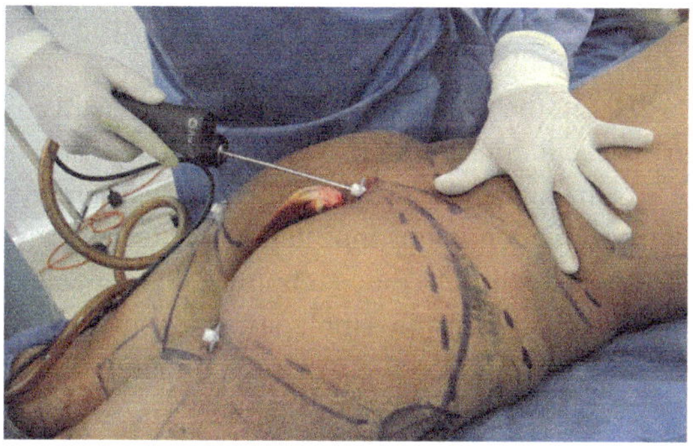

Fig. 15.15 Deep extraction on the green and red zones

solution infiltrated, but remember that the clinical endpoint is loss of tissue resistance.

Extraction

Deep Extraction

Deep liposuction is performed using a 3 mm cannula over the marked areas. The intergluteal crease incision is used to access the lower back and upper gluteal area. It is important to do a careful extraction and not to overresect the red area to ensure a smooth transition from the green zone into the trochanteric depression (Fig. 15.15).

Accessing from the infragluteal midpoint (IGM), begin the extraction of the lower and the lateral gluteal areas and especially the inner thigh area. This area needs to be extracted from distal (upper limit of the adhesion zone) to proximal to achieve a smooth transition into the buttocks.

Superficial Framing

As stated before, the only area for framing is the sacral dimples. These are created by superficial liposuction using a 3 mm suction cannula. The compression technique with the nondominant hand over the tip of the cannula is used to remove almost all subcutaneous fat at the dimples. The midline can be deepened with the 3 mm cannula between the paralumbar muscles as far inferiorly as an imaginary line between the sacral dimples.

Negative Spaces

The sacral triangle, the waistline, and the extensive blending between the green and red zones are addressed in this step. The idea is to merge the aggressive extraction from the green zone into the red zone, especially at the hip area, next to the trochanteric depression. This area is difficult to access from the central intergluteal incision, so special cannulae have been designed for this purpose (4.6 mm and 3.0 mm curved cannulae) (Fig. 15.16).

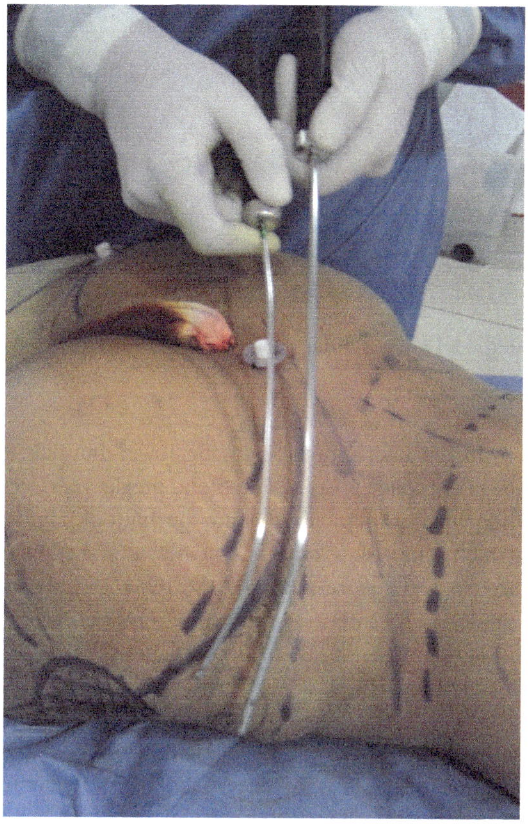

Fig. 15.16 Curved cannulae showing the area that can be reached over the hip

Warning!

It is imperative to work on the hip area with the special curved cannulae and to remove the fat with caution to avoid overresection that will lead to a masculine appearance. If the surgeon is not sure about the endpoint for this area, it is always better to leave a little more fat than expected. A touch-up is always an option later, but overresection is very difficult to correct.

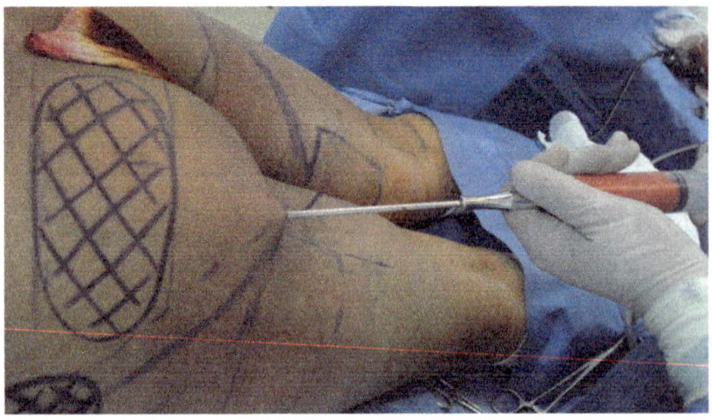

Fig. 15.17 Fat grafting

In the lateral portion of the lower buttock, a negative space is created to blend the deep extraction in the lateral thigh and the buttock shape, which is more curved. The line between the lower trochanteric depression and the IGM serves as a guideline for intermediate extraction to eliminate the step created by the deep extraction.

The inner thigh is suctioned through the IGM incision. The upper inner thigh is blended with the middle third of thigh, using conservative and cautious lipoplasty over the adhesion zone to avoid irregularities.

Warning!
Remember to start the inner thigh extraction from distal to proximal to avoid an unwanted overresection on the midportion on the inner thigh (the adhesion zone). Most of the times, extraction of the midportion of the thigh is not needed.

Fat Grafting

Fat tissue is harvested with a 3 mm blunt cannula to an empty, sterile bottle trap. Use decantation to separate the fat cells from the saline and serosanguinous components. Through the mid inferior gluteal incision, insert the cannula and start placing the grafts with a fanning motion from deep to superficial. Most of the graft is placed in the middle third of the gluteus, with additional graft placed to upper or lower poles if needed (Fig. 15.17) [6–9].

Warning!
Begin the fat grafting procedure by placing the cannula parallel to the surgical table, from intramuscular into the gluteus maximus and medius muscles and later more superficial in the supramuscular level. Always infiltrate small strips of fat and inject the fat on the way out so there is no elevation in the compartment pressure. This may minimise the risk of fat embolism.

Postoperative Care

Mild compression is recommended in the buttock area to prevent reabsorption of the grafted fat. In the thighs, a normal compression garment is required to prevent swelling. The garment should be used for a period of 2 months.

Therapeutic manual lymphatic drainage massage is used over the thigh areas, directed to the inguinal lymph nodes at the inner thigh. Buttocks are one of the most rewarding areas to treat in high-definition body sculpting (Figs. 15.18, 15.19, 15.20, 15.21, and 15.22).

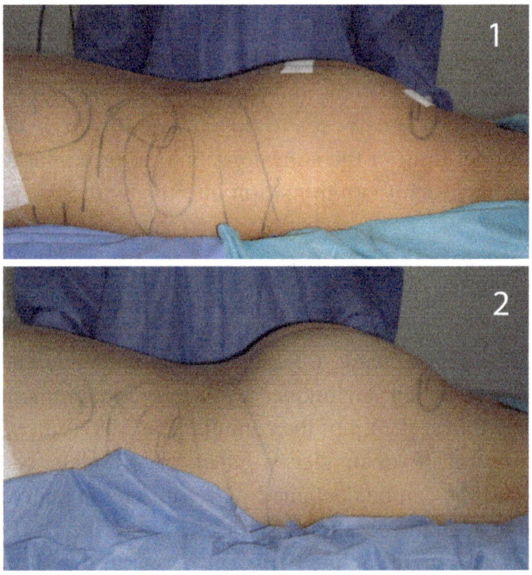

Fig. 15.18 Intraoperative images: (*1*) preoperative, (*2*) immediate results after liposuction and fat grafting of 350 ml per side

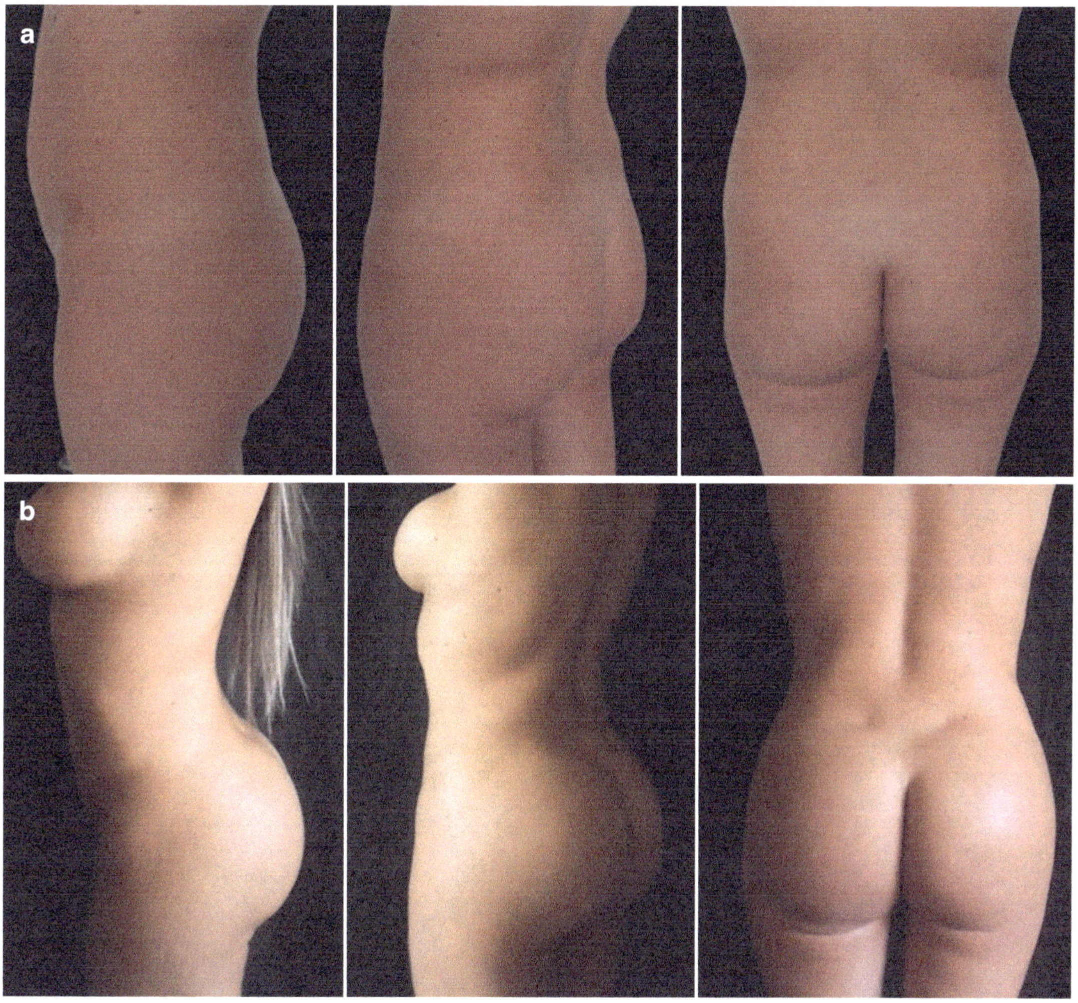

Fig. 15.19 A 28-year-old female patient preoperative (**a**) and 4 years postoperative (**b**). 500 ml was grafted on each side

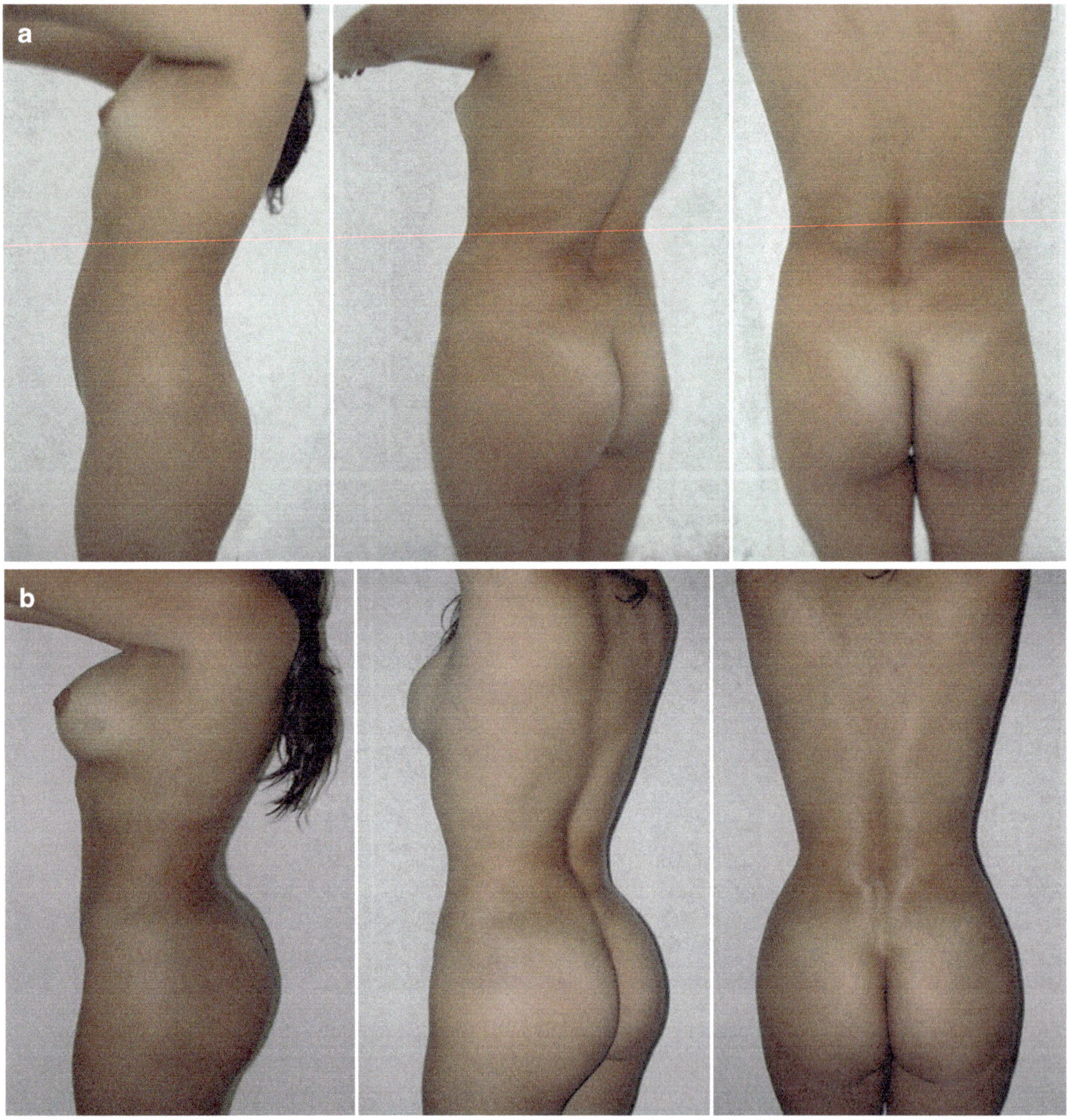

Fig. 15.20 A 20-year-old female patient preoperative (**a**) and 1 year postoperative (**b**). 400 ml was grafted on each side

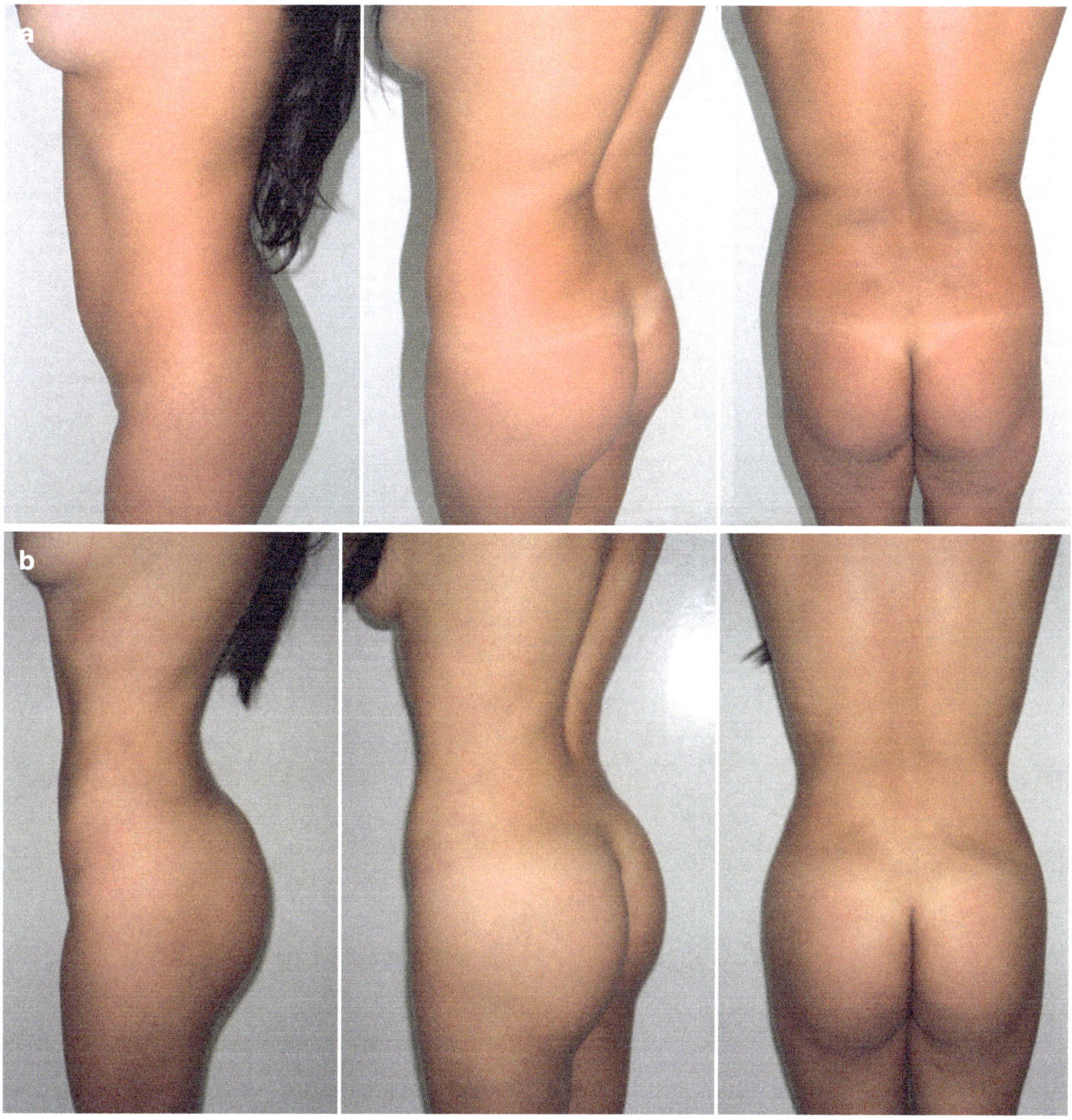

Fig. 15.21 A 29-year-old female patient preoperative (a) and 1 year postoperative (b). 400 ml was grafted on each side

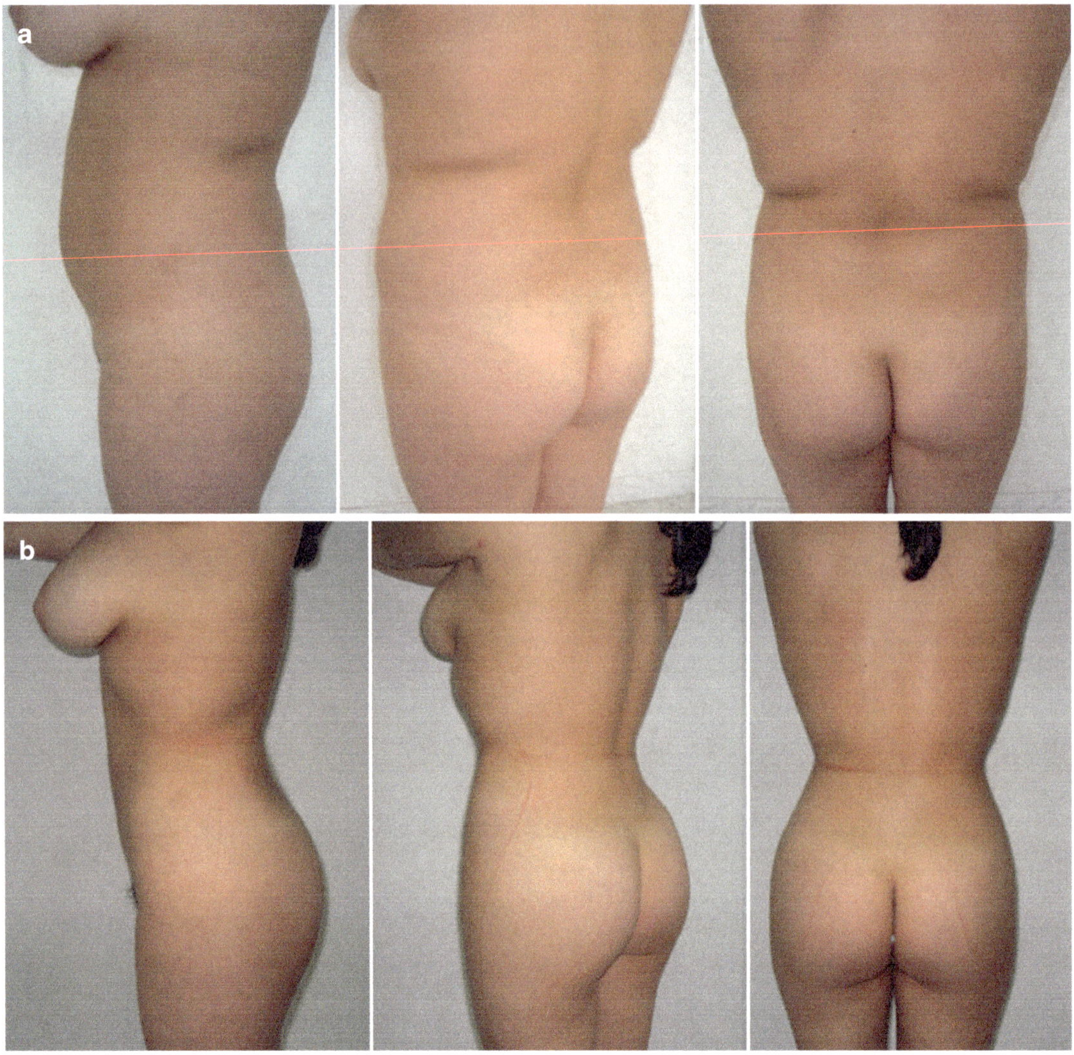

Fig. 15.22 A 24-year-old female patient preoperative (**a**) and 1 year postoperative (**b**). Asymmetric grafting was done: 250 ml was grafted on the left buttock and 350 ml on the right side

References

1. Roberts TL, Weinfeld AB, Bruner TW, Nguyen K (2006) "Universal" and ethnic ideals of beautiful buttocks are best obtained by autologous micro fat grafting and liposuction. Clin Plast Surg 33(3):371–394
2. Hoyos AE, Millard JA (2007) Vaser-assisted high definition lipoplasty. Aesthetic Surg J 27:594–604
3. Mendieta CG (2011) The art of gluteal sculpting, Quality Medical Publishing, Inc St Louis, Missouri
4. Mendieta CG (2003) Gluteoplasty. Aesthetic Surg J 23(6):441–455
5. Mendieta CG (2006) Intramuscular gluteal augmentation technique. Clin Plast Surg 33(3):423–434
6. De Pedroza LV (2000) Fat transplantation to the buttocks and legs for aesthetic enhancement or correction of deformities: long-term results of large volumes of fat transplant. Dermatol Surg 26(12): 1145–1149
7. Harrison D, Selvaggi G (2007) Gluteal augmentation surgery: indications and surgical management. J Plast Reconstr Aesthet Surg 60(8):922–928
8. Nicareta BB, Pereira LHL, Sterodimas AA, Illouz YGY (2011) Autologous gluteal lipograft. Aesthetic Plast Surg 35(2):216–224
9. Pereira LH, Radwansky H (1996) Fat grafting of the buttock and lower limbs. Aesthetic Plast Surg 20:409

16 Female Breasts

Introduction

There is a rising demand for aesthetic enhancement of the breast (Fig. 16.1). The use of implants is still considered the gold standard to improve the volume and shape of the female breast. However, many patients who desire augmentation still have reservations and concerns about the use of silicone or saline implants. Autologous fat provides an alternative to implants for moderate augmentation and contouring of the breast [1].

Fat was first proposed as a filling material by Neuber in 1893. The concept rapidly gained momentum, and subsequent work by Guerrero Santos, Bircoll, Coleman [2], and others has shown that it is possible and safe to harvest and graft fat for rejuvenation of the face and contouring of the body, provided it is handled with care [1, 3].

Fat has many attributes of the ideal filler. It is natural, soft, and safe and has the potential for permanence if it acquires a new blood supply following placement in the recipient site. Since

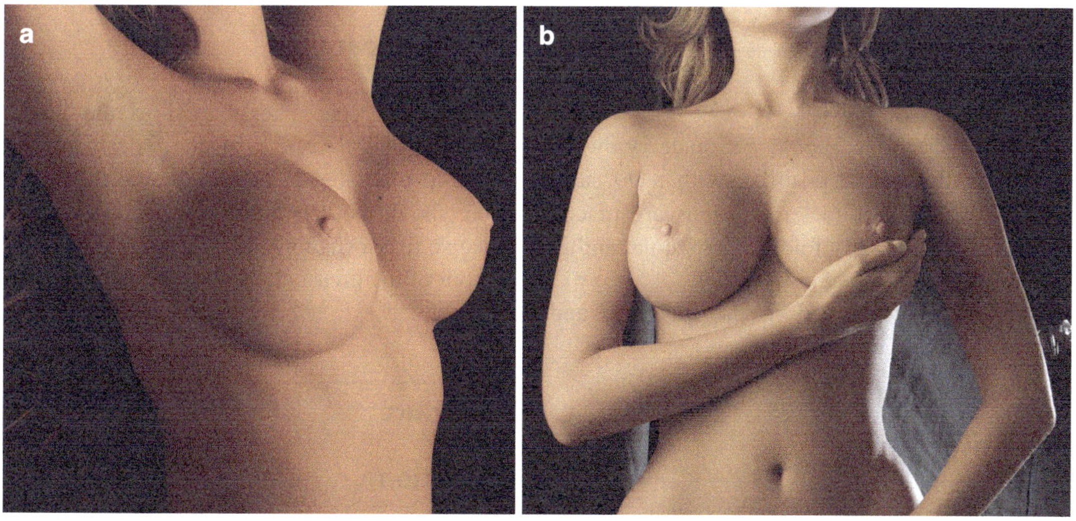

Fig. 16.1 Aesthetically ideal female breasts (**a**, **b**)

A.E. Hoyos, P.M. Prendergast, *High Definition Body Sculpting*,
DOI 10.1007/978-3-642-54891-8_16, © Springer-Verlag Berlin Heidelberg 2014

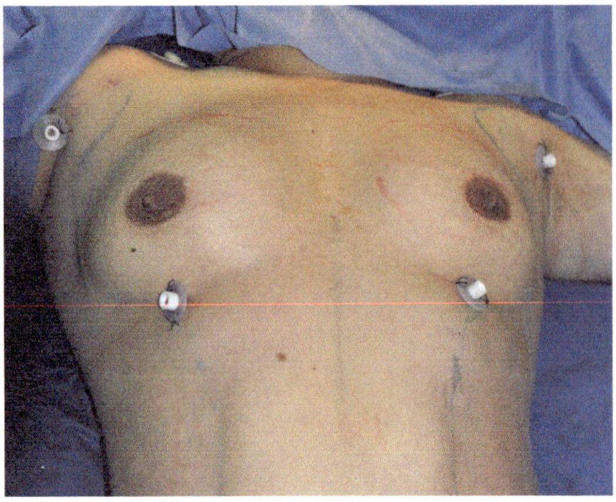

Fig. 16.2 Incisions with ports at the anterior axillary fold and in the inframammary fold

breast fat grafting is technique dependent, the long-term results are variable [4–6]. We use VASER ultrasound to emulsify fat before extraction, a process that does not compromise viability of the adipocytes.

The breast has a rounded shape defined by the breast gland contour. The anatomical features surrounding the breast gland enhance its shape and projection. The triangular area between the clavicle and the anterior insertion of the deltoid muscle; the axillary portion of the gland, or Spence's tail; and the negative space lateral to the gland, should follow a lazy "S."

Stealth Incisions

The ideal incisions should be made with the patient in the supine position, with a 90° arm abduction. Five-millimeter incisions are placed in the anterior axillary fold, in the areola, and in the inframammary fold.

The ports are placed in the incisions and sutured in place (Fig. 16.2).

The Use of Drains

Drains are not necessary in the breast. The fat injections are performed by accessing the breast tissue through the anterior axillary fold incisions. These incisions should be closed to avoid leakage of fat following the procedure.

Marking

Deep Markings

With the patient in the standing position, outline the gland. Mark the areas that need more projection. This is usually the upper poles of the breast. Most of the fat will be injected in these areas. Mark the surrounding area of the breast, from the axilla lateral to Spence's tail to the lower portion of the lateral chest wall (Fig. 16.3). These surrounding areas will be treated with thorough fat removal in order to enhance the relative size and shape of the breast itself.

Framing

Little framing is needed in the breast area. However, a slight delineation of the pectoralis border at the upper limit of the breast enhances the breast shape and increases muscular definition. The lateral "S" is marked to define the smooth contours of the breast.

Negative Space

The negative space lies lateral to the breast, from the lateral aspect of the inframammary crease to the anterior axillary line at the axilla. There should be very little fat remaining in this space so that a shadow is created, enhancing the contour of the breast along the "S".

Procedure

Infiltration

Proceed to infiltrate using tumescent solution with 1,000 ml of normal saline, 50 ml of 1 %

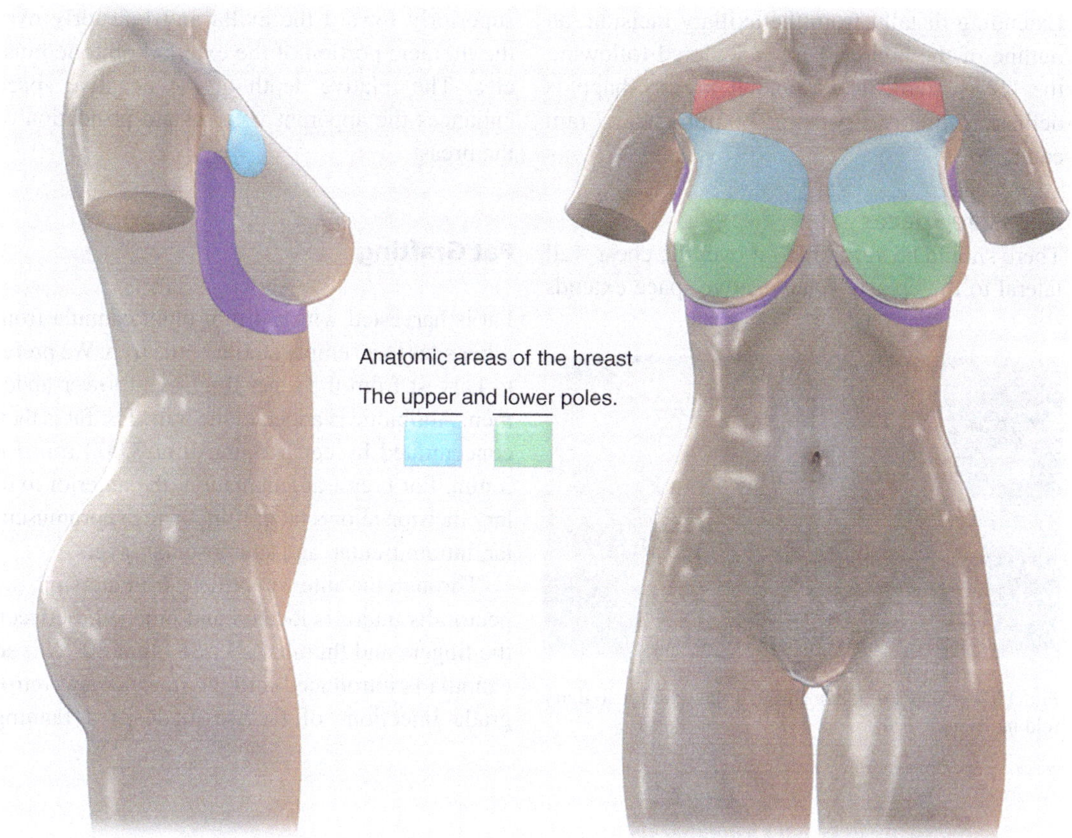

Fig. 16.3 Anatomical areas of the breast, upper and lower poles (*green* and *blue*), the subclavicular triangle (*red*), the peripheral area around teh breast (*purple*). On the lateral view, note the tail of Spence extending towards the axilla

lidocaine, 12.5 ml of sodium bicarbonate, and 1 ml of epinephrine 1:1,000. The ratio of infiltrate to volume of fat removed is approximately 2:1.

Emulsification

To enhance the breast, superfluous fat near the axilla and around the breast is emulsified and removed using VASER. Beginning in the superficial layer, smooth even strokes are used with the ultrasound set to pulsed mode at 80 %. Pulsed mode halves the energy delivered to the tissues and reduces the risk of excessive heat generation under the thin skin around the axilla and breast. Never forget to protect the skin from burning by using a double-layered wet towel around the port and under the probe. The axillary site is prone to burns due to the angulation required in this area.

Additional VASER time is required in the framing areas where thorough fat removal and sculpting are performed to create shadows.

Extraction

Deep Extraction

Through the anterior axillary fold incision, the axillary fat pad and the extra fat surrounding the lateral breast are extracted using a 3.7 mm cannula (Fig. 16.4).

Superficial Framing

In the superficial layer, aspiration along the upper pectoralis muscle line near the axilla is performed.

Extending distally from the axillary incision, an outline of the breast gland is sculpted following the "S" pattern. The rounded breast shape is delineated in this way using 3.0 mm and 3.7 mm cannulae.

Negative Spaces

There should be very little fat over the chest wall lateral to the breast. This negative space extends superiorly toward the axilla and inferiorly over the thoracic portion of the external oblique muscles. The relative depth of the negative space enhances the apparent volume and projection of the breast.

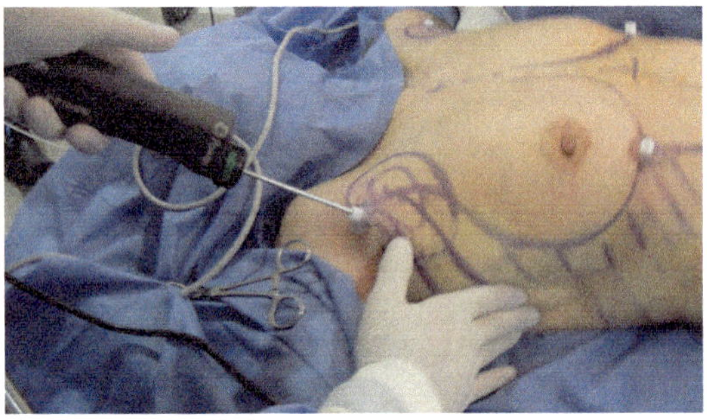

Fig. 16.4 Deep extraction through the anterior axillary fold incision

Fat Grafting

Fat is harvested with a 4 mm blunt cannula from other sites to an empty sterile bottle trap. We prefer to harvest from the inner thighs and lower abdomen. Antibiotic is added to the trap. The fat is then concentrated by centrifuging it at 3,000 rpm for 3 min. For breast augmentation, the anterior axillary incision allows fat grafting in the supramuscular, intramuscular, and submuscular layers.

Through the anterior axillary fold incision, the pectoralis major is located and pinched, between the fingers and thumb. A 3 mm blunt 30° curved cannula is introduced into the muscle, and retrograde injections of fat are made in a fanning

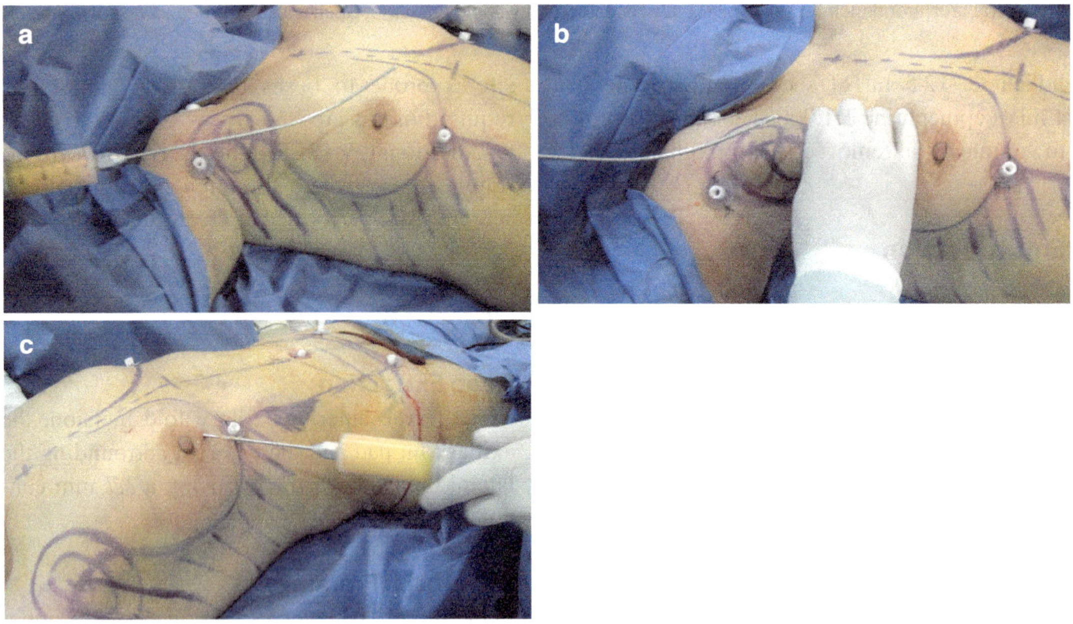

Fig. 16.5 Breast fat grafting: (**a**) the curved cannula for axillary access. (**b**) Pinching technique and injection through the anterior axillary incision. (**c**) Fat injection though the areolar incision

motion, first in the intramuscular plane and later in the submuscular plane (Fig. 16.5). Once these layers are full, a 16-gauge needle or cannula is used with 5 ml syringes for supramuscular fat grafting into the fat around the breast gland and in the subdermal tissues. Small strips of fat are placed in a fanning motion from deep to superficial (Fig. 16.6). The average volume of fat grafting is 100–300 ml per side.

Fat grafting is used during high-definition body sculpting [3] to provide a moderate augmentation of the breasts (Figs. 16.7, 16.7, 16.8, 16.9, and 16.10).

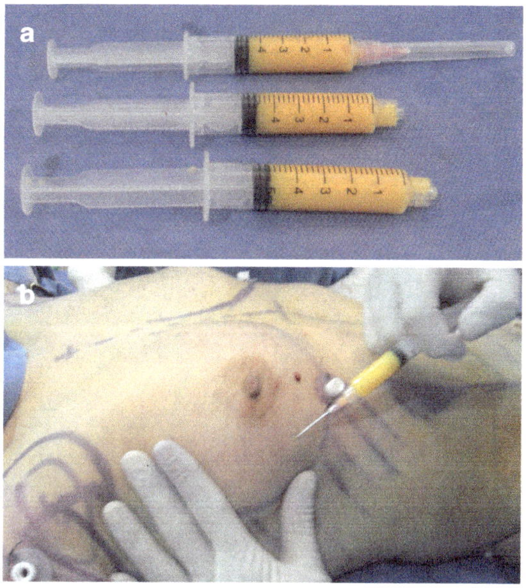

Fig. 16.6 Supramuscular-subdermal tissue fat grafting. (**a**) 5 mm syringes with the fat for grafting. (**b**) Injection technique

Warning!
Avoid the use of drains in the breasts when fat is grafted to the area.

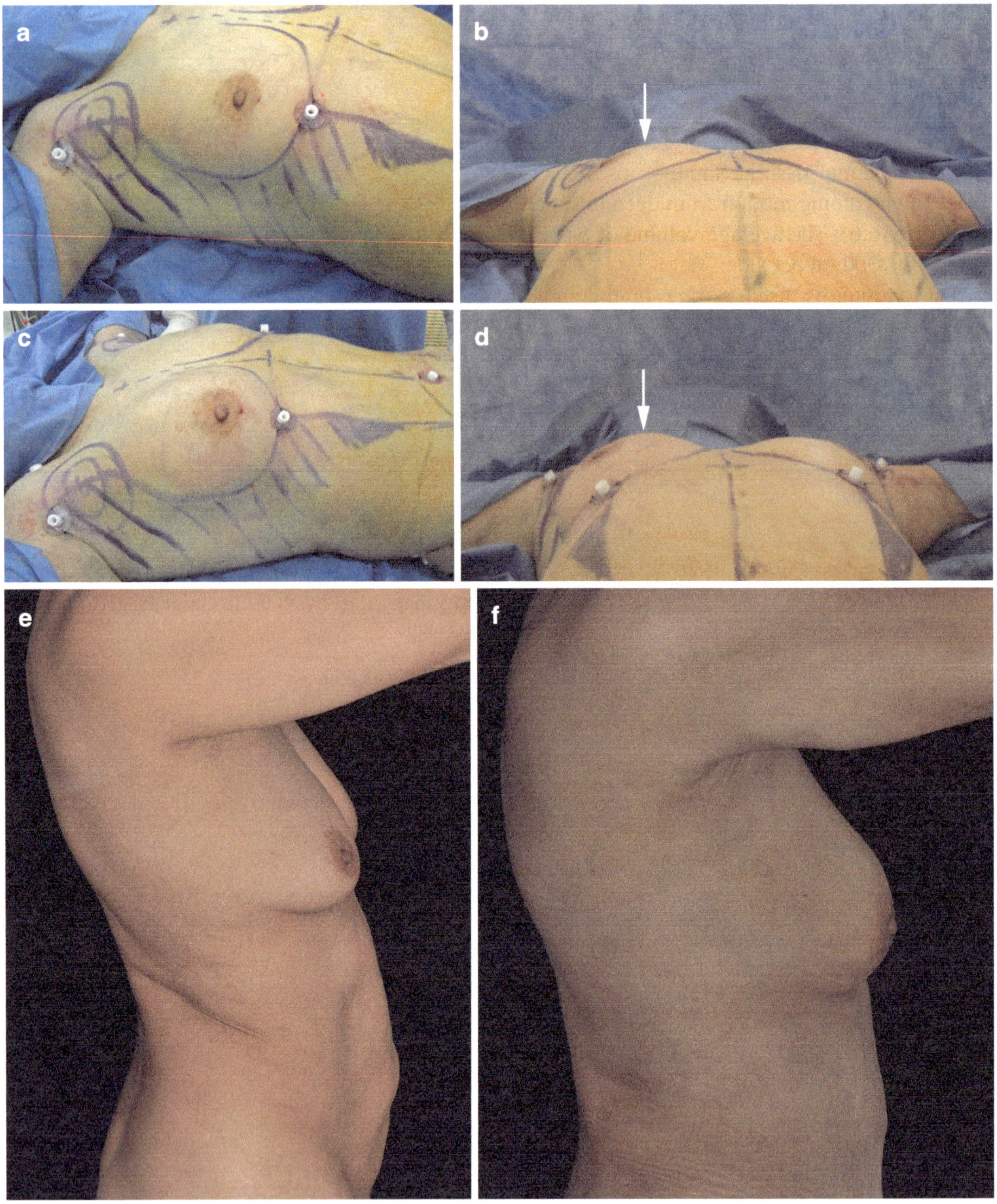

Fig. 16.7 Grafting: before (**a**, **b**,) and after (**c**, **d**) the fat injection. Notice the change of volume between the two images (*arrows*). (**e**) Preoperative, (**f**) 6 months postoperative

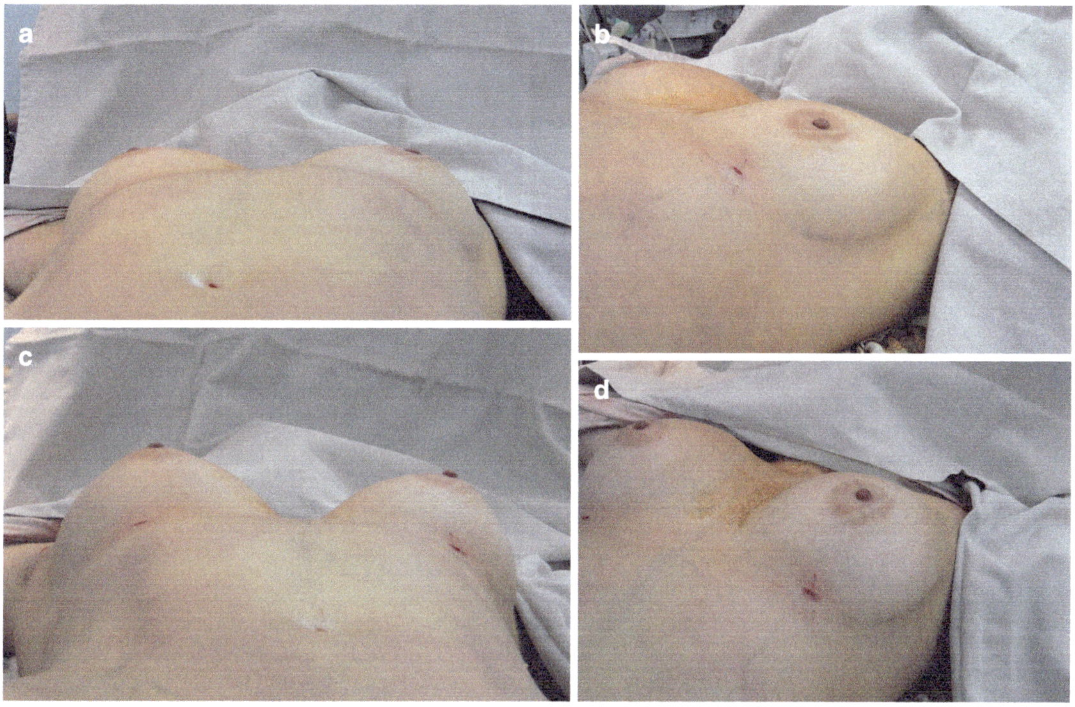

Fig. 16.8 Grafting: before (**a**, **b**) and after (**c**, **d**) the fat injection

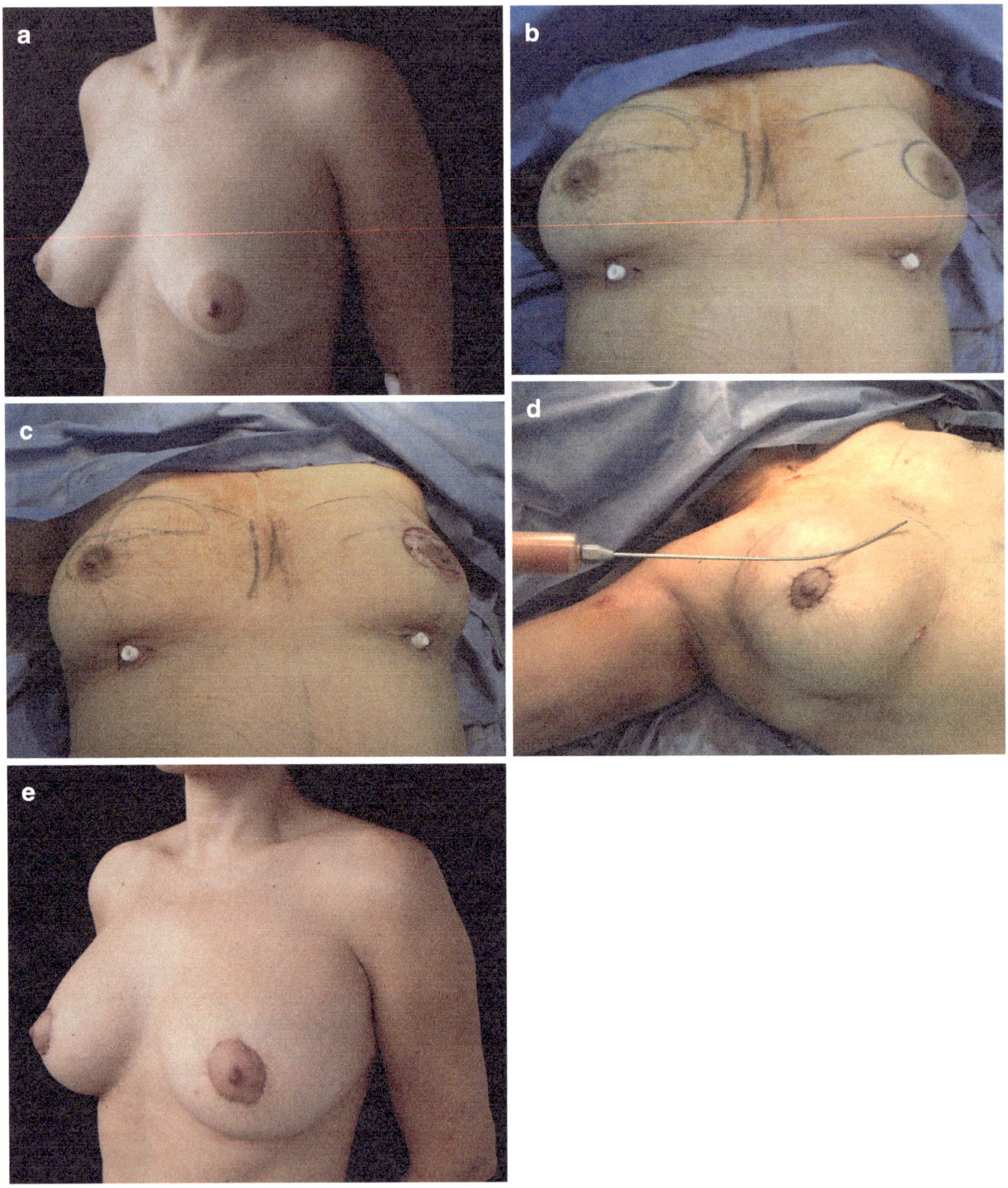

Fig. 16.9 Mastopexy and fat grafting: preoperative (**a**). Intraoperative (**b**), after deepithelialization (**c**), curved cannula over the breast showing the area reached for fat grafting (**d**), and postoperative results after one month (**e**)

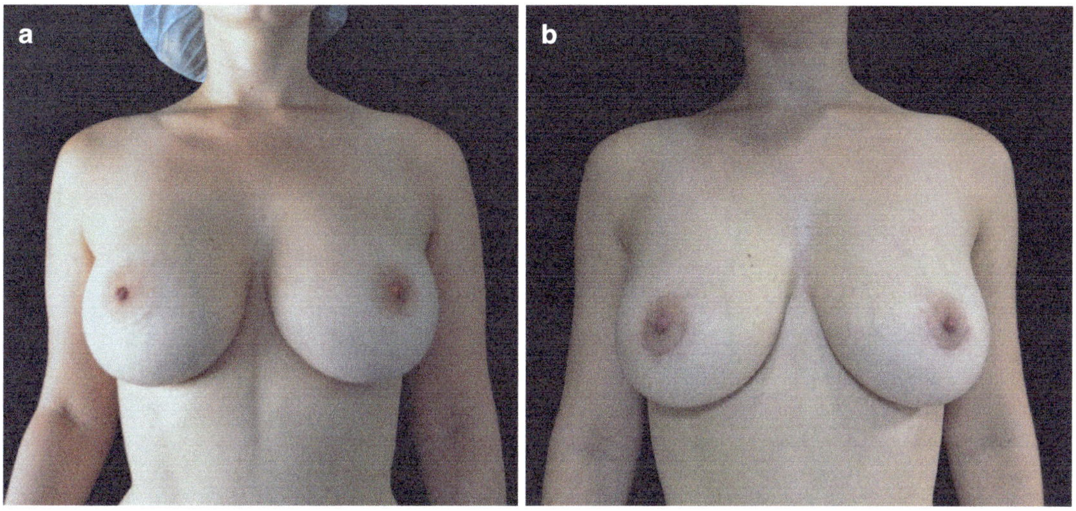

Fig. 16.10 A 28-year-old patient who had previous breast augmentation surgery (400 cc implants). The patient wanted the implants removed, a small reduction, but not a long scar. Preoperative (**a**), postoperative (**b**) after implants were removed and fat grafting to preserve part of the volume

References

1. Chajchir A (1996) Fat injection: long-term follow-up. Aesthetic Plast Surg 20(4):291–296
2. Coleman SR, Saboeiro AP (2007) Fat grafting to the breast revisited: safety and efficacy. Plast Reconstr Surg 119(3):775–785; discussion 786–7
3. Hoyos AE, Millard JA (2007) Vaser-assisted high definition lipoplasty. Aesthetic Surg J 27:594–604
4. De Blacam C, Momoh AO, Colakoglu S, Tobias AM, Lee BT (2011) Evaluation of clinical outcomes and aesthetic results after autologous fat grafting for contour deformities of the reconstructed breast. Plast Reconstr Surg 128(5):411e–418e
5. Illouz YG, Sterodimas A (2009) Autologous fat transplantation to the breast: a personal technique with 25 years of experience. Aesthetic Plast Surg 33(5):706–715
6. Kamakura T, Ito K (2011) Autologous cell-enriched fat grafting for breast augmentation. Aesthetic Plast Surg 35(6):1022–1030

Female Arms

17

Introduction

The beautiful female arm displays a subtle balance between slimness, softness, and definition. The arm should appear slim but not skinny, and certain muscles should be visible, but not others. For instance, the deltoid outline is desirable, and some definition of the biceps is acceptable. However, a developed triceps is perceived as a masculine feature, so it is not appropriate to display and define this muscle in the female arm (Fig. 17.1).

Although the aesthetic ideal described above is generally accepted as the goal in lipoplasty of the female arm, each patient has her own conception of beauty [1]. Some women want very slim arms with little muscular definition and others want accentuation of the deltoid shape, while others want a masculine look. The preoperative assessment plays a crucial role in determining the wishes and expectations of the patient. During the consultation, it is helpful to ask the patient about some of their favorite star's arm shape. Some will mention Angelina Jolie (slim), while others would say Jessica Biel or Cameron Diaz (toned, deltoid outlined) and others will say Madonna (very athletic, deltoid and biceps outlined, almost masculine).

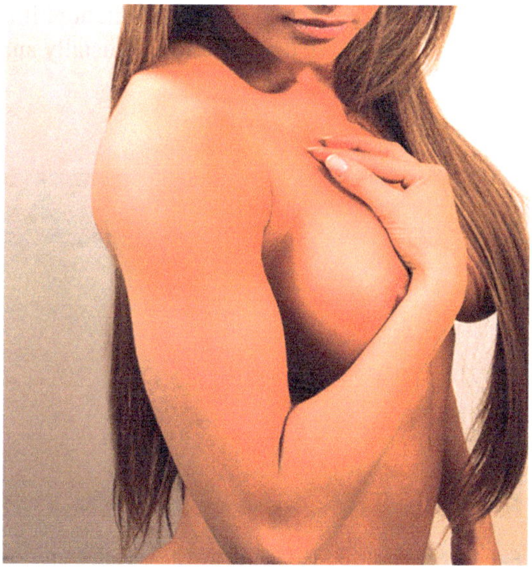

Fig. 17.1 Athletic slim female arms

Stealth Incisions

The incisions are made with the patient in the prone position, with a 90° arm abduction, 90° elbow flexion, and complete external rotation.

Three 5 mm incisions are used: in the posterior axillary crease, in the anterior axillary fold, and at the elbow over the olecranon tip (Fig. 17.2).

The Use of Drains

Drains are not needed. As in the male approach, the distal incisions at the elbows are left open for permissive drainage. Early postoperative massage should be implemented to facilitate drainage.

A.E. Hoyos, P.M. Prendergast, *High Definition Body Sculpting*,
DOI 10.1007/978-3-642-54891-8_17, © Springer-Verlag Berlin Heidelberg 2014

Markings

The markings are best drawn with the patient in the standing position. Compared to the markings in the male patient, the female arm markings are relatively easy.

Deep Markings

With the patient's arm in adduction, first, the excess fat over the posterior aspect of the arm is marked. In some women, significant fat deposits are located in the internal portion of the arm [2]. These are marked with the arm in abduction. It is important to mark all the posterior fat distally and proximally and mark the mid posterior arm for cautious extraction.

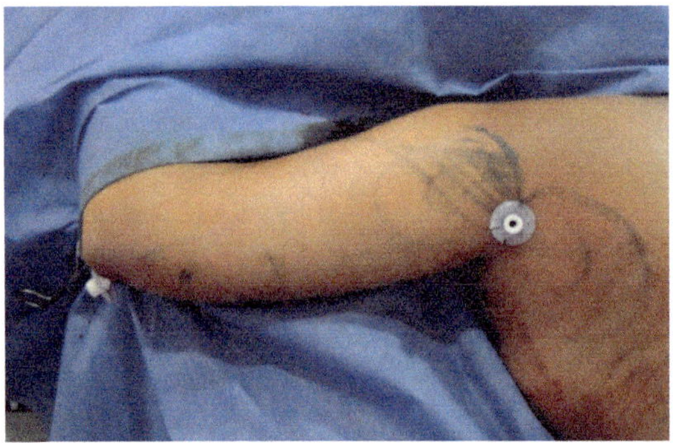

Fig. 17.2 Female posterior arm incisions with ports

The Youth Angle

As in male patient, the inferior border of the female arm with the arm in 90° abduction forms the "youth angle." The more acute the angle is, the more pronounced the triceps muscle mass and the younger the arm looks. In obese and older people, the angle tends to be obtuse due to the presence of extra fat and/or laxity of skin (Fig. 17.3).

Framing

With the arm in 90° abduction and 90° elbow flexion, mark the posterior deltoid muscle sulcus. The triceps is not marked, as the ideal female arm does not have significant muscle mass in that area. In some patients, the intermuscular crease between the biceps and triceps is marked, both anteriorly and posteriorly.

Negative Spaces

A triangle is formed between the curved line of the posterior sulcus of the deltoid, the tip of the insertion of the deltoid in the humerus, and the point in the posterior axillary fold. This triangle forms a negative space area that is marked for extraction (Fig. 17.4).

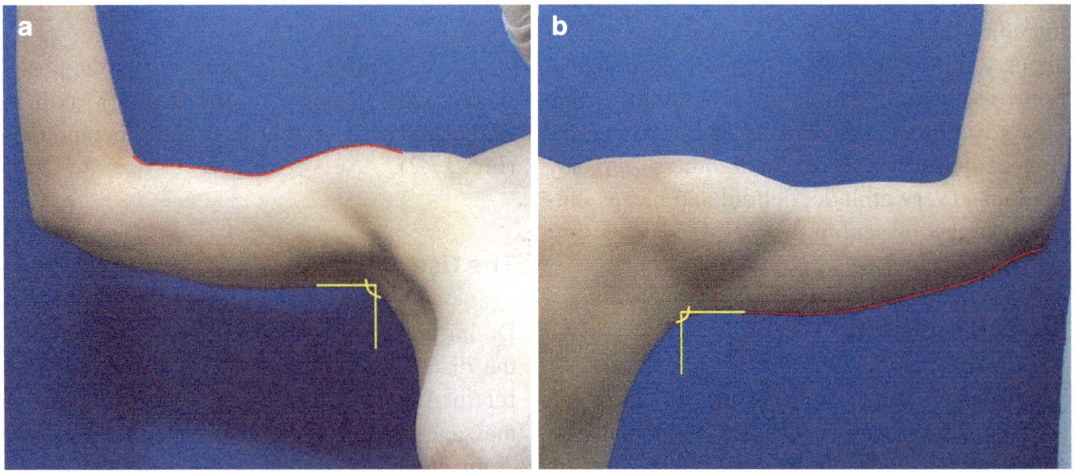

Fig. 17.3 Female youth angle in the anterior (a) and posterior (b) views

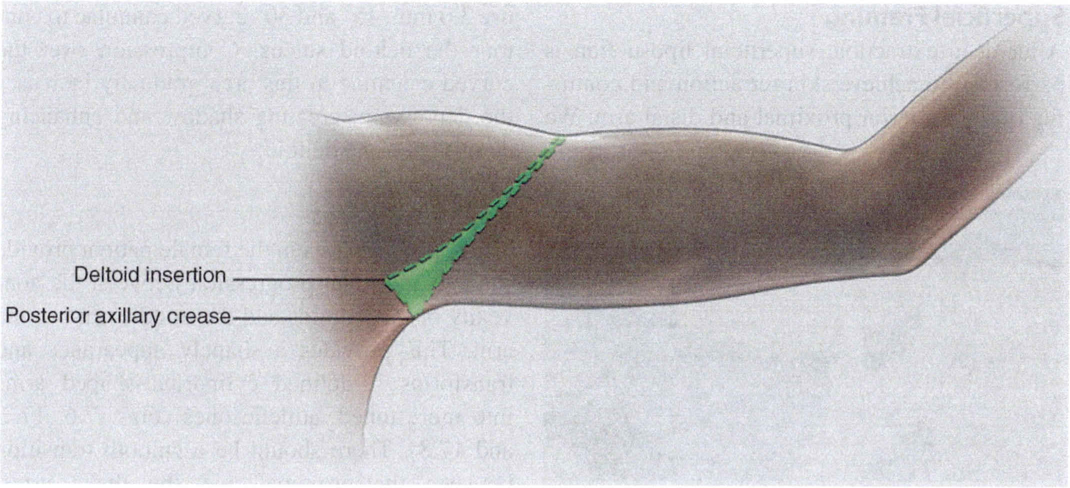

Fig. 17.4 Posterior markings: negative space in female is a curved triangle comprehended between the posterior axillary fold, the posterior insertion of the deltoid following tis curvature into the trochiter insertion

Procedure

Place the patient in the prone position with 90° arm abduction and 90° elbow flexion.

Most of the deep fat extraction is performed in the deep layer of the posterior arm. Both deep and superficial extractions to define the muscular landmarks in women can be achieved with the patient in the prone position [3–5].

Infiltration

Tumescent solution is used to uniformly infiltrate the fat layers, starting in the deep layer and ending in the superficial layer. The solution consists of 1,000 ml of normal saline, lidocaine 100 ml 1 %, 12.5 ml of 8.4 % w/v sodium bicarbonate, and a 1 ml vial of 1:1,000 epinephrine. Lidocaine doses can be significantly reduced when the procedure is performed under general anesthesia. The total dose administered should not exceed the maximum safe dosage based on the patient's weight. The analgesia effects of tumescent local anesthesia last for several hours following the procedure; this is particularly advantageous for delicate areas such as the arms. The ratio of infiltration to suction should be 2:1.

Emulsification

Emulsification is performed using third-generation ultrasound emulsification. The average time of emulsification is 2 min per 100 ml of tumescent solution infiltrated, but the clinical endpoint is loss of tissue resistance. Start in the superficial layer in pulsed mode, using a 3.7 mm, 2-groove probe. For the deep layer, emulsification is performed in continuous mode.

Extraction

Deep

Deep liposuction is performed with a 3 mm cannula in marked areas, mostly in the posterior arm. The extraction should start from distal to proximal, and the middle third should be left for last, since overresection must be avoided in this area (Fig. 17.5).

> **Warning!**
> Fat extraction in the distal upper arm must be thorough and blend with the rest of the arm. Leaving distal fat in the arm creates a deformity that we call the "Popeye" look.

Superficial Framing

After deep extraction, superficial liposuction is performed to achieve skin retraction and conturing of the posterior proximal and distal arm. We use 3.0 mm, 45° and 30° curved cannulae to contour the deltoid sulcus. Compression over the curved cannulae in this area gradually increases the depression, creating shadow and enhancing definition of the deltoid.

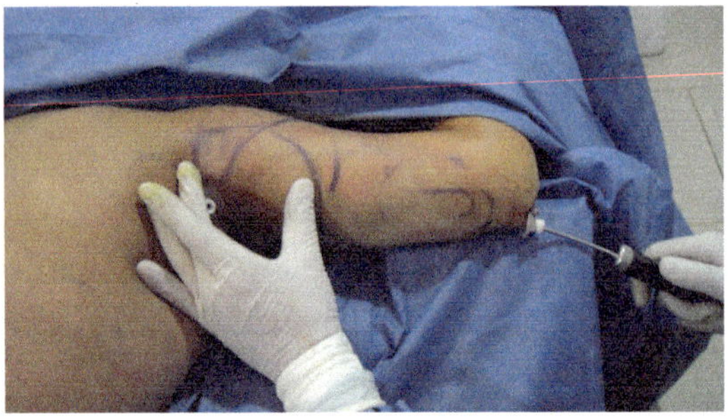

Fig. 17.5 Proximal fat extraction on the posterior arm through the elbow incision

Negative Spaces

The negative spaces in the female patient provide shadow and tonal progression between the convexity of the deltoids and the middle third of the arm. This provides a shapely appearance and transforms ill-defined cylindrical-shaped arms into more toned, athletic ones (Figs.17.6, 17.7, and 17.8). There should be a smooth transition between the proximal and the distal arms, although overresection in the middle third of the arm should be avoided. Later, sculpt the negative

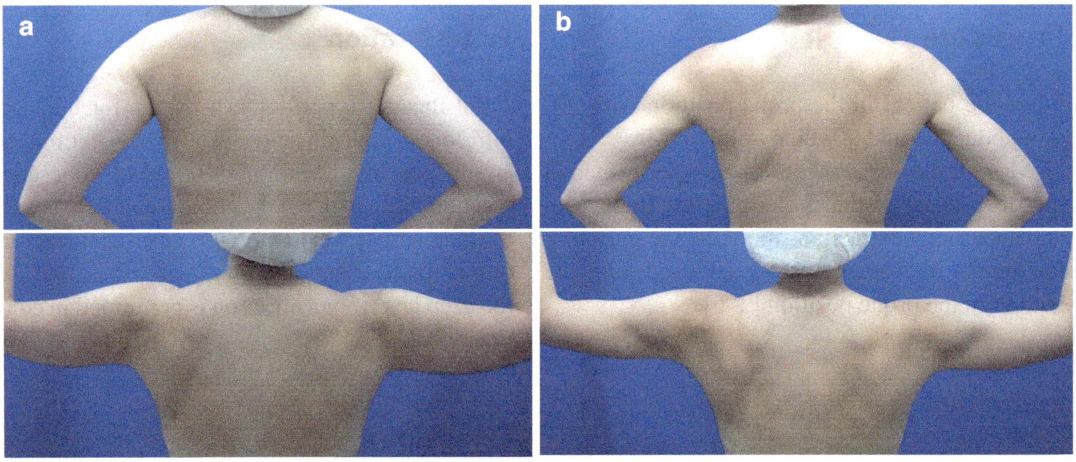

Fig. 17.6 A 29-year-old woman, preoperative (**a**) and postoperative posterior views (**b**). Note the contour improvement due to the deltoid definition

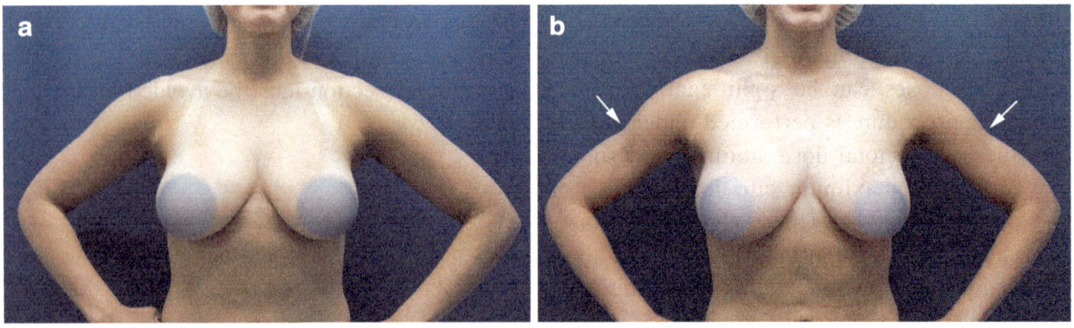

Fig. 17.7 A 29-year-old woman, preoperative (**a**) and postoperative (**b**). Note the slimmer curvature of the arm, along with the indentation of the deltoid (*arrows*)

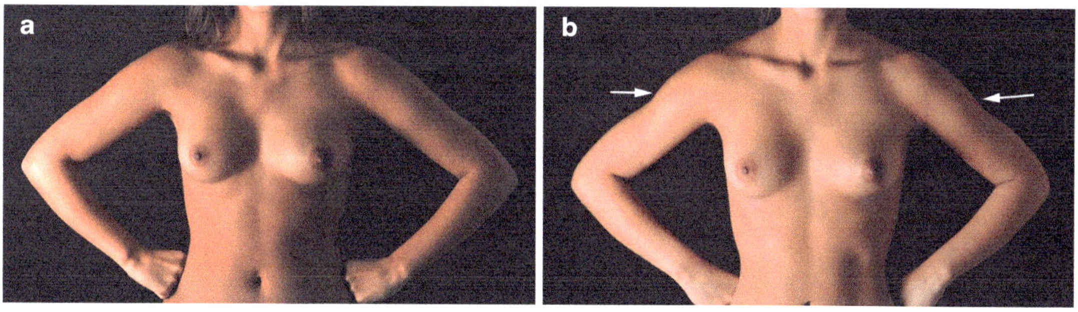

Fig. 17.8 A 26-year-old slim female patient. Preoperative (**a**) and 1-year postoperative (**b**) anterior view: notice the trochiter definiton and slight volume increase of the deltoid after 40cc of fat injection on both sides. Also, the trochiter indentation of the deltoid distal insertion into the humerus that gives and athletic appearance (*arrows*)

space triangle between the curved line of the posterior sulcus of the deltoid, the tip of the insertion of the deltoid in the humerus, and the point in the posterior axillary fold. Since enhancing the triceps is not desirable in females, the triangle reaches the axillary fold.

Warning!
All the arm liposuction must be done with small 3 mm cannulae to avoid unwanted contour irregularities. When contouring the deltoid and triceps, a special curved cannula must be used.

Fat Grafting

Use decantation to separate the fat from aqueous components. Then, extract the infranatant and add antibiotic solution. The fat grafting is performed using a curved, 3 mm cannula. Inject between 50 and 100 ml of fat intramuscularly in the mid fascicle of the deltoid via the posterior axillary incision. The free hand of the surgeon must control the direction and depth of the tip of the cannula.

The aim of the graft is to enhance the deltoid outline and obtain a better definition of the lateral curvature of the arm [6].

Postoperative Care

After the procedure is completed, the axillary fold incisions are closed with subdermal sutures. The elbow incision is left open for drainage and covered with a sterile gauze pad.

Lymphatic drainage massage is indicated to reduce the swelling and bruising. External ultrasound should be applied to prevent the formation of excessive fibrosis, since this is an area prone to do so. Also, stretching exercises are recommended to prevent retractions.

References

1. Glanz S, Gonzalez-Ulloa M (1981) Aesthetic surgery of the arm: part I. Aesthetic Plast Surg 5:1
2. Avelar J (1989) Regional distribution and behavior of the subcutaneous tissue concerning selection and indication for liposuction. Aesthet Surg J 13:155–165
3. Appelt EA, Janis JE, Rohrich RJ (2006) An algorithmic approach to upper arm contouring. Plast Reconstr Surg 118:237–246
4. Duncan DI (2012) Improving outcomes in upper arm liposuction: adding radiofrequency-assisted liposuction to induce skin contraction. Aesthet Surg J 32(1): 84–95
5. Hoyos AE, Millard JA (2007) Vaser-assisted high definition lipoplasty. Aesthet Surg J 27:594–604
6. Hoyos A, Perez M (2012) Arm dynamic definition by liposculpture and fat grafting. Aesthetic Surg J 32(8): 974–987

Female Lower Limb: Thighs and Calves

18

Introduction

Beautiful, slim, and shapely female legs are synonymous with sex appeal. Although long, toned, or slightly muscular women's legs might be generally perceived to be attractive, there is little consensus of what exact shapes and contours an attractive leg should have (Fig. 18.1). The curves, shapes, and spaces between the legs all contribute to the aesthetics of the lower limb.

Since the lower extremity is an area of high exposure in females, body contouring requires precision because there is little room for error. One of the challenges is that there are multiple adhesion zones and danger areas for liposuction in the lower limb [1, 2].

Some surgeons do not perform liposculpture of the legs due to artistic and/or technical difficulties. There is a scarcity of published medical data pertaining to beauty standards, aesthetic ideals, and surgical techniques for the lower limb [3]. We are now describing a form of ultrasound-assisted lipoplasty that represents a safe, effective, and reproducible technique for enhanced definition of the lower limb.

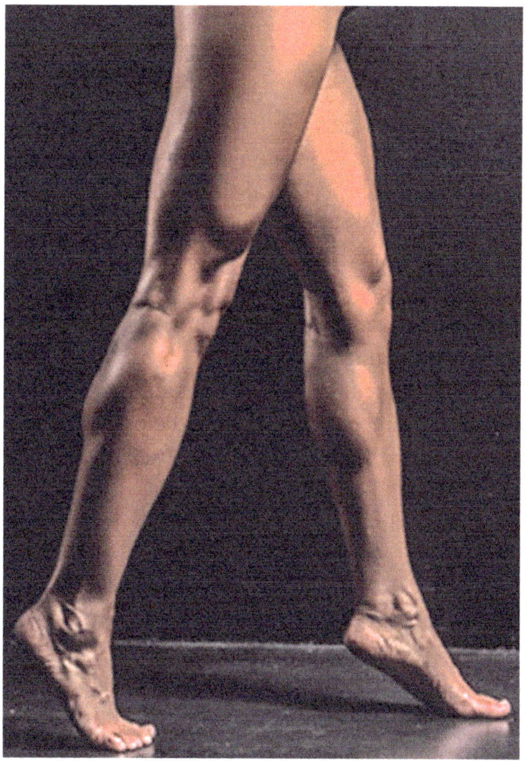

Fig. 18.1 Athletic female legs

The Ideal Leg

The author describes a simple method to delineate the perfect leg following a series of convexities and concavities. Anterior and posterior contours, as well as medial and lateral ones are defined by muscular shape and volume, localized fat pads and bony prominences. All these components in balance define atractive legs.

Medial

Starting proximally, there should be a visible "rhomboid of light" between the upper inner thighs. The superior borders of the rhomboid are

A.E. Hoyos, P.M. Prendergast, *High Definition Body Sculpting*,
DOI 10.1007/978-3-642-54891-8_18, © Springer-Verlag Berlin Heidelberg 2014

formed by the most medial aspect of the gluteal crease; the inferior borders by the inner thigh. Moving distally, the inner thigh forms a slight convexity, followed by a subtle concavity in the middle third. This concavity defines an adhesion zone and an area prone to contour irregularities. Below the zone of adherence, the lower limb has a gentle convex-concave-convex curvature that the author refers to as the double "S" shape: convex due to the femur and the knee fat pad, concave in the proximal calf, and convex over the medial gastrocnemius.

The distal calf has a slight concave line following the gastrocnemius shape toward the calcaneus bone.

Lateral

An important part of the female silhouette is formed by the smooth convex transition between the hip fat and the lateral thigh. Ideally, the trochanteric depression should not be visible in the female patient. The lateral thigh contour follows the shape of the quadriceps muscle and continues distally as a slight concavity, marking the site of the zone of adherence.

At the knee there is a continuation of the concavity and smooth transition to the proximal convexity of the leg over the lateral gastrocnemius, creating a "C" curve, followed by a subtle concavity distally towards the heel (Fig. 18.2).

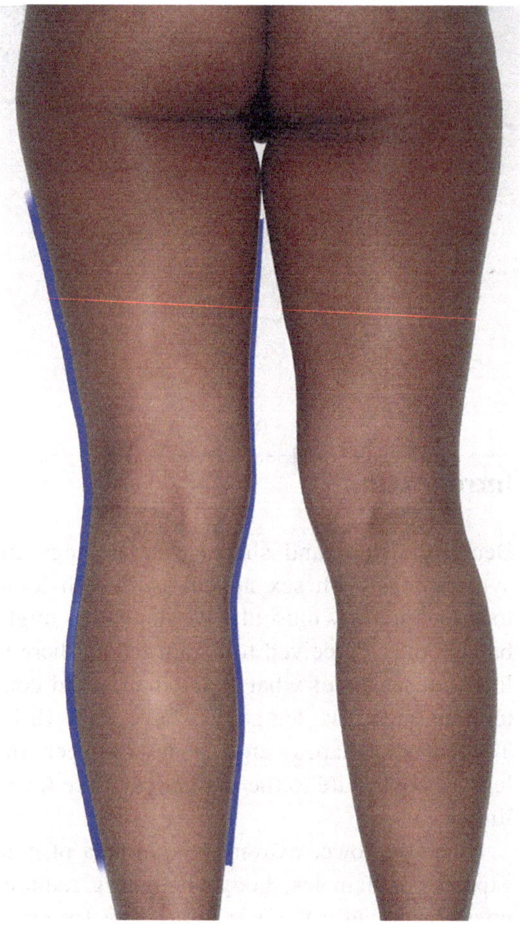

Fig. 18.2 Aesthetically ideal leg: good skin tone, balanced muscles in volume and shape, smooth curvilinear silhouette

Stealth Incisions

The legs play an important role in female physical attractiveness. Since they are regularly exposed, the incisions need to be as concealed as possible. Moreover, the neurovascular anatomy in the lower limb forbids us to make access incisions in certain areas [4–6]. The incisions for lower limb liposculpture are:

1. Infragluteal crease midpoint (IGM): This incision provides access to the lower half of the buttocks, posterior and inner thigh, banana roll, and lateral thigh.
2. Pubic incision: This allows access to the anterior leg and the inner anterior thigh. With the use of long cannulae, the lower thigh can also be reached.
3. Knee incision: An incision over the upper portion of the patella provides access to the lower leg, medial thigh, medial knee fat pad, and the lateral thigh.
4. Posteromedial knee point (PMK): This incision provides access to the middle, lower, and medial posterior thigh as well as the upper portion of the posterior and medial calf. Do not cross to the lateral side from this site to avoid neurovascular injury [5].
5. Posterolateral knee point (PLK): From this incision we can access the middle and lower lateral thigh as well as the lateral and posterior calf. Again, to avoid neurovascular injury, avoid crossing to the medial side form this access incision [6]. Special care should be taken to avoid the common peroneal nerve [4].

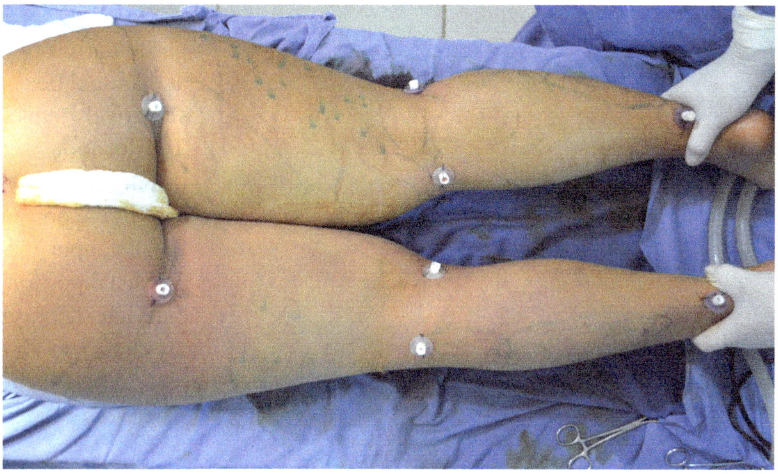

Fig. 18.3 Posterior lower limb incisions with ports

6. Achilles tendon incision: An incision in the skin over the tendon provides access to the medial and lateral aspects of the lower and middle calf. The incision should be placed above the level of the superior borders of the malleoli to avoid inadvertent injury to vascular and neural structures (Fig. 18.3) [6].

The Use of Drains

Drains are not necessary for thighs or calves, but lower incisions can be left open for permissive drainage. Drainage through the PMK and PLK incisions is facilitated by gravity and external compression.

Markings

Deep Markings

The general markings will start from proximally in zones 3 and 4 in the subgluteal area (Fig. 18.4).

Zone 3 is marked to delineate the upper inner thigh fat. The markings extend inferiorly over the middle third of the inner thigh so that there is a smooth transition form the slight convexity of the upper inner thigh to the flattened or slight concave area at the zone of adherence.

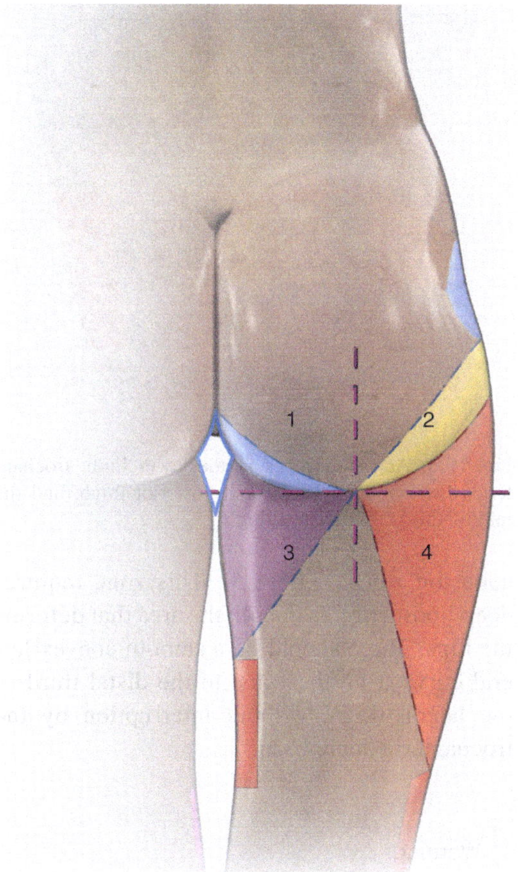

Fig. 18.4 Inferior perigluteal and leg zones: *1* lower internal angle (*blue*); *2* transition zone between the lateral thigh and the external gluteal fold (*yellow*); *3* inner thigh (*purple*); *4* lateral thigh (*red*)

Zone 4, the outer thigh, extends from the lateral portion of the buttocks (described in Chap. 15) to the inferior limit of the trochanteric depression superiorly and inferiorly to the distal third of the lateral thigh where there is an

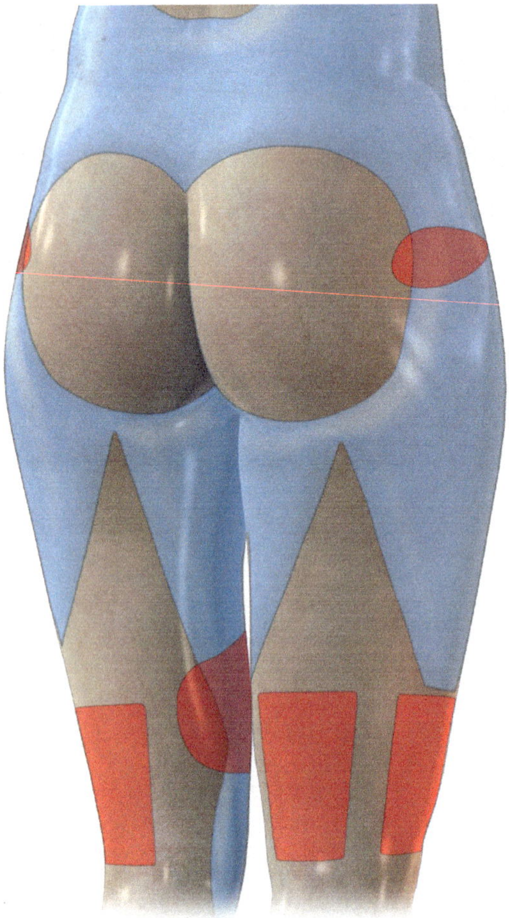

Fig. 18.5 Adhesion zones in the lower limb: trochanteric, distal third of lateral and posterior thigh, and the middle-third of the medial thigh

adhesion zone (Fig. 18.5). This zone requires deep liposuction to debulk the area that deforms the hips. There should be a smooth convex lateral curve from the waist to the distal third of the lateral thigh, without interruption by the trochanteric depression.

Warning!

Special attention should be paid to the adhesion zones that are present in the lower limb. In these zones, there is a union of the superficialis fascia with the muscular fascia, with only a layer of superficial subcutaneous fat. The zones of adherence are particularly prone to contour irregularities and should be avoided or treated very conservatively and cautiously with liposuction. The location of the zones of adherence is usually fairly constant:

1. Middle portion of the medial thigh
2. Distal portion of the lateral thigh
3. Distal portion of the posterior leg
4. Gluteal crease

The zones should be marked in different ink, preferably red, to remind the surgeon where the suction should be cautious.

We divide the inner thigh into thirds: proximal, middle, and distal (Fig. 18.6). Extra fat deposits are marked in the standing position over the proximal and distal thirds. We recommend doing so with the patient standing up in slight hip abduction.

In the knee area, we mark the extra fat, usually above the patella, that obscures the knee shape. In the calves, extra fat is typically located in the anterior-medial portion over the tibia, laterally and medially over the calves, and distally surrounding the Achilles tendon. Histologically, the fat in the calf area appears as superficial fat. It is dense and prone to contour irregularities.

The common peroneal nerve (CPN) is derived from the sciatic nerve (SN) in the popliteal region. The tibial nerve (TN) and CPN leave the common SN sheath at variable distances from the popliteal crease (usually about 100 mm from it). The TN travels deep in the posterior leg, while the CPN wraps around the head of the fibula at the level of the knee joint. Then, it divides into two branches: the superficial peroneal nerve (SPN) and the deep peroneal nerve (DPN). The SPN runs superficial, lateral, and anterior in the leg, while the DPN runs deeply on the anterior surface of the interosseous membrane.

The CPN and the SPN are located in danger zones for liposuction, as trauma to these structures can result in foot drop, dysesthesias, or walking disorders [4–6].

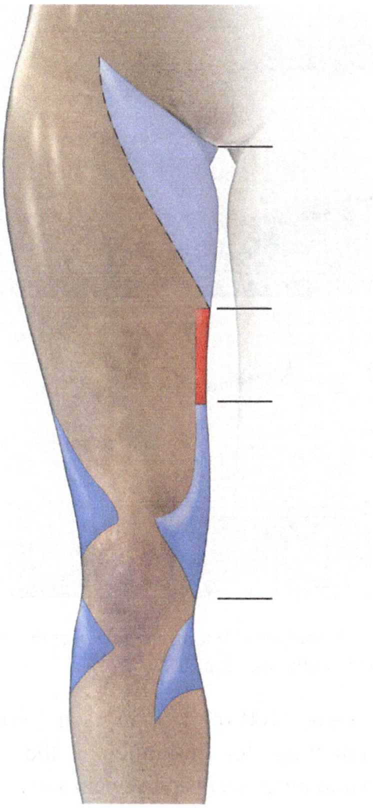

Fig. 18.6 Leg markings. The inner thigh is divided into thirds: proximal, middle, and distal. The proximal and distal areas (*blue*) require thorough extraction, while the middle (*red*) contains an adhesion zone and should be treated with caution. Notice the areas to fat extraction around the inner thigh and the knee (*blue*)

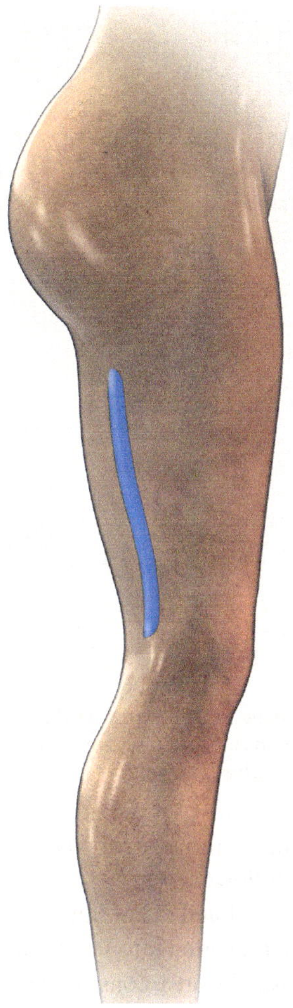

Fig. 18.7 The lateral marking of the thigh for framing (*blue zone*). The space between the iliotibial tract and the lateral edge biceps femoris is marked for superficial fat removal to create a shadow (*blue*)

Warning!
The anatomy of the common and superficial peroneal nerves should be known in order to minimize the likelihood of inadvertent injury leading to significant complications.

The incision over the Achilles tendon is placed above the level of the malleoli to avoid the neurovascular structures that are intimately related to the malleoli on both sides.

Framing

Few areas are marked for framing in the female lower limbs, except the lateral intermuscular space between the iliotibial tract and the lateral biceps femoris. Sculpting along this linear marking provides gentle definition to the muscle groups and a toned appearance to the thighs (Fig. 18.7).

Negative Spaces

Depending on the patient's preference, increased muscularity of the legs can be achieved by removing more fat in the negative spaces, revealing the definition of the underlying and surrounding

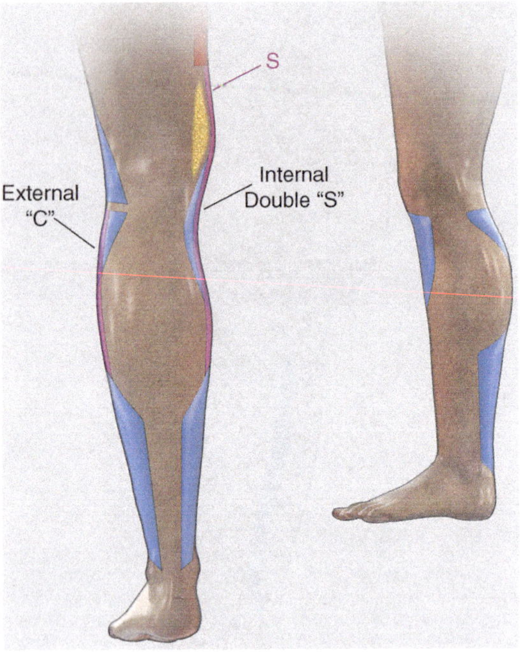

Fig. 18.8 Female leg showing aesthetic "C" and "S" curves. Notice the areas of fat extraction in order to create this curvatures (*blue*)

muscles. The main negative spaces in the lower limb are as follows:

1. The proximal and distal inner thigh, ensuring a smooth transition into the middle third.
2. The peripatellar area, consisting of four wedges of extraction that "clean" the fat around the knee (Fig. 18.6). A distal continuation into the medial calf creates an internal "double S" feature (Fig. 18.8). In the lateral knee, these wedges continue distally to form the "C" shape of the lateral proximal calf.
3. In the distal calf, two wedge areas are located at each side of the Achilles tendon, with a smooth transition into the proximal calf.

Procedure

Infiltration

We begin the infiltration in the thigh and later proceed to the calf. Start in the deep and later in the superficial layers with standard tumescent solution. Uniform distribution needs to be achieved in order to predict uniform skin retraction. We prefer to use lidocaine (100 ml 1 % in each 1,000 ml of tumescent fluid) for infiltration in the calves in order to minimize postoperative pain and encourage prompt activity (walking) following surgery.

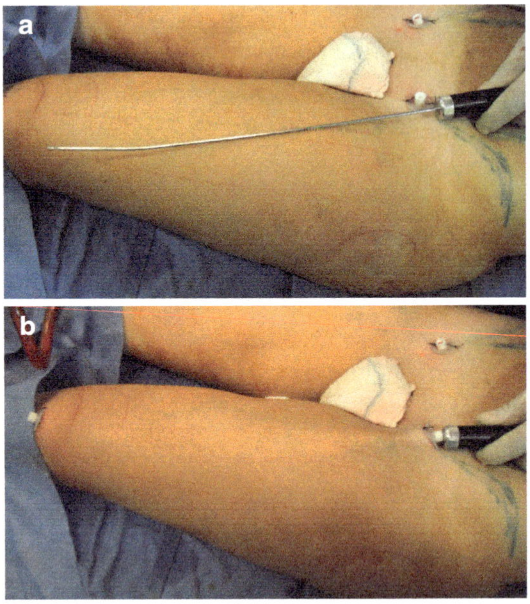

Fig. 18.9 Intraoperative long cannula over the leg (**a**) and through the pubic incision (**b**)

Emulsification

Fat emulsification is performed with third-generation ultrasound; a 3.7 mm 2-ring VASER probe is used for most of the thighs and a 2.9 mm 3-ring probe for the knees, banana rolls, and most of the calves. VASER is used in 80 % pulsed mode in the superficial and intermediate layers, while in the deep layer, it is used at 80 % continuous mode for more rapid emulsification and debulking.

Extraction

Deep Extraction

Deep lipoplasty is performed over the large fat deposits, avoiding adhesion zones. Perform thorough deep liposuction over the large fat pads of the thighs with long cannulae (4.6 mm, 3.7 mm) (Fig. 18.9). The lateral thigh area is suctioned using 4.6 mm, 3.0 mm curved, and semi-curved VentX cannulae. The special curved cannulae

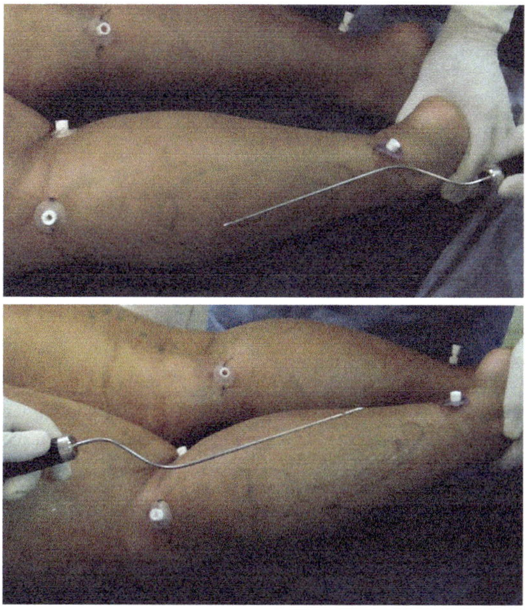

Fig. 18.10 Curved, S-type cannula over the calf showing access from the knee incision and from the Achilles incision

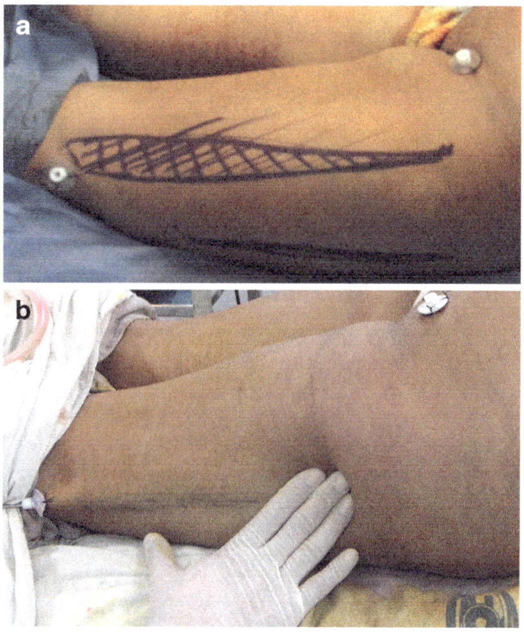

Fig. 18.11 Intraoperative image of the lateral intermuscular space: (**a**) marking, (**b**) framing procedure

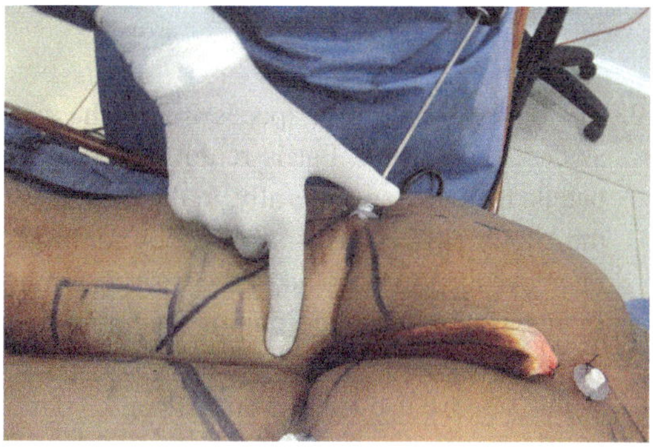

Fig. 18.12 Intraoperative image showing the inner thigh extraction. Remember to work from distal to proximal to avoid contour irregularities

allow us to follow the natural anatomical curves of the thighs.

In the knee, the suction is performed using the 3.0 mm short cannula.

The calf area is treated using a combination of a 3.0 mm curved cannula and a specially designed "S"-shaped cannula that allows more freedom of motion over the Achilles and the posterior knee incisions (Fig. 18.10).

Superficial Framing

The degree of sculpting performed to obtain definition in the thigh depends on the patient's wishes and the preoperative muscularity of the lower limb. Superficial framing is limited since excessive intermuscular liposuction could masculinize the female thigh or look unnatural. The main specific framing zone is the lateral intermuscular space between the iliotibial tract and the biceps femoris, which divides the anterior and posterior leg. This can be performed with a 3.0 mm 34 cm cannula from the lateral posterior knee incision (Fig. 18.11).

Negative Spaces

The main objective of this step is to provide smooth transitions between the deep liposuction areas and the adhesion zones and to contour the ideal shape of the leg. As we stated before, the aesthetically appealing female leg does not need sharp intermuscular indentations. The negative spaces are as follows:

1. The inner thigh proximally to enhance the rhomboid of light. Fat is removed from distally to proximally to avoid steps over the middle third adhesion zone. This is performed using 3.7 and 3.0 mm long cannulae (Fig. 18.12).

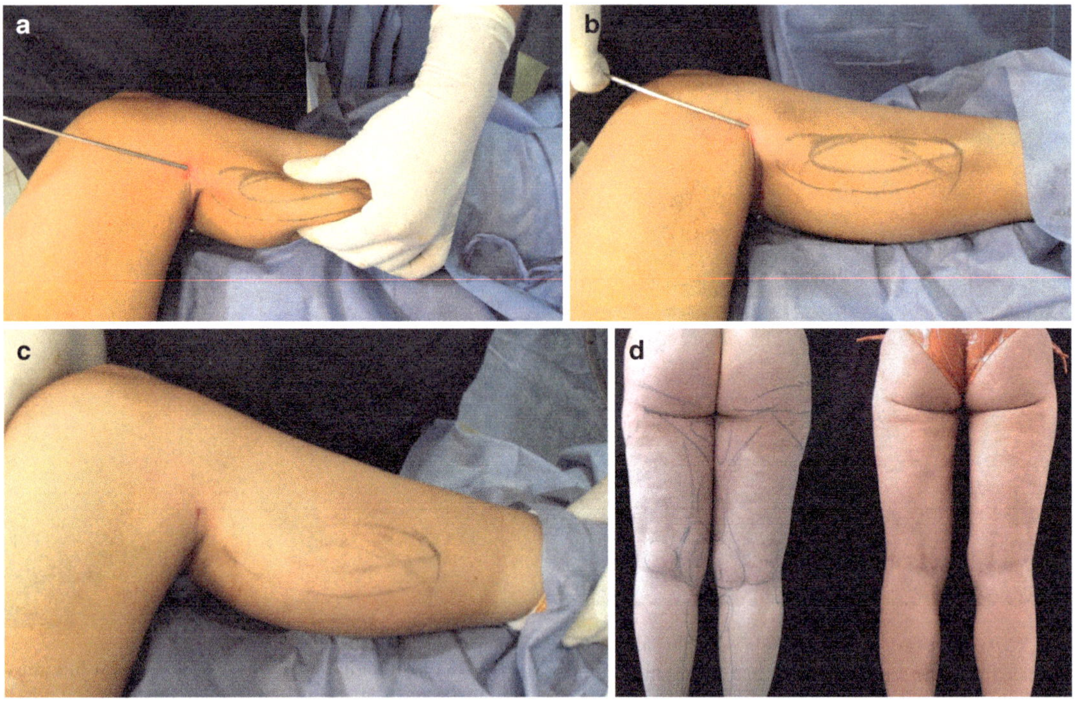

Fig. 18.13 Fat grafting: (**a**) pinching technique with the cannula through the PMK incision, (**b**) grafting procedure, (**c**) final result, (**d**) before and after

2. There are four negative spaces around the knee as described above. Fat is removed above the patella medially and laterally. In the medial leg, the "double S" curve is sculpted by removing fat above the medial head of the gastrocnemius. In the lateral leg, the sculpting continues to form a "C" curve over the lateral proximal calf. In this step we use 3.0 mm straight and 3.0 mm semi-curved cannulae.
3. To define the distal calf, two wedge areas are located at each side of the Achilles tendon, with a smooth transition into the proximal calf. This area is very awkward to work with standard cannulae, so specially designed 3.0 mm curved, 3.0 mm semi-curved, and 3.0 mm "S"-shaped cannulae are used.

Fat Grafting

Fat grafting in the thigh is seldom necessary. In the calves, in selected cases intramuscular gastrocnemius fat grafting is performed to produce volume enhancement. Fat grafting is performed through a 3.0 mm blunt-tipped cannula from the posterior knee incisions. The average volume of infiltration is 50–100 cc, mostly inside the medial head of the gastrocnemius muscle (contrary to men, in whom we infiltrate both medial and lateral heads). A pinching maneuver is made to locate the muscle belly, and fat is injected retrogradely in small strips and in a fanning motion from deep to superficial (Fig. 18.13). Since the calf is an area of high mobility, we do not recommend supramuscular fat grafting due to the high rate of reabsorption.

Postoperative Care

Incisions should be closed in the pubis, IGM, and anterior knee using subdermal sutures. The posterior knee and distal Achilles incisions can be left open for permissive drainage.

A properly fitting compression garment is recommended when lipoplasty is performed proximal to the knee. When liposuction is also performed distal to this point, the addition of thromboembolic deterrent (TED) compression stockings (18 mmHg) is recommended. The use of garment and stockings should extend to at least 4–6 weeks.

Lymphatic drainage massage should be performed daily for up to ten (thighs only) to twenty sessions (in the cases of calf liposuction). In the immediate postoperative period, normal massage is employed to "milk" the pooled tumescent fluid toward the open incisions or drains. This is followed by formal manual lymphatic drainage (MLD) by a trained MLD therapist to accelerate healing and soften tissues. The use of extended leg-calf-feet pressotherapy is also helpful to reduce the swelling (Fig. 18.14).

Lipoplasty of the calves results in prolonged postoperative edema. The patient must be advised preoperatively that the final results in the legs will be seen only after 6 months following surgery, although visible results will be appreciated sooner (Figs. 18.15, 18.16, and 18.17).

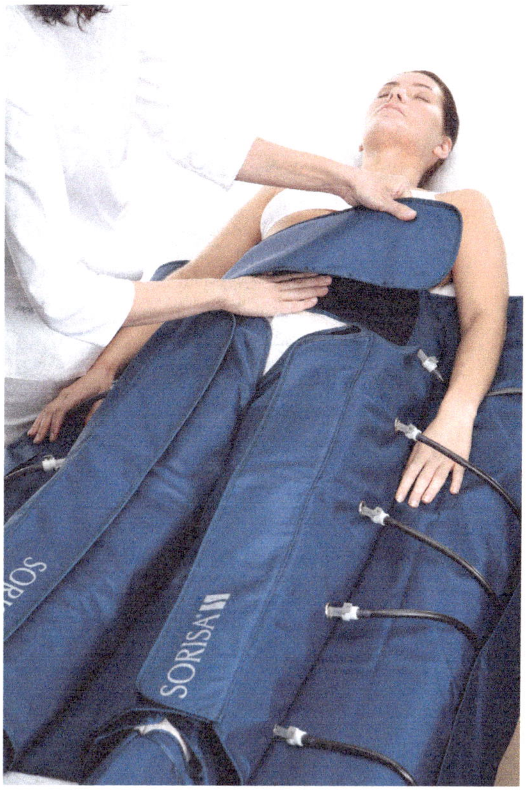

Fig. 18.14 Pressotherapy in progress showing the patient with compression stockings

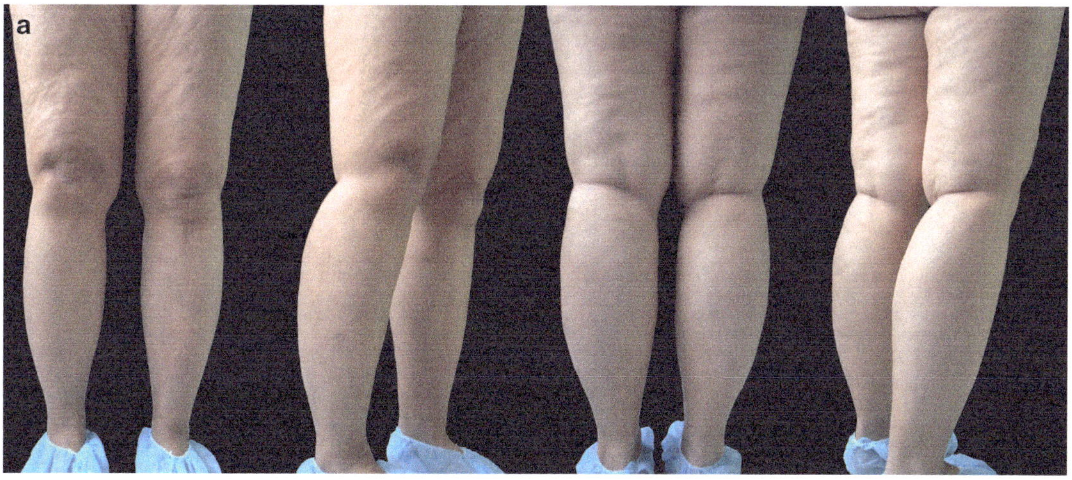

Fig. 18.15 A 46-year-old female. Preoperative (**a**) and 6 months postoperative (**b**)

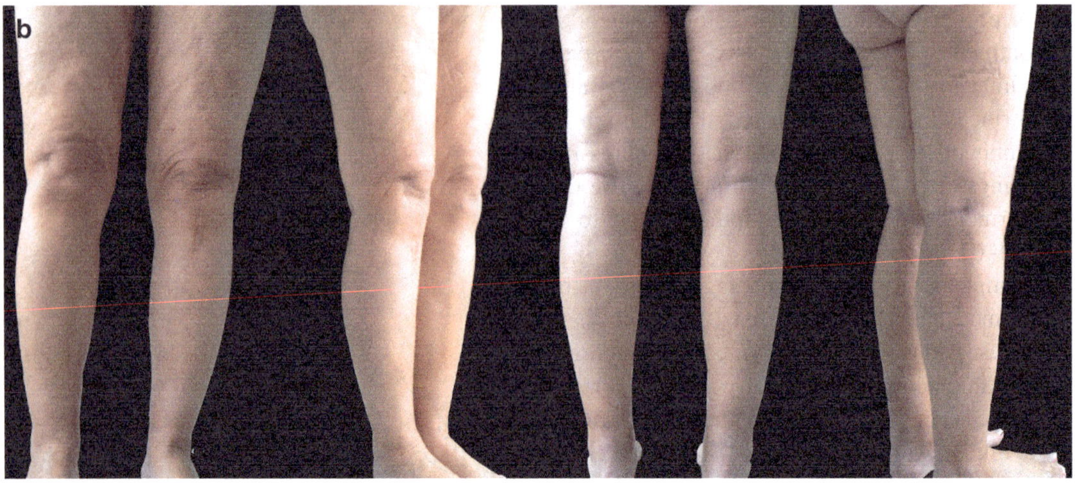

Fig. 18.15 (continued)

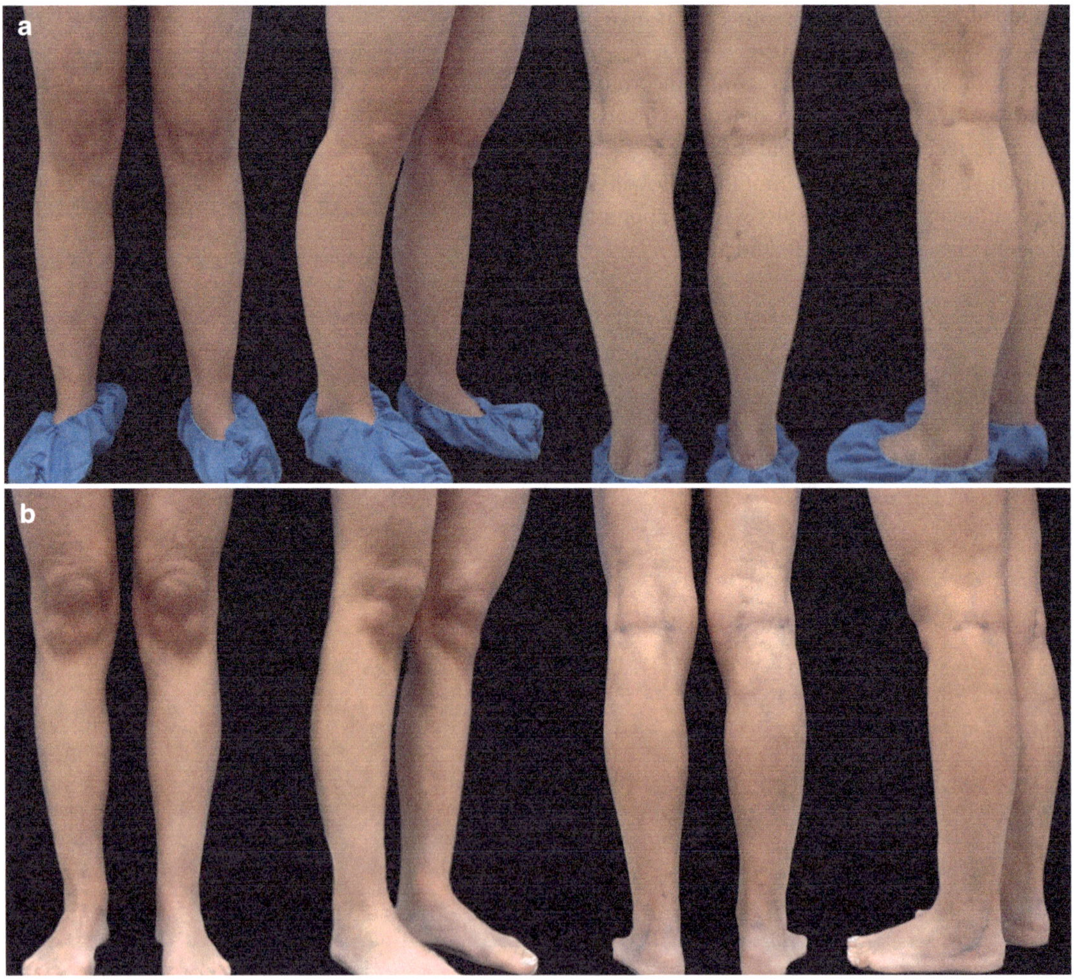

Fig. 18.16 A 29-year-old female. Preoperative (**a**) and 6 months postoperative (**b**)

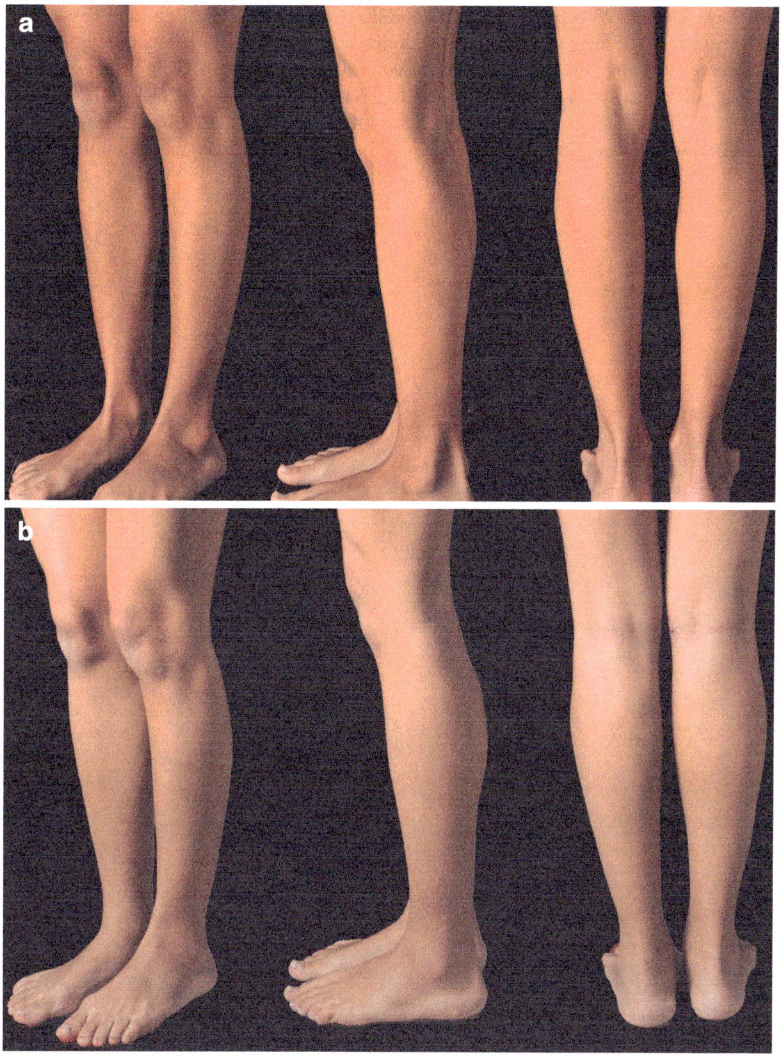

Fig. 18.17 A 25-year-old female. Preoperative (**a**) and 15 days postoperative, including fat grafting to the calves (**b**)

Warning!

The presence of asymmetric swelling or unilateral posterior calf pain following surgery should raise the suspicion of deep venous thrombosis (DVT). The usual swelling and bruising post-liposuction can confound the signs of DVT. If there is any suspicion, a DVT must be ruled out by performing leg duplex ultrasonography.

References

1. de Souza Pinto EB, Indaburo PE, Da Costa Muniz A, Martinez YP, Gerent KMM, Iwamoto H, Marão Miziara AC (1996) Superficial liposuction: body contouring. Clin Plast Surg 23(4):529–548
2. Hoyos AE, Millard JA (2007) Vaser-assisted high definition lipoplasty. Aesthet Surg J 27:594–604
3. De Pedroza LV (2000) Fat transplantation to the buttocks and legs for aesthetic enhancement or correction of deformities: long-term results of large volumes of fat transplant. Dermatol Surg 26(12):1145–1149

4. Deutsch A, Wyzykowski RJ, Victoroff BN (1999) Evaluation of the anatomy of the common peroneal nerve. Defining nerve-at-risk in arthroscopically assisted lateral meniscus repair. Am J Sports Med 27(1):10–15
5. Saleh HA, El-fark MM, Abdel-Hamid GA (2009) Anatomical variation of sciatic nerve division in the popliteal fossa and its implication in popliteal nerve blockade. Folia Morphol (Warsz) 68(4):256–259
6. Solomon LB, Ferris L, Tedman R, Henneberg M (2001) Surgical anatomy of the sural and superficial fibular nerves with an emphasis on the approach to the lateral malleolus. J Anat 199(Pt 6):717–723

Part IV

Postoperative Considerations

19 Postoperative Care

In order to achieve excellent results and minimize complications in high-definition body sculpting, a comprehensive postoperative care regimen should be prescribed. Complications and suboptimal results arising from internal ultrasound, extensive superficial and deep lipoplasty, and large-volume fat transfer can be avoided or reduced by implementing a plan of appropriate care and therapies in the postoperative period. These include advice, medications, drainage, compression, massage, and external energy-based procedures. To ensure success, the importance of compliance with postoperative care and attending postoperative visits must be explained to the patient during preoperative consultations. It is useful to remind the patient that results are obtained not only by the operative procedure but also by adhering to a laborious recovery care schedule.

Targets of Postoperative Care

1. Treat the signs and symptoms of postsurgical bruising and edema.
2. Monitor and promote the healing process.
3. Prevent and treat fibrosis, adhesions, or undesirable scar tissue.
4. Ameliorate visible scars, hypertrophic scars, and keloids.
5. Provide continuous care advice to the patient to optimize healing.
6. Identify complications.

Drainage

The most common adverse sequelae of lipoplasty procedures in the postoperative period include swelling, bruising, and pain. These arise following the accumulation of excessive fluid and blood in the extracellular space. Liposuction edema and ecchymosis occur when there is a mechanical disruption of capillaries and lymphatics, increased capillary hydrostatic pressure, and extravasation of blood, water, and large molecular weight substances into the interstitium, resulting in an increase in the extravascular osmotic pressure [1]. These pathophysiologic processes are exacerbated by closing incisions and trapping pooled interstitial fluid, injudicious intravenous fluid administration, and excessive, prolonged postoperative compression. Open drainage is encouraged to reduce postoperative swelling and pain and reduce the systemic absorption of lidocaine where the concentration in tumescent fluid is high. Silicone drains are placed in dependent sites such as the pubic and sacral incisions to keep them patent for the duration of the drainage postoperatively (Fig. 19.1). In the anterior abdomen, the drain tubing is conveniently placed along the gulley that defines the linea semilunaris. Alternatively, small adits may be placed in dependent areas using a 1.5 mm or 2.0 mm biopsy punch. These remain open longer than slit incisions that tend to heal quickly and impede drainage. Although closed drains (e.g., Jackson-Pratt) may also be used,

A.E. Hoyos, P.M. Prendergast, *High Definition Body Sculpting*,
DOI 10.1007/978-3-642-54891-8_19, © Springer-Verlag Berlin Heidelberg 2014

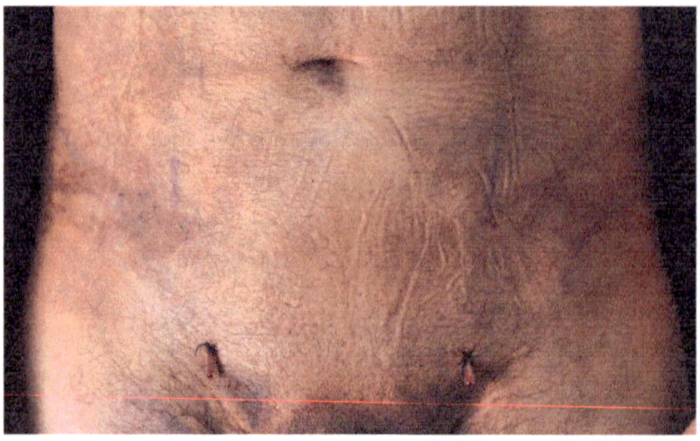

Fig. 19.1 Pubic drains in place in a male patient

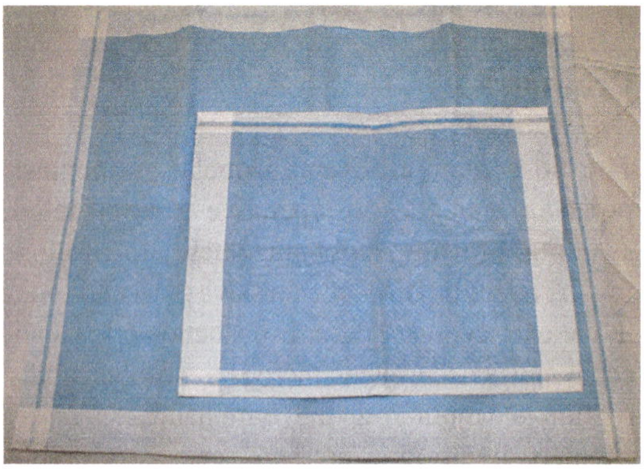

Fig. 19.2 Absorbent pad (HK Surgical Inc. San Clemente CA) designed for absorbing large volumes of tumescent fluid and evenly distributing the garment's compression over the skin

large drainage volumes require frequent emptying. With open drainage, superabsorbent pads are placed over the drain or adit to improve patient comfort and protect against messy leakage of blood-tinged tumescent fluid. Absorbent pads or sponges are also designed to evenly distribute the compressive force of the overlying vest or garment (Fig. 19.2). Drainage following high-definition body sculpting usually ceases after 1–3 days at which time the open drain can be removed. Closed drains are removed once there is under 30 ml of drainage in 24 h.

Compression

At the end of the lipoplasty procedure, a compression garment is applied in order to reduce liposuction edema, provide hemostasis, close potential spaces, provide patient comfort, and facilitate smooth even skin redraping and retraction. Adherent foam dressings have been used extensively under the compression garment to distribute the compressive force of the garment, overcome capillary pressure, and stabilize the skin [2]. In the past, Reston™ foam has been recommended to significantly reduce postoperative ecchymosis and swelling [2, 3]. These adherent foam sheets are cut into the required shapes to fit the body contours and placed directly on the skin. Significant problems have arisen as a result of crimping of the dermis, including avascular bullae and postinflammatory hyperpigmentation [4]. Silicone foams such as Epi-foam™ (Biodermis Inc. Henderson NV) and TopiFoam® (Byron Medial, Inc. Tucson AZ) have been designed specifically for lipoplasty patients to ameliorate excessive pressure on the dermal capillaries. The problems resulting from foam directly adhering to the skin have been overcome by incorporating foam into material vests. Hoyos, in association with the Marena Group Inc. (Lawrenceville, GA), has developed a foam vest specifically designed for high-definition body sculpting (Fig. 19.3). The vest compresses the torso circumferentially and is placed either directly on the skin or over absorbent pads. Variable compression is achieved using Velcro straps. In addition, a semirigid board is placed in the front of the vest to restrict flexion of the abdomen so that the skin does not crease excessively. A compressive garment is placed over the foam vest (Fig. 19.4). The foam vest with garment should be worn for at least 2 weeks, followed by the garment alone for an additional 2–4 weeks.

The purpose of compression in the first few postoperative days is to ensure adequate hemostasis and facilitate open drainage. After that, the compression garment should not be excessively tight. Moderate compression only is required to elevate hydrostatic pressure in the interstitium, promote reabsorption of water, and allow the skin to retract smoothly. The compression also provides a comfortable support for the patient. After a few days, an overly tight compression garment may compromise lymphatic flow and prolong edema. Flow through lymphatic vessels is promoted by intermittent external elevations of

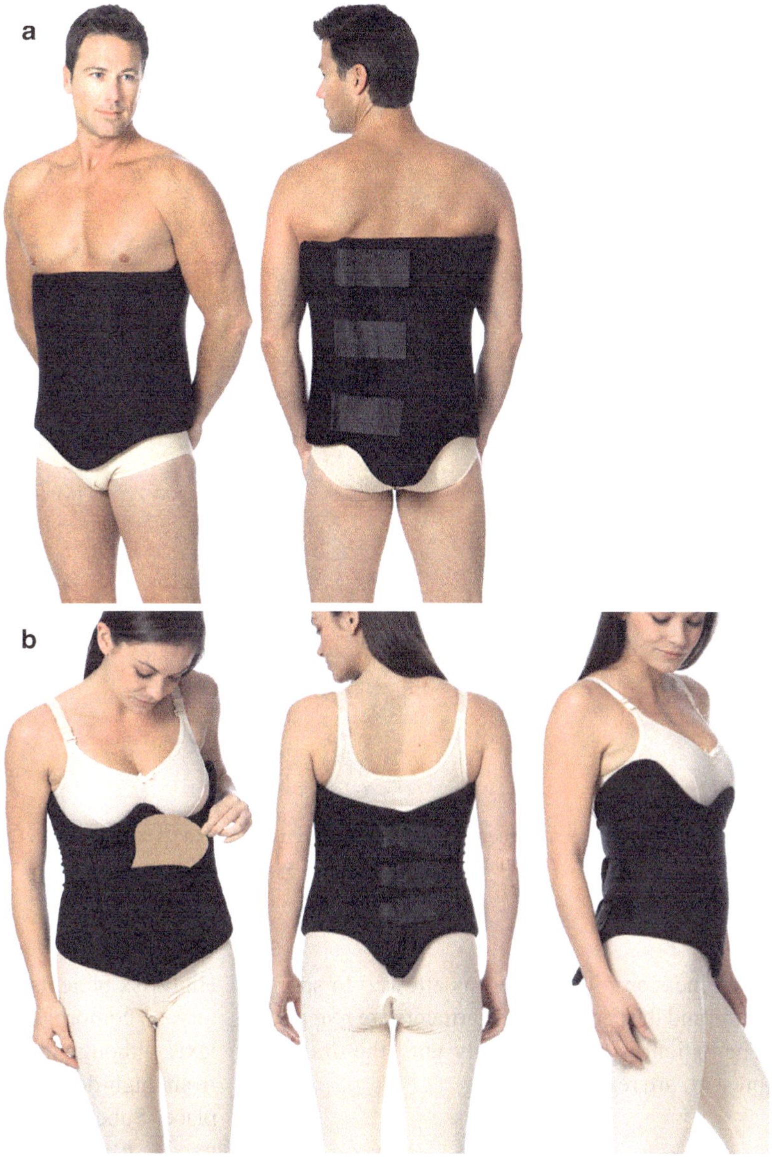

Fig. 19.3 Specialized foam vest (4D vest, Marena Group Inc. Lawrenceville, GA) for high-definition body sculpting. Anterior and posterior view: (**a**) male, (**b**) female (notice that the foam vest is applied directly over the skin, the model has a skin-toned garment underneath for modesty purposes)

pressure up to 2 mmHg, such as occurs with arterial pulsations and muscular contractions. Excessive compression closes proximal lymph valves and impedes flow. Bimodal compression refers to the strategy of reducing compression after 5–7 days and is easily achieved by altering the adjustable Velcro straps on the foam vest. Less compressive 2nd-stage compression garments are also available for this purpose. The ideal compression garment should be optimally compressive and elastic for patient comfort, soft, durable, and antimicrobial. The material should also be breathable and should wick away moisture and sweat from the patient's skin. Marena Group's F7 fabric achieves these aims using premium yarns such as Invista LycraSoft® spandex, Tactel®MultiSoft nylon, and Invista's Coolmax® fibers. Halogenated phenoxy compounds provide antimicrobial protection and F7 material also provides ultraviolet protection (UVP50).

The compression garment and vest are removed after 24 h to change the dressings, check the condition of the skin, and gently massage trapped subcutaneous fluid toward the drains or

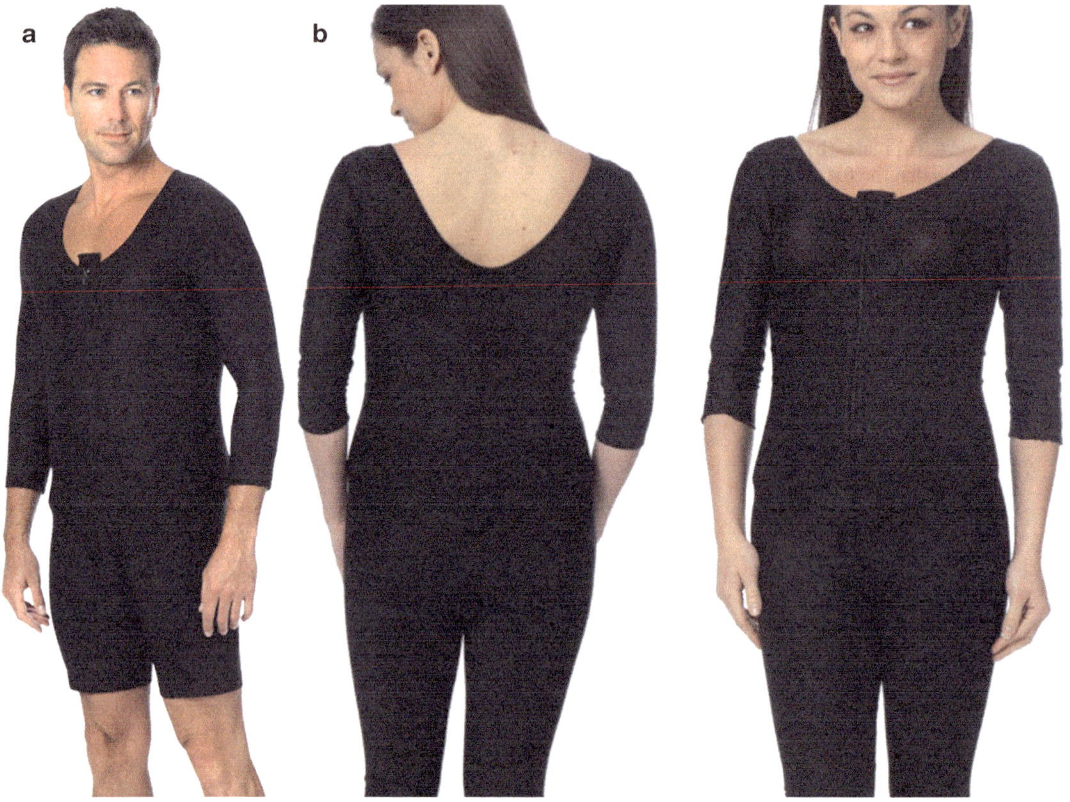

Fig. 19.4 Compression garment (4D garment, Marena Group Inc. Lawrenceville, GA). The garment is placed over the compression foam vest: (**a**) male, (**b**) female

open incisions. The patient is allowed to sponge bathe and the compression garments are reapplied. The patient is reviewed daily until the drains, if present, are removed.

Ambulation

The benefits of lipoplasty under tumescent local anesthesia include intraoperative patient mobility and immediate postoperative ambulation. Extensive high-definition lipoplasty is usually performed under general anesthesia or intravenous sedation. For these patients, early ambulation is recommended to reduce venous stasis and help prevent venous thromoboembolism. Low molecular weight heparin (LMWH) should be considered if large volumes are removed or in patients who have combined lipoplasty and abdominoplasty [5]. High-risk patients based on previous medical history or comorbidity should also receive prophylaxis, although these patients are usually excluded from high-definition body sculpting in the first place. Subcutaneous enoxaparin can be administered 1 h after surgery without precipitating significant bleeding [5]. A dose of 40 mg per day for 6–11 days is appropriate, although the optimum timing and duration of chemoprophylaxis is still uncertain [6]. In recent years, a large number of plastic surgeons have adopted multimodal thromboembolism prophylaxis, including LMWH, thromboembolic deterrent (TED) stockings, and intra- and postoperative intermittent pneumatic compression boots [7]. In 2011, the American Society of Plastic Surgeons Task Force compiled recommendations for thromboembolism prophylaxis in patients undergoing plastic surgery procedures, including major body contouring [8].

Table 19.1 Risk factors for venous thromboembolism based on the 2005 Caprini Risk Assessment Model

1 point for each risk factor	2 points for each risk factor	3 points for each risk factor
Age 41–60 years	Age 60–74 years	Age over 75 years
Minor surgery planned	Malignancy (previous or present)	History of DVT/PE
History of prior major surgery (<1 month)	Major surgery (>45 min)	Family history of thrombosis
Varicose veins	Patient confined to bed (>72 h)	Positive factor V Leiden
History of inflammatory bowel disease	Central venous access	Positive prothrombin 20210A
Swollen legs (current)		Elevated serum homocysteine
Obesity		Positive lupus anticoagulant
Sepsis (<1 month)		Elevated anticardiolipin antibodies
Serious lung disease (>1 month)		Heparin-induced thrombocytopenia
Abnormal pulmonary function (COPD)		Other congenital or acquired thrombophilia
Other risk factors		
For women only:		
Oral contraceptives or hormone replacement therapy		
Pregnancy or postpartum (<1 month)		
History of unexplained stillborn infant, recurrent spontaneous abortion, premature birth with toxemia or growth-restricted infant		

Table 19.2 Measures to prevent venous thromoboembolism in patients undergoing high-definition body contouring performed under general anesthesia lasting more than 60 min

2005 Caprini RAM score	Recommendations
3–6	Should consider the option to use postoperative LMWH or unfractionated heparin
3 or more	Should consider the option to utilize mechanical prophylaxis throughout the duration of chemical prophylaxis for nonambulatory patients
7 or more	Should strongly consider the option to use extended[a] LMWH postoperative prophylaxis

[a]Extended therapy for up to 4 weeks

For patients undergoing high-definition body sculpting under general anesthesia, the 2005 Caprini Risk Assessment Module can be used to assess the risk of venous thromboembolism (VTE) (Table 19.1). The score obtained guides evidence-based perioperative VTE prophylaxis (Table 19.2). Evidence from the studies reviewed by the Task Force suggests that combined use of LMWH or unfractionated heparin plus mechanical prophylaxis is more effective in preventing VTE in patients than either alone.

CARE System of Postoperative Care

The CARE (Cosmetic Active Recovery) system is designed to accelerate healing in the postoperative period and shorten the recovery time for the patient. This regimen incorporates several therapies and modalities that work synergistically to improve patient comfort, optimize results, and reduce complications. It is sometimes used before surgery to prepare the tissues for intervention.

Some general effects of the CARE system:

- Activates the lymph and lymphatic circulation
- Improves blood circulation
- Enhances immune system function
- Stimulates the parasympathetic nervous system (relaxation effect)
- Promotes healing processes (reduces hypertrophic scars and keloids)
- Reduces fibrosis after liposuction

Treatment Protocol:

1. Manual lymphatic drainage
2. External ultrasound
3. Pressotherapy
4. Diathermy
5. Radiofrequency
6. Wet heat
7. Other energy-based devices

Manual Lymphatic Drainage

Manual lymphatic drainage (MLD) plays an integral role in the postoperative healing process following high-definition body sculpting. Most contemporary MLD techniques are based on the techniques originally pioneered by Emil Vodder in the 1930s. Therapists performing postoperative lymphatic drainage should have specific training in MLD to understand and perform the delicate hand movements required to mobilize fluid, increase lympho-motoricity, and soften fibrosis [9]. These movements include pump, scoop, stationery circle, and rotary (Fig. 19.5). The slow, repetitive, movements of MLD stretch the skin and provide superficial compression, achieving transient pressures of approximately 30 mmHg, followed by rest phases where the skin is allowed to return to its normal position. The strategically induced change in pressure in the subcutaneous tissues enhances filling and emptying of initial lymphatics, increases the rate of contraction of lymphatics, and increases lymphatic transport capacity [10]. Firmer, deeper movements may be employed in localized areas to soften hardened tissue due to fibrosis or fibrosclerosis, but excessively deep, diffuse pressure is avoided to minimize capillary filtration.

There are several benefits of MLD. These include:

1. Stimulation of the circulation and lymphatic flow. Improved dermal perfusion reduces side effects such as cutis marmorata, thinning of the skin, and ulceration.
2. Stimulation of the immune system. The passage of lymph in the lymph nodes stimulates humoral and cellular immunity.
3. Manual lymphatic drainage stimulates the parasympathetic nervous system with relaxation and anti-spastic effects. Constant stimulation of C-fiber mechanoreceptors also has inhibitory, analgesic effects. Perineural edema is also lessened with MLD, further reducing pain.
4. Reduction in fibrosis. Following liposuction, edema (swelling) is an excessive accumulation of fluid (hydrocolloids) in the interstice. Similarly, lymphedema occurs when there is impaired removal of lymph from the interstice. This accumulation of protein-rich fluid in the tissues eventually becomes organized, resulting in fibrosis. Manual lymphatic drainage helps reduce this process and soften tissues.
5. Improved cellular nutrition and tissue recovery. Since swelling increases the distance between the tissues and blood, the reduction in swelling following MLD increases the ease with which cells are oxygenated and receive vital nutrients.

In addition to enhancing lymphatic flow, MLD has been shown to improve microcirculation, further ameliorating postoperative pain, swelling, and ecchymosis [11].

The postoperative course of MLD commences in the early postoperative period, usually 2–3 days after surgery, after standard drainage massage on the first and second postoperative to eliminate residual tumescent fluid. The patient should receive MLD every 2–3 days for the first 2 weeks and as required thereafter until tissues soften and edema resolves. The intensity and frequency of treatments is tailored for each patient. Patients who have undergone very superficial lipoplasty may benefit from daily treatments for up to 10 days, followed by 5–10 further treatments at intervals until tissues have softened. The author recommends a session of MLD 1–2 days preoperatively as well to prime the lymphatic system. Typically, the MLD therapist begins proximally in the neck before moving distally. Ipsilateral and contralateral lymphatics are treated, as well as lymph territories outside the zone of lipoplasty in order to bypass injured lymphatics and nodes. Following high-definition lipoplasty, breathing techniques with simultaneous external massage may also be incorporated into the MLD session to encourage drainage in the deep abdominal lymphatic vessels and nodes. The duration of lymphatic drainage should be approximately 45 min.

Patients should be reassured that the MLD treatments are not painful, but gentle, relaxing, and effective. Deep massage maneuvers (kneading friction) are contraindicated during the first few weeks to avoid inadvertent injury to the delicate lymphatics, exacerbating edema.

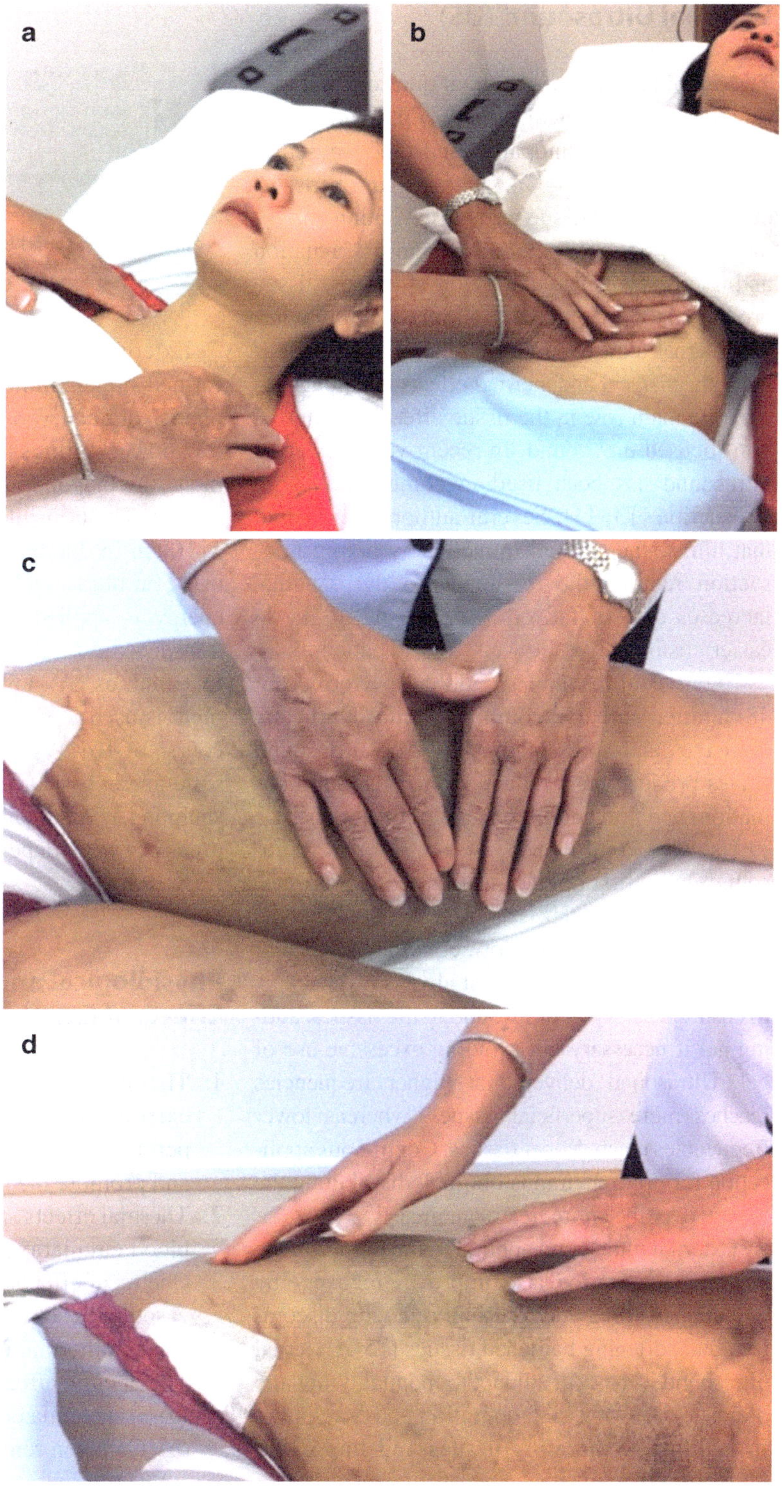

Fig. 19.5 (**a**) Manual lymphatic drainage commences in the neck, (**b**) drainage of deep abdominal vessels, (**c**, **d**) lymph drainage of the thighs using superficial skin stretching techniques

MLD, pressotherapy, and external ultrasound can be combined. These postoperative modalities are not limited to lipoplasty procedures. Patients undergoing facial cosmetic surgery, abdominoplasty, and breast surgery will also benefit from these therapies.

External Ultrasound (US)

The use of non-focused external ultrasound is well established in physical therapy for treating soft tissue injuries, tendinopathy, and other musculoskeletal conditions [12]. Ultrasound exerts its effects on adipose tissue through cavitation, micromechanical disruption, and heating. Cavitation and micromechanical disruption of adipose tissue predominates in a medium of tumescent fluid during internal ultrasound-assisted lipoplasty, whereas micromechanical and thermal effects are thought to play the main role in the tissue effects of external non-focused ultrasound. In recent years, external ultrasound has been used in combination with liposuction [13, 14]. Several authors have found that ultrasound applied immediately before liposuction reduces the resistance to the cannula, increases ease of fat removal, and results in an easier postoperative recovery for the patient.

External ultrasound should be performed at 48 h after surgery, combined with lymphatic drainage and pressotherapy. The ultrasound waves produce heat, reduce pain, reduce inflammation, and prevent the formation of fibrosis.

Using external non-focused ultrasound, ultrasound gel is first applied to the treatment areas. A frequency of 3 MHz is appropriate, applying the transducer to the skin in slow, continuous, circular movements. The contact must always be checked, to ensure delivery of ultrasound to the tissues, adding gel if necessary but avoiding excessive use of gel. Ultrasound delivered at higher frequencies reaches more superficial tissues, whereas lower frequencies reach deeper tissues. Continuous application for up to 25 min is optimal, distributing the energy over the entire treatment area.

External ultrasound applied to the tissues in the postoperative period also improves recovery by reducing swelling and bruising, relieving discomfort, and softening hardened tissues [15]. External ultrasound is a useful adjunct to manual lymphatic drainage following high-definition body sculpting. In addition to warming tissues and improving tissue circulation, the micromechanical effect loosens remaining subdermal fat lobules and helps soften tissue. External ultrasound therapy may also facilitate skin retraction [16].

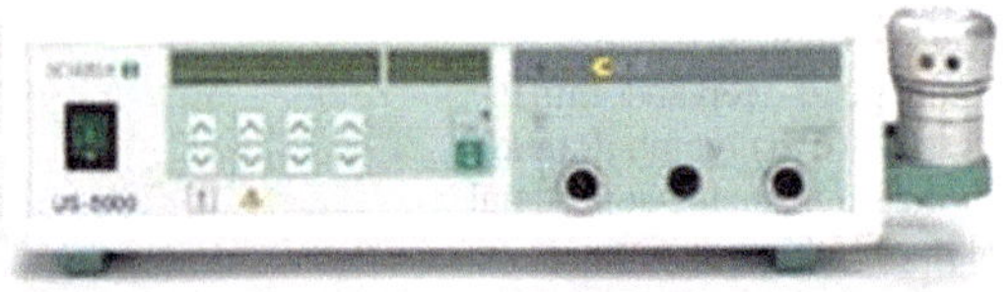

Fig. 19.6 Ultrasound equipment (Sorisa US 5000)

External ultrasound treatments can be performed either immediately before manual lymphatic drainage or at alternate visits. Using low-power settings (10–15 W) at 1 MHz, a treatment on the abdomen and flanks takes about 20 min. The transducer heads usually range from 5–10 cm in diameter and are applied to the skin using an ultrasound coupling gel or lotion. More energy is applied to areas of firmness, but the transducer must always be in motion to avoid thermal injuries. A slow, expanding circular movement is used to treat the entire treatment area. A course of 10–20 sessions accelerates healing and softening of tissues following high-definition body sculpting. These can be performed daily or 2–3 times per week depending on the clinical scenario (Fig. 19.6).

Physiological and Therapeutic Effects of External Ultrasound

1. The micromechanical effects produced by external ultrasound increase cell membrane permeability, improve cellular metabolism, and promote the release of adhesions.
2. Thermal effects stimulate cell metabolism and blood circulation and hyperemia.
3. Chemical effects occur through the release of vasodilator substances, stimulated by mechanical and thermal insults.
4. Therapeutic effects:
   (a) Hyperemia enhances cellular metabolism.
   (b) Collagen remodeling and induction.
   (c) Increased cell membrane permeability produces an anti-inflammatory effect.
   (d) Micro-massage softens fibrotic tissue.
   (e) Analgesia and muscle relaxation.

Precautions Using External Ultrasound

1. Do not apply over the ears, eyes, ovaries, testes, or heart.
2. Do not apply the ultrasound over areas where there is evidence of thrombophlebitis, to avoid embolization.
3. Avoid treating over the thoracic area in patients with a pacemaker.

Pressotherapy

Pressotherapy is a therapeutic method widely used in cosmetic surgery, physiotherapy, aesthetic medicine, and oncology for drainage and reduction of venous and lymphatic edema. Pressotherapy activates the venous and lymphatic circulation, stimulating interstitial fluid reabsorption and lymphatic drainage centrally.

A pressotherapy system incorporates a compressor that insufflates air to a boot-shaped pneumatic bag or pouch in which the extremities are placed. The air pouches are made as double-walled compartments so that each compartment can be separately insufflated. This allows the use of synchronized graded pressures that imitate the natural venous drainage in limbs. Pressotherapy does not replace lymphatic drainage; on the contrary, they are two independent techniques that work in complementary ways.

Pressotherapy has a powerful diuretic effect, so you must advise the patient to empty the bladder before the treatment to avoid discomfort. When performing pressotherapy, the patient should be in the supine position with the legs slightly elevated with respect to the trunk, promoting venous return by gravity. The treatment is usually 30–35 min, performed three times per week.

For optimal postoperative care, the authors recommend using ultrasound first, followed by manual lymphatic drainage, and ending with pressotherapy (Fig. 19.7).

Physiologic and Therapeutic Effects of Pressotherapy

1. Promotes reabsorption of interstitial fluid and clearance of toxins
2. Stimulates lymphatic and venous drainage

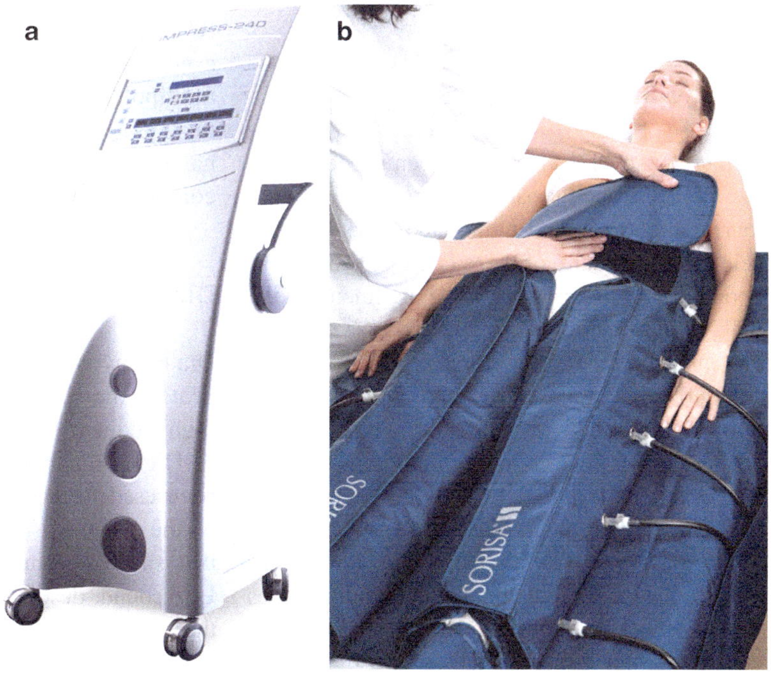

Fig. 19.7 Pressotherapy equipment (Impress 240): (**a**) Intelligent 6-mode handling console. (**b**) Full-body garments for pressotherapy

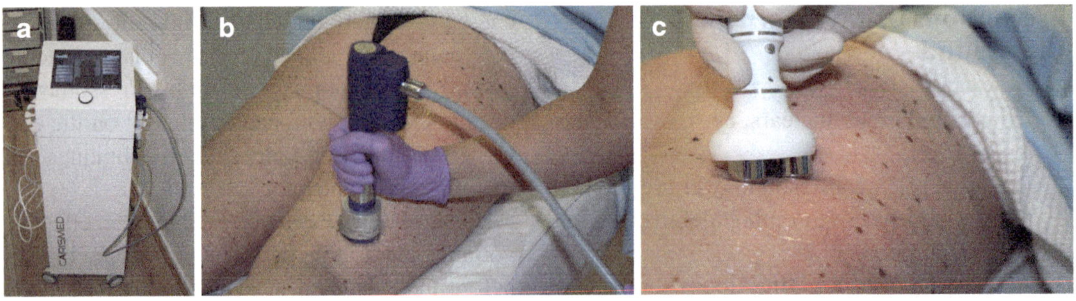

Fig. 19.8 The LipoKontur platform (Carismed GmbH, Germany). This technology softens tissues and improves healing using the SHYLD (shockwaves, hyperthermia, lymphatic drainage) concept. (**a**) LipoKontur platform. (**b**) Radial shockwave handpiece. (**c**) Multipolar radiofrequency handpiece

3. Increases the elasticity and vitality of reactive tissue
4. Exhibits analgesic and relaxing effects

Contraindications to Pressotherapy

1. Recent thrombophlebitis or phlebothrombosis
2. Significant or tortuous varicose veins
3. Skin infections
4. Cardiac failure
5. Uncontrolled hypertension
6. Acute inflammation
7. Neoplasm
8. Significant renal or respiratory failure

Energy-Based Therapies

Numerous novel devices have been introduced to the market to noninvasively improve body contour, tighten skin, and reduce the appearance of cellulite [17]. Many of these can safely be incorporated into the postoperative regimen in the high-definition lipoplasty patient to ease recovery and enhance further the appearance of the skin and surface contour. Ultrasound and pressotherapy are described above. Multipolar radiofrequency (RF) devices are commonly used to improve cellulite, shrink fat cells, and tighten skin [18]. The radiofrequency energy heats subcutaneous tissues, improves microcirculation, and stimulates collagen remodeling. Combination devices have been introduced to provide synergy and confer multiple benefits such as skin tightening, volume reduction, and lymphatic drainage [19, 20]. VelaShape II (Syneron, Inc. Irvine CA) incorporates bipolar RF, infrared, and mechanical tissue manipulation with vacuum and rollers. SmoothShapes XV (Cynosure Inc. Westford, MA) combines a 915 nm continuous wave diode laser and LED energy along with mechanical manipulation. Radial or non-focused extracorporeal shockwave therapy (ESWT) is becoming increasingly popular to treat cellulite, for body contouring, and to improve skin elasticity [21, 22]. Shockwaves have been shown to improve wound healing by stimulating angiogenesis, cell migration and proliferation, and collagen synthesis [23–25]. The author uses Lipokontur (Carismed GmbH, Hohen Neuendorf, Germany), a novel combination platform that incorporates multipolar radiofrequency and radial ESWT, in most patients after the course of MLD and external ultrasound is completed to smooth and soften contours (Fig. 19.8).

Diathermy

Diathermy is a therapeutic method that produces heat in the tissues by passing through them a high-frequency oscillating current.

High-frequency electromagnetic currents have been used for electrotherapy since the beginning of the twentieth century, based on observations that showed its main effect is to produce heat. Ultrasound, described above, is one form of diathermy, or electrically induced heat. Short wave diathermy and microwave are also used in physical therapy to heat tissues. The heat is not produced on the surface, but is generated within the tissues and spreads to the surrounding area.

The therapeutic effects of diathermy include:

1. Temperature augmentation
2. Increased metabolic cellular reactions
3. Increased consumption of oxygen and nutrients
4. Elimination of toxins
5. Regeneration of tissue and remodeling of collagen

In addition, hyperthermia ameliorates chronic inflammatory processes, enhances muscle fiber relaxation, and has antispasmodic and analgesic effects.

Wet Heat

Wet heat or moist heat is used in physical therapy to induce vasodilatation and improve blood flow to tissues. It has anti-inflammatory and analgesic effects and contributes to the reduction and softening of fibrosis.

Wet heat is particularly useful following lipoplasty of the arms, where superficial liposuction under thin skin to induce skin retraction increases the chance of palpable fibrosis.

Carboxytherapy

Carboxytherapy involves the application of carbon dioxide for medical purposes. It is a minimally invasive medical procedure with minimal risks and complications. Filtered carbon dioxide gas is insufflated into the subcutaneous tissues through fine 30-gauge needles. The maximum volume of gas that can be applied in a single session according to international consensus is 2,000 ml. Also, the volume of gas applied in various treatments is dosed per kilogram of weight and per treatment area.

Carboxytherapy works by stimulating tissue oxygenation, and so we achieve an improvement in the quality of skin and in the microcirculation of the tissues. It is indicated in cellulite, striae, skin laxity, fibrosis, and post-liposuction adhesions.

Conclusion

The purpose of a thorough postoperative care regimen in patients undergoing high-definition body sculpting is to avoid complications and optimize the aesthetic result. In the immediate postoperative phase, blood-tinged tumescent fluid is evacuated by compression and open drainage. Bimodal compression, using specialized foam and garments, reduces swelling, ecchymoses, and liposuction edema. After 2–3 days, manual lymphatic drainage commences in order to accelerate healing. External ultrasound and pressotherapy can be used during the same treatment session as MLD to provide synergy and further accelerate healing. Various other energy-based modalities, including radiofrequency and radial extracorporeal shockwave therapy, are useful adjuncts after 4–6 weeks, particularly if there is any fibrosis, reduced skin tone, or cellulite.

References

1. Klein JA (1999) Post-tumescent liposuction care: open drainage and bimodal compression. Dermatol Clin 17(4):881–889
2. Schlesinger SL, Kazcynski AJ (1993) Use of Reston foam in liposuction. Aesthetic Plast Surg 17(1):49–51
3. Grazer F (1989) Expert commentary. Plast Surg 2:44–50
4. Klein JA (2000) Miscellaneous complications. In: Klein JA (ed) Tumescent technique. Mosby, St. Louis, pp p46–p47
5. Newall G, Ruiz-Razura A, Mentz HA, Patronella CK, Ibarra FR, Zarak A (2006) A retrospective study on the use of low-molecular-weight heparin for thromboembolism prophylaxis in large volume liposuction and body contouring procedures. Aesthetic Plast Surg 30(1):86–95
6. Reish RG, Damjanocic B, Colwell AS (2012) Deep venous thrombosis prophylaxis in body contouring: 105 consecutive patients. Ann Plast Surg 69(4): 412–414
7. Conroy FJ, Thornton DJ, Mather DP, Srinvasan J, Hart NB (2006) Thromboembolic prophylaxis in plastic surgery: a 12-year follow-up in the UK. J Plast Reconstr Aesthet Surg 59(5):510–514
8. Murphy RX Jr, Alderman A, Gutowski K, Kerrigan C, Rosolowski K, Schechter L, Schmitz D, Wilkins E (2012) Evidence-based practices for thromboembolism

prevention: summary of the ASPS venous thromboembolism Task Force Report. Plast Reconstr Surg 130(1):168e–175e
9. Kasseroller RG (1998) The Vodder School: the Vodder method. Cancer 83(12):2840–2842
10. Williams A (2010) Manual lymphatic drainage: exploring the history and evidence base. Br J Community Nurs 15(4):S18–S24
11. Hutzschenreuter P, Brümmer H, Ebberfeld K (1989) Experimental and clinical studies of the mechanisms of effect of manual lymph drainage therapy. J Lymphol 13(1):62–64
12. Tsai WC, Tang ST, Liang FC (2011) Effect of therapeutic ultrasound on tendons. Am J Phys Med Rehabil 90(12):1068–1073
13. Gasperoni C, Salgarello M (2000) The use of external ultrasound combined with superficial subdermal liposuction. Ann Plast Surg 45(4):369–373
14. Mendes FH (2000) External ultrasound-assisted lipoplasty from our own experience. Aesthetic Plast Surg 24(4):270–274
15. Cook WR Jr (2006) External ultrasound before and after tumescent liposculpture. In: Shiffman MA, Di Giuseppe A (eds) Liposuction. Prinicples and practice. Springer, Berlin/Heidelberg, pp 276–279
16. Rubin A, Hoefflin S, Rubin M (2002) Treatment of postoperative bruising and edema with external ultrasound and manual lymphatic drainage. Plast Reconstr Surg 109(4):1469–1471
17. Mulholland RS, Paul MD, Chalfoun C (2011) Noninvasive body contouring with radiofrequency, ultrasound, cryolipolysis, and low-level laser therapy. Clin Plast Surg 38(3):503–520
18. Kaplan H, Gat A (2009) Clinical and histopathological results following TriPollar radiofrequency skin treatments. J Cosmet Laser Ther 11(2):78–84
19. Winter ML (2009) Post-pregnancy body contouring using a combined radiofrequency, infrared light and tissue manipulation device. J Cosmet Laser Ther 11(4):229–235
20. Lach E (2008) Reduction of subcutaneous fat and improvement in cellulite appearance by dual-wavelength, low-level laser energy combined with vacuum and massage. J Cosmet Laser Ther 10(4): 202–209
21. Adatto MA, Adatto-Neilson R, Novak R, Krotz A, Haller G (2011) Body shaping with acoustic wave therapy AWT/EPAT: randomized, controlled study on 14 subjects. J Cosmet Laser Ther 13(6):291–296
22. Christ C, Brenke R, Sattler G, Siems W, Novak P, Daser A (2008) Improvement in skin elasticity in the treatment of cellulite and connective tissue weakness by means of extracorporeal pulse activation therapy. Aesthet Surg J 28(5):538–544
23. Contaldo C, Högger DC, Khorrami Borozadi M, Stotz M, Platz U, Forster N, Lindenblatt N, Giovanoli P (2012) Radial pressure waves mediate apoptosis and functional angiogenesis during wound repair in ApoE deficient mice. Microvasc Res 84(1):24–33
24. Chow DH, Suen PK, Fu LH, Cheung WH, Leung KS, Wong MW, Qin L (2012) Extracorporeal shockwave therapy for treatment of delayed tendon-bone insertion healing in a rabbit model: a dose-response study. Am J Sports Med 40(12): 28622871
25. Yoo SD, Choi S, Lee GJ, Chon J, Jeong YS, Park HK, Kim HS (2012) Effects of extracorporeal shockwave therapy on nanostructural and biochemical responses in the collagenase-induced Achilles tendinitis animal model. Lasers Med Sci 27(6): 1195–1204

20 Complications of High-Definition Body Sculpting

Introduction

Effective high-definition body sculpting employs advanced techniques and extensive superficial lipoplasty and should not be attempted by beginners. If the procedure is not planned and performed with great attention to detail and with proper postoperative care, the complication rate will be higher. The patient should be made aware during informed consent that high-definition lipoplasty is different to conventional lipoplasty. During the procedure, controlled irregularities are deliberately created to enhance definition. Patients who may not be motivated to attend frequent postoperative visits should be excluded since postoperative therapies play an important role in optimizing results and minimizing complications. The patient must also understand the importance of constant compression with foam vests and garments in the postoperative period. Most of the complications associated with high-definition body sculpting can also arise following conventional lipoplasty techniques. They are described in this chapter. The use of third-generation ultrasound-assisted lipoplasty (VASER) technology is important for successful high-definition lipoplasty and may also reduce excessive blood loss, prolonged edema, as well as stimulate skin retraction [1, 2].

General Liposuction Complications

The following general complications are not specific to high-definition lipoplasty and may arise following any form of surgical fat removal.

Bleeding

Excessive bleeding during or following high-definition body sculpting is rare. Using the tumescent technique, saline causes profound vasoconstriction so the emulsification and removal of fat is occurring in an almost bloodless field. Although a creamy, bloodless aspirate is typical during tumescent VASER lipoplasty, a bloody aspirate may be produced in very fibrous areas such as the back, upper abdomen, or male breasts. If the aspirate is excessively bloody, the area should be avoided or more tumescent fluid should be infiltrated.

To exclude patients who potentially have a bleeding abnormality, the preoperative investigations should include at least a full blood count including platelet count, liver function tests, prothrombin time (PT), and activated partial thromboplastin time (APTT). Any abnormality should be repeated and the patient should be referred to a hematologist for further investigation. A positive family history of bleeding diathesis also warrants detailed coagulopathy studies. Preoperatively, patients should not take any medications, vitamins, herbals, or supplements with antiplatelet effects for at least 7–10 days. These include aspirin, nonsteroidal anti-inflammatory drugs, vitamin E, ginseng, ginger, ginkgo biloba, and garlic.

Sequelae of intraoperative and postoperative bleeding depend on the volume of blood loss, condition of the patient, treatment area, and presence of drains and compression. Open or closed drains serve to reduce the likelihood of hematoma by

A.E. Hoyos, P.M. Prendergast, *High Definition Body Sculpting*,
DOI 10.1007/978-3-642-54891-8_20, © Springer-Verlag Berlin Heidelberg 2014

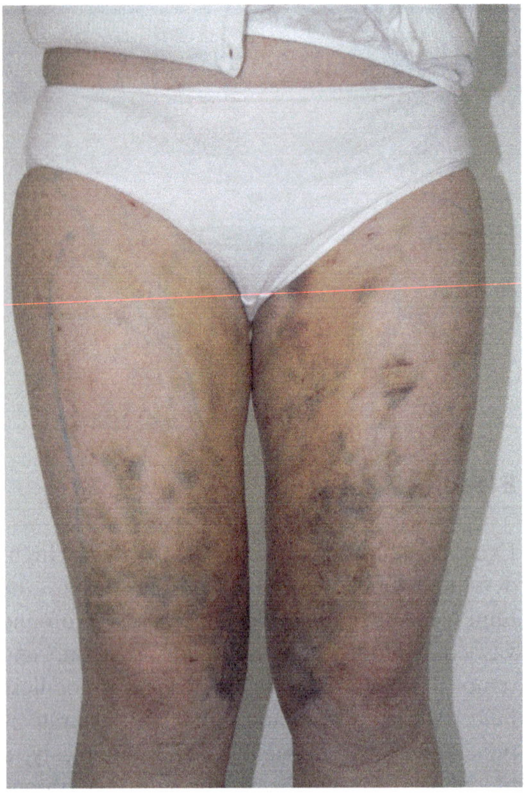

Fig. 20.1 Extensive bruising over the thighs following ultrasound-assisted lipoplasty

evacuating blood. The application of compression garments is essential immediately postoperatively in order to facilitate hemostasis and compress small vessels. Although some ecchymosis is normal, extensive ecchymosis may occur in areas more prone to have bruising, particularly in the thighs (Fig. 20.1). Resolution of ecchymosis occurs without intervention, although oral or topical arnica Montana may accelerate healing [3]. A small hematoma may resolve without intervention. A large hematoma can be evacuated or aspirated once it liquefies. Untreated, a large hematoma will become organized and form a mass, seroma, and chronic pseudocyst requiring aspiration [4].

Infection

Infection is unusual following lipoplasty and high-definition body sculpting. Sterile technique using properly sterilized instruments in appropriately selected patients serves to keep the incidence of infection very low. The components of tumescent fluid (lidocaine, epinephrine, and sodium bicarbonate) also have antimicrobial effects on bacteria, mycobacteria, and fungi [5]. Despite this, serious, life-threatening infections following liposuction have been reported [6, 7].

Patients who are immunocompromised will have an increased risk of infection and should either be excluded from treatment or their condition controlled and closely monitored in the perioperative period. Preoperative investigations to identify these pathologies like diabetes or human immunodeficiency virus (HIV) include fasting glucose, testing for HIV I and HIV II, and hepatitis C. Patients taking systemic corticosteroids are contraindicated from high-definition body sculpting, since the risks of impaired healing and infection outweigh the benefits. Smokers should be advised not to smoke for at least 1 month before and for 1 month after surgery. Prophylactic antibiotics, such as a cephalosporin, should commence before surgery and be continued for 5 days. An alternative can be used for patients allergic to penicillin. Some surgeons prefer intravenous antibiotics at the time of surgery.

A superficial infection around the incision site following high-definition body sculpting will manifest as blanching erythema, heat, and tenderness. The offending organism is usually staphylococcus or streptococcus. Fluid, exudate, or pus should be sent for culture and sensitivity in order to ensure appropriate antibiotic coverage. A swollen, red, mass that appears weeks or even months after surgery should raise the suspicion of an atypical mycobacterial infection. These masses may require drainage or excision and prolonged antibiotic therapy. Necrotizing fasciitis represents a severe life-threatening streptococcal group A infection or mixed bacterial infection that leads to thrombosis of the subcutaneous vessels and spreading gangrene. Timely treatment with antibiotics, surgical debridement of necrotic tissue, and hyperbaric oxygen therapy may prove curative.

Necrosis

Necrosis of tissue and skin may occur following aggressive superficial lipoplasty if the subdermal vascular plexus is compromised. This is more likely if the patient is a smoker, in secondary cases, or if sharp cannulae are used. If the ultrasonic probe is not continuously moving in the tissues, or if it is activated in dry tissues, mechanical energy will be converted to heat and a burn may result. In order to minimize the incidence of necrosis, very superficial maneuvers such as pinching or compression should be limited to areas where shadows are required such as over the linea alba or linea semilunaris and not performed extensively over the abdomen. Additionally, a burn or necrosis is rare when pulsed ultrasonic delivery to the superficial tissues is used using a gentle dynamic technique in wet tissues. The postoperative compression foam and garment should be tailored to fit the patient properly to avoid excessive compression that may compromise perfusion to the skin and superficial tissues.

Seroma

A seroma is an abnormal collection of fluid in the subcutaneous tissues that occurs as a result of trauma, burns, or friction following lipoplasty. It is usually an inflammatory exudate, but may also be comprised of lymph [8]. An untreated hematoma may also become a seroma over time. Seromas are more common in overweight or obese patients with large abdomens. Large seromas are uncommon following high-definition body sculpting because the patients are usually not obese [9]. Diagnosis is either by clinical examination or ultrasound examination. Early seromas can be drained by needle aspiration followed by compression. Drainage may be required every few days until it resolves. A chronic seroma that persists longer than 1 month may require aspiration and injection of room air into the cavity, curettage, or formal excision. Ultrasound-guided drainage is more accurate than blind aspiration [10].

Thromboembolism

Risk factors for deep venous thrombosis (DVT) and pulmonary embolism (PE) should be identified during the consultation and assessment. These include age over 40 years, obesity, previous history of thromboembolism, cancer, smoking, and estrogen therapy. Prolonged surgery and postoperative immobilization also increase the risk. For lengthy procedures performed under intravenous sedation or general anesthesia, perioperative antithrombotic prophylaxis will reduce the risk of DVT and PE. In general, if the procedure is performed purely under tumescent local anesthesia where the patient is moving during the procedure, prophylaxis is not required. Patients should mobilize as soon as possible postoperatively and stay well hydrated. Measures to reduce the risk of thromboembolism associated with high-definition body sculpting include discontinuing estrogens for 3 weeks before and after surgery, ensuring the patient wears thromboembolic deterrent (TED) or antiembolic/antithrombotic stockings, subcutaneous low molecular weight heparin toward the end of the procedure and postoperatively for patients undergoing procedures estimated to last longer than 1 h under sedation or general anesthesia, and excluding high-risk patients from treatment. A DVT may manifest as calf swelling, tenderness, or pain on passive dorsiflexion of the foot. A duplex scan should be performed to assess the deep venous system and make the diagnosis. Symptoms and signs of PE include tachycardia, dyspnea, tachypnea, and pleuritic chest pain. Several cases of fatalities due to pulmonary embolism associated with liposuction have been reported [11, 12]. If suspected, therapy may be commenced even before a definitive diagnosis is made with imaging such as ventilation-perfusion lung scan and CT pulmonary angiography.

Pulmonary Edema

The preoperative history and examination should identify patients with preexisting cardiac disease. An electrocardiogram, chest X-ray, and echocardiogram can be used to investigate cardiac function. Patients with cardiac failure should not undergo tumescent lipoplasty due to the large volumes of fluid infiltrated during the procedure. Even in healthy patients, injudicious use of intravenous fluids as well as large volumes of subcutaneously infiltrated fluid can cause fluid overload and pulmonary edema [13]. Fluid balance should be monitored carefully during high-definition body contouring where large surface areas are being treated and large volumes of tumescent fluid are required. Usually intravenous fluids are not required except to maintain a patent intravenous line.

Lidocaine Toxicity

Lidocaine can be administered safely in tumescent anesthesia in doses up to 55 mg/kg [14]. Reducing the maximum dose to 45 mg/kg is prudent in order to reduce the incidence of lidocaine toxicity. Toxicity occurs when lidocaine is absorbed systemically and appears as perioral tingling, numbness of the tongue, dizziness, nausea, and vomiting. With increasing plasma levels, cardiac toxicity can occur. The treatment of lidocaine toxicity is supportive. It is important to remember that since lidocaine is absorbed very slowly from the fat compartment, peak plasma concentrations occur only 12–18 h after administration. Drugs that are metabolized through the cytochrome P450-3A4 enzyme pathway compete with lidocaine and have the potential to increase toxicity [15]. These medications should be discontinued for at least 2 weeks before tumescent anesthesia. During tumescent anesthesia, the rapid infiltration of fluid may increase serum levels of lidocaine since it takes 12–15 min for epinephrine to cause full vasoconstriction. A lidocaine concentration of 0.05–0.1 % is safe and effective for most areas and indications. For high-definition body sculpting under local anesthesia, a concentration of 0.1 % (1,000 mg lidocaine in each 1 L bag physiologic saline) is often required in the superficial tissues to ensure full anesthesia during detailed sculpting. If the procedure is performed under general anesthesia, the lidocaine dose is reduced to about 25 % or even less. Lidocaine administered to patients under general anesthesia provides postoperative analgesia for several hours due to the lipophilic nature of the lidocaine molecule.

Apart from lidocaine toxicity, allergies to lidocaine, and even anaphylaxis, can occur [16, 17]. Any previous adverse reactions to local anesthetic should be identified preoperatively. Treatment of allergic reactions includes oxygenation, circulatory support, antihistamines, and steroids.

Perforation

Penetration of the probe or cannula through the abdominal wall can occur during any lipoplasty procedure on the abdomen, particularly if the procedure is performed under intravenous sedation or general anesthesia. Several cases of intestinal perforation following abdominal lipoplasty have been reported [18–20]. Intestinal perforation causes peritonitis and may lead to septic shock, necrotizing fasciitis, and death. A perforation can be the result of the cannula passing through a defect in the abdominal wall, into an undiagnosed abdominal wall hernia, or careless movement of the cannula in a vertical, rather than horizontal, direction. An ultrasound scan of the anterior abdominal wall should be performed preoperatively if an hernia is suspected or if a scar from previous surgery appears tethered or depressed [18]. The peritoneum could be adherent to the skin in such cases. Intraoperatively, the nondominant hand should always feel the tip of the probe or cannula as gentle strokes are made through the tissues. Particular care should be taken near the costal margin to avoid penetration of the thoracic cavity. Treating the upper abdomen using access incisions in the inframammary crease ensures the cannula is oriented inferiorly over the costal margin, reducing the risk of inadvertent intrathoracic penetration. Care should also be taken to protect the posterior costal margin when treating the flanks or back. As well as perforation of a viscus, vessels may be injured causing intra-abdominal or retroperitoneal bleeding [21]. Care should be taken accessing the abdominal fat using incisions that are inferiorly placed near the groin. The probes and cannulae should be guided superficially to the abdomen to avoid passing under or through the inguinal ligament. Definition over the linea alba is made by sculpting superficially, not deeply over it. Particular care should be taken to stay in the superficial plane around the umbilicus and near the xiphoid process.

If a patient experiences excessive abdominal pain during or after abdominal lipoplasty, perforation should be suspected. A patient with peritonitis will typically have tachycardia, fever, pain, and rebound abdominal tenderness. An emergency exploratory laparotomy is required. Penetration of the thorax causes a pneumothorax with chest pain and dyspnea, requiring prompt tube thoracostomy. Necrotizing fasciitis is a severe infective sequela of intestinal perforation that requires cardiovascular support and surgical debridement and may require abdominal wall reconstruction [20].

Fat Embolism

Fat embolism occurs when both fat and the vasculature are disrupted or injured mechanically, resulting in mobilization of fat droplets into the systemic circulation. Although lethal cases of fat embolism are rare, some degree of embolization may commonly occur during lipoplasty [22]. Combined lipoplasty and autologous fat grafting may increase the likelihood of fat emboli [23]. Fat embolism syndrome is an uncommon condition affecting the pulmonary system, cardiovascular system, central nervous system, and skin [24]. The patient develops dyspnea, fever, tachycardia, and a petechial rash. The pathophysiology of fat embolism syndrome includes an inflammatory reaction on the endothelium caused by release of fatty acids from adipocytes by lipase [25]. Treatment of clinically significant fat emboli and fat embolism syndrome is supportive, with fluids, electrolyte balance, and oxygenation or ventilation if required. Systemic steroids such as methylprednisolone may ameliorate the inflammatory response and improve respiratory status in some cases [26].

Specific Energy-Assisted Liposuction Complications

As mentioned previously, energy-assisted liposuction technologies aim to improve the efficiency of fat removal and reduce trauma to the tissues. Ultrasound-assisted liposuction emulsifies fat through cavitation. The vibratory excursion of the tip of the ultrasonic probe can also generate heat, particularly if it comes in contact with the skin or if the probe is not in constant motion through the tissues. As such, the most notable specific complications of ultrasound-assisted lipoplasty relate to burns.

Depending on the port location, burns can be divided as follows:

(a) Pre-port burn (Fig. 20.2): If the proximal end of the probe rests on the skin during ultrasound delivery, the vibration of the probe can lead to significant burns. A wet sterile towel, folded and soaked in sterile water, should always be placed between the probe and the skin during the VASER procedure.
(b) Port burn: Transmission of vibrations from the probe, through the skin port onto the skin can result in a burn around the incision site. To avoid this complication, the port should be sutured securely into the incision. Also, torquing of the probe should be avoided. To move the probe to a different area, it should be withdrawn almost entirely before redirecting it.
(c) Post-port burn: This type of burn is produced when the probe tip abuts the dermis of the skin from inside. This can occur by an end-hit or a parallel-hit. An end-hit results when the probe tip is forced injudiciously against the dermis. A parallel-hit results when the probe lies very superficially where there is either excessive power utilized or insufficient tumescent fluid around the probe. Post-port burns can be prevented by proper technique, adequate tumescent infiltration superficially, using pulsed mode in the subdermal plane, and always being aware of the location of the tip of the probe.

Complications Related to High-Definition Body Sculpting

High-definition body sculpting requires great attention to detail, from the preoperative assessment and marking to the intraoperative technique and postoperative care. The sculpting techniques required to produce a beautifully defined and

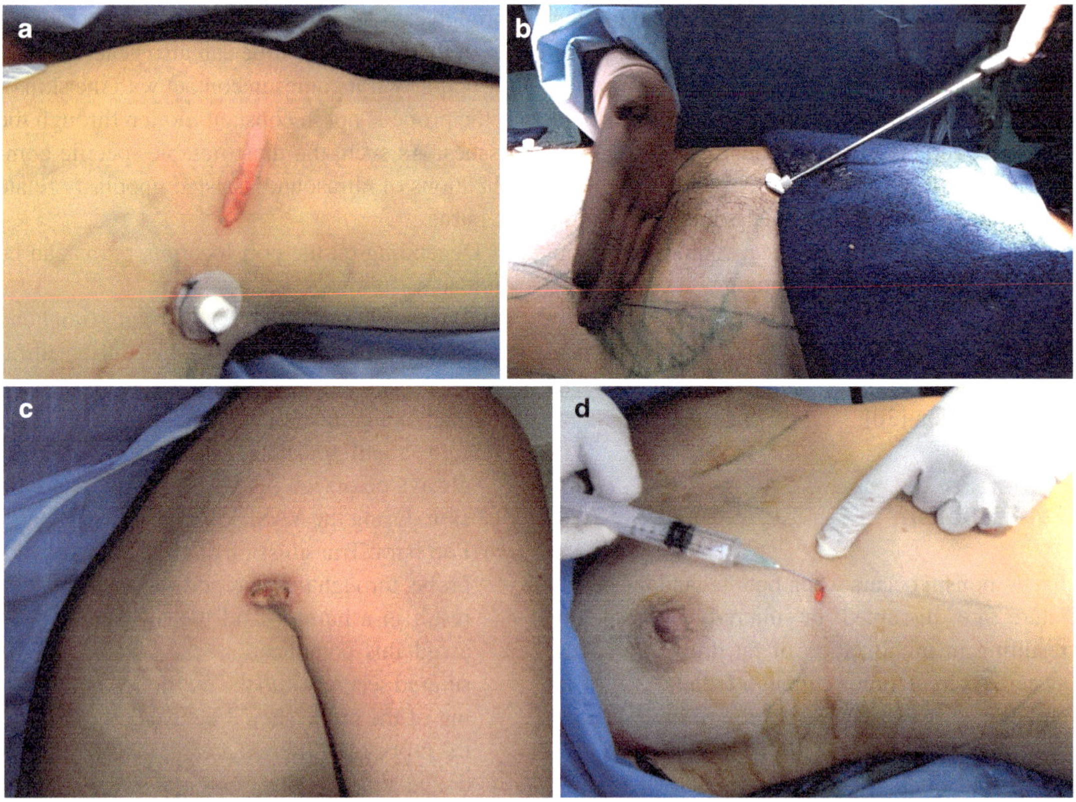

Fig. 20.2 Burns: (a) Pre-portal VASER burn. (b) Safe technique includes careful skin protection with double-layered wet surgical towel. (c) Skin burn on the incision site due to inadequate infiltration technique or probe torquing. (d) Adequate infiltration at the incision site

natural result are unforgiving. Too much or too little may lead not only to a suboptimal result at best but also to complications.

Contour Irregularities

Preoperative photographs document preexisting irregularities, cellulite, scars, and asymmetry. Preoperative markings must be precise, since this will guide the surgeon during the procedure. If marking is inaccurate, a concavity, depression, or groove will be sculpted in the wrong area. The result is an unsightly defect rather than improved muscular definition. Unwanted contour irregularities may occur if excessive fat removal is performed superficially. On the other hand, if an even thorough emulsification of fat is not performed superficially, irregularities may also appear and the skin will not retract and redrape properly.

The procedure can be repeated to thoroughly remove superficial fat and eliminate the irregularities (Fig. 20.3). To contour the body evenly and smoothly, several access incisions should be placed such that probes and cannulae reach the treatment areas from different angles. The cannulae used in the superficial layers should be small (3.0 mm), while larger cannulae may be used initially in the deeper layers for debulking before refined sculpting. The use of vented cannulae (VentX) may reduce irregularities by reducing the avulsion forces created when the cannula is in the patient. Applying suction with the cannula in one position without movement should be avoided. Minor irregularities may improve with smooth even postoperative compression garments and manual lymphatic drainage. Larger defects require either lipectomy around the defect or autologous fat transfer to fill the defect. If extensive contour irregularities are present following

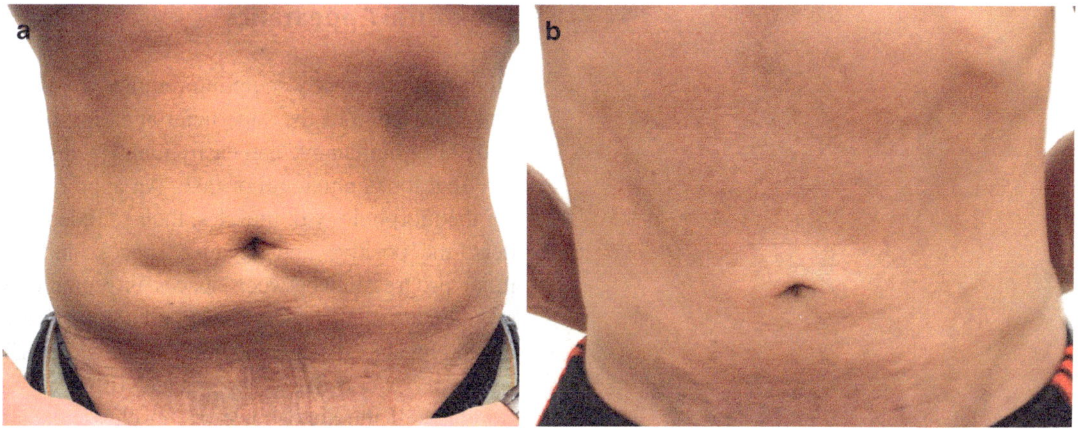

Fig. 20.3 Contour irregularities: (a) After lipoplasty where fat removal in the superficial layer was not sufficiently thorough. (b) Following touch-up procedure to thoroughly treat the superficial layer, allowing the skin to redrape

an incomplete fat removal procedure, thorough superficial lipoplasty may be required to reduce the uneven contours and allow the skin to redrape smoothly and evenly.

Skin Retraction

Although controlled, uniform skin retraction is one of the key elements in high-definition body sculpting, it can also lead to unwanted physical defects. Unwanted skin retraction may occur when garments and foam are not routinely used and the patient does not correctly follow postoperative instructions. The areas that are more prone to developing abnormal fibrosis include areas of thin skin such as the inner thighs, the posterior arms, and the axillae and lateral pectoral areas (Fig. 20.4). External compression from belts or tight clothes should be avoided during the early postoperative period to prevent skin creases or folds that become tethered to the underlying tissues.

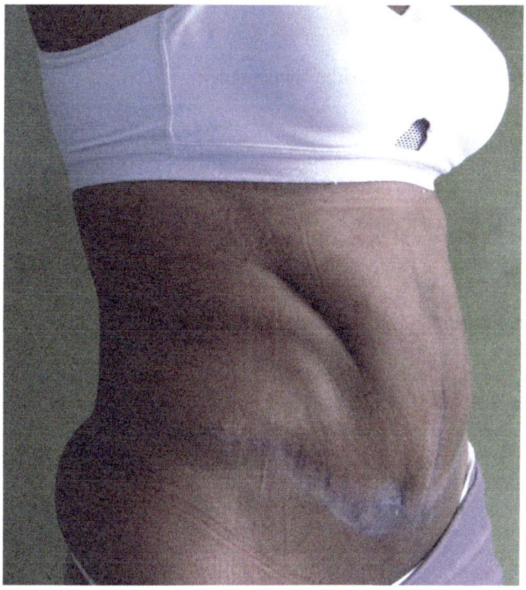

Fig. 20.4 Undesired skin retraction

Asymmetry

If there is symmetry preoperatively, then efforts should be made intraoperatively to remove equal volumes of fat from each side. Preoperative asymmetries should also be documented and brought to the attention of the patient. Asymmetry due to uneven fat distribution can be improved or corrected by removing more fat on the larger side or shifting fat to areas where it is deficient. Skeletal abnormalities may also cause asymmetries. Although these cannot be corrected with lipoplasty, an illusion of symmetry can sometimes be created by lipoplasty. If an asymmetry is caused in contour or definition by the procedure itself, a repeat procedure should be performed to correct this. Excess fat can be removed, whereas areas that have been excessively removed may require autologous fat injections.

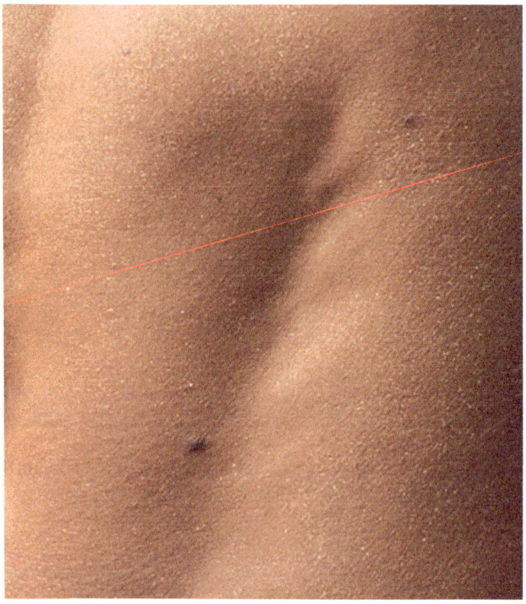

Fig. 20.5 "Wood-like" appearance

Unnatural Appearance

High-definition body sculpting requires an excellent knowledge of the superficial anatomy of the body. The human eye can easily identify any feature that looks unnatural or fake. An appreciation for the morphology or muscles, their rounded borders, the positive and negative spaces, and the tonal progression between spaces is required to produce a natural result. Simply creating a frame around muscle groups with linear depressions will cause a "wood-like" appearance (Fig. 20.5). Similarly, if the appearance of muscles is etched upon an abdomen in an overweight patient, the result is the so-called "ninja turtle" man (Fig. 20.6). Patients who are overweight or obese are not ideal candidates for high-definition body sculpting. Usually it is appropriate to treat the torso circumferentially, including the upper arms, to obtain a harmonious and natural appearance. This can be performed in staged procedures if necessary.

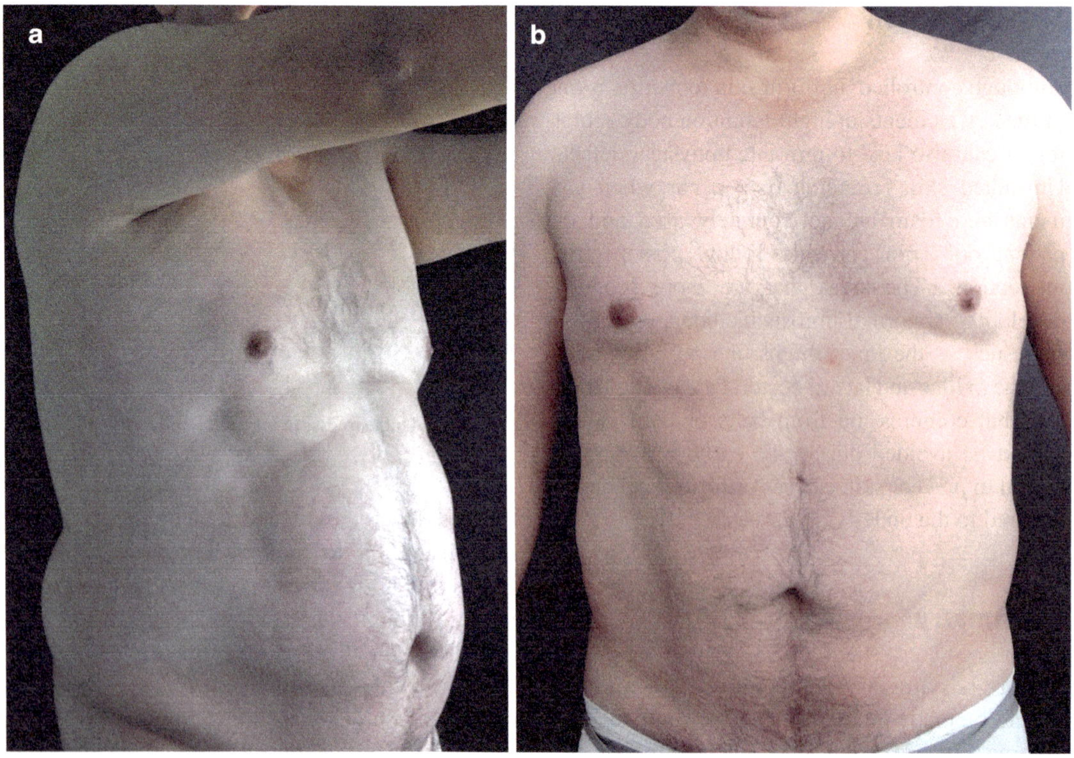

Fig. 20.6 "Ninja turtle" man as a result of contouring around muscle groups in the presence of abdominal protrusion or obesity. (**a**) oblique view, (**b**) anterior view

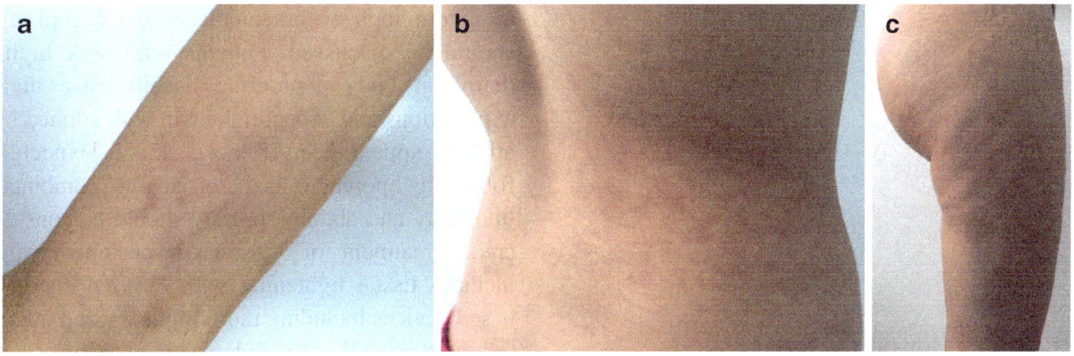

Fig. 20.7 Mottled skin appearance on the arms (**a**), dorsum (**b**), and thighs (**c**)

Aggressive, prolonged, and widespread superficial liposuction may cause permanent damage to the subdermal vascular plexus. This can result in an unusual mottled or blotchy appearance to the skin, resembling cutis marmorata (Fig. 20.7) [27].

Fibrosis and Nodularity

During the postoperative healing process, the skin and soft tissues feel firm. Some inflammatory and fibrotic reaction is inevitable following ultrasound-assisted superficial high-definition lipoplasty. This can be kept to a minimum by avoiding unnecessary or excessive delivery of ultrasound to the tissues, as well as minimal use of traumatic cannulae or aggressive technique. The compression garment should be smoothly placed over the skin to prevent subcutaneous fibrosis leading to irregularities. Subcutaneous nodularity or masses may be inflammatory, or the result or seromas or hematomas. These can be assessed with the use of external ultrasound. Although fibrosis normally softens over 6 months without intervention, postoperative lymphatic massage, external ultrasound, radiofrequency, diathermia, and mechanical massage are useful modalities to soften tissues and accelerate healing. The patient should be made aware preoperatively that it is normal for the skin to feel firm for a number of weeks during the healing phase. Patchy dysesthesias and sensory loss may also occur in the treatment areas. This is almost always a transient phenomenon due to neuropraxia caused by mechanical injury to the sensory nerves. If a discrete mass is present, needle aspiration can be performed to diagnose a seroma or hematoma. Ultrasound guidance facilitates diagnosis and therapy. An erythematous, tender mass indicates an infective process and should be assessed and treated appropriately with ultrasound, drainage, culture, and antibiotics. Persistent fibrosis may be treated with conservative doses of intralesional steroids such as triamcinolone.

Unsightly Scars

Consideration should be given to the placement of incisions for high-definition body sculpting, particularly in patients who are prone to hypertrophic scars or postinflammatory hyperpigmentation. Usually incisions can be hidden in the pubic area, umbilicus, axillary creases, inframammary folds, and natal cleft. Some patients with dark skin types have a propensity to postinflammatory hyperpigmentation. The incision sites appear brown and this can take several months, or even years, to fade (Fig. 20.8). Topical lightening agents such as 4 % hydroquinone, kojic acid, or azelaic acid may be used to lighten the skin. Patients should be advised to wear sunscreen and avoid sun exposure for 6 weeks following the procedure. Various treatments can be used to try to improve hypertrophic scars including topical silicone gel or sheeting, topical 5 % imiquimod, vitamin E, and pressure/massage therapies [28].

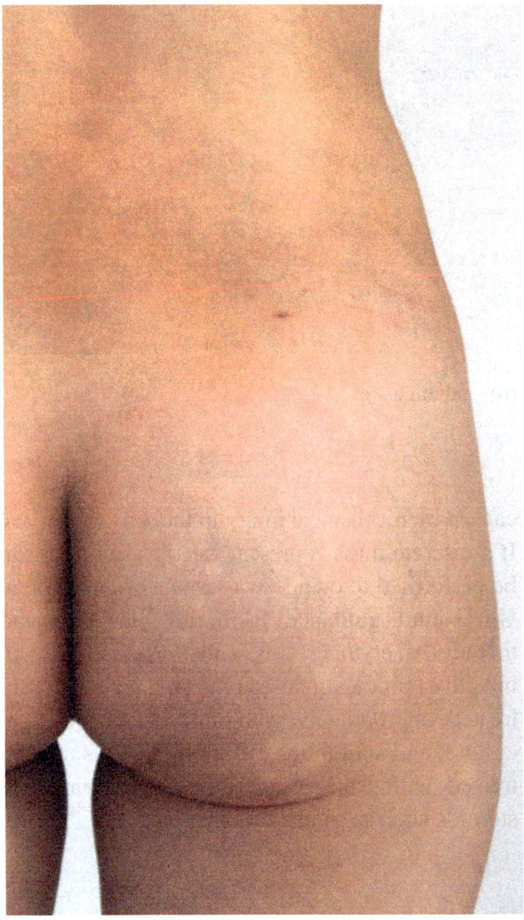

Fig. 20.8 Postinflammatory hyperpigmentation of lipoplasty incision site. The brown linear scar is seen above the right buttock. The suture marks are also visible

Loose Skin

Skin laxity following any form of lipoplasty may occur if the skin does not fully retract to fit the new contours when subcutaneous fat is removed. This is more likely in certain areas, including the lower abdomen, periumbilical area, upper arm, and above the knees. The use of energy-based devices may improve skin retraction, as has been shown in studies with third-generation ultrasound-assisted lipoplasty [2]. The risk of skin laxity and looseness should be explained to the patient during the preoperative consultation. Patients with poor skin tone, striae, and large volumes of fat are at increased risk of postoperative looseness. Alternative excisional procedures such as abdominoplasty, brachioplasty, and thighplasty should be discussed. Patients who seek high-definition body contouring usually have high expectations and expect tight skin with a toned or athletic appearance. If loose skin is expected following lipoplasty in these patients, combined lipoplasty and abdominoplasty should be considered. Treatment of loose skin postoperatively includes tissue tightening with external energy-based devices including radiofrequency and infrared light, as well as secondary skin excision.

Burns

Pre-port, port, and post-port burns are possible complications of high-definition body sculpting using ultrasound-assisted lipoplasty (Fig. 20.2). The need for thorough superficial and deep emulsification of fat means the energy delivered to the tissues is substantial. However, it should not exceed 2 min of ultrasound delivery per 100 ml of tumescent fluid infiltrated. Maintaining the probe tip in a fluid-filled fat compartment at all times helps reduce the incidence of burns. Other measures include skin protection with wet towels, use of pulsed mode in the superficial plane, and avoidance of torquing of the probe in the port.

References

1. Garcia O, Nathan N (2008) Comparative analysis of blood loss in suction-assisted lipoplasty and third-generation internal ultrasound-assisted lipoplasty. Aesthet Surg J 28(4):430–435
2. Nagy MW, Vanek PF (2012) A multicenter, prospective, randomized, single-blind, controlled clinical trial comparing VASER-assisted lipoplasty and suction-assisted lipoplasty. Plast Reconstr Surg 129(4): 681e–689e
3. Shiffman MA (2011) Arnica Montana. In: Prendergast PM, Shiffman MA (eds) Aesthetic medicine: art and techniques. Springer, Berlin/Heidelberg, pp 289–294
4. Shiffman MA (2006) Prevention and treatment of liposuction complications. In: Shiffman MA, Di Giuseppe A (eds) Liposuction. Principles and practice. Springer, Berlin/Heidelberg, pp 333–334
5. Igra H, Lanzer D (2005) Avoiding complications. In: Hanke CW, Sattler G (eds) Procedures in cosmetic dermatology. Liposuction. Elsevier/Saunders, Philadelphia, p 133

6. Alexander J, Takeda D, Sanders D, Goldberg H (1988) Fatal necrotizing fasciitis following suction-assisted lipectomy. Ann Plast Surg 29(6):562–565
7. Gibbons MD, Lim RB, Carter PL (1998) Necrotizing fasciitis after tumescent liposuction. Am Surg 64(5):458–460
8. Andrades P, Prado A (2007) Composition of postabdominoplasty seroma. Aesthetic Plast Surg 31(5):514–518
9. Kim J, Stevenson TR (2006) Abdominoplasty, liposuction of the flanks, and obesity: analyzing risk factors for seroma formation. Plast Reconstr Surg 117(3):773–779
10. Stebbins WG, Hanke CW, Peterson J (2011) Ultrasound-guided drainage of a seroma following tumescent liposuction. Dermatol Ther 24(1):121–124
11. Platt MS, Kohler LJ, Ruiz R, Cohle SD, Ravichandran P (2002) Deaths associated with liposuction: case reports and review of the literature. J Forensic Sci 47(1):205–207
12. Lehnhardt M, Homann HH, Daigeler A, Hauser J, Palka P, Steinau HU (2008) Major and lethal complications of liposuction: a review of 72 cases in Germany between 1998 and 2002. Plast Reconstr Surg 121(6):396–403
13. Gilliland MD, Coates N (1997) Tumescent liposuction complicated by pulmonary edema. Plast Reconstr Surg 99(1):215–219
14. Ostad A, Kageyama N, Moy RL (1996) Tumescent anesthesia with a lidocaine dose of 55 mg/kg is safe for liposuction. Dermatol Surg 22(11):921–927
15. Shiffman MA (1998) Medications potentially causing lidocaine toxicity. Am J Cosmet Surg 15(3):227–228
16. Kennedy KS, Cave RH (1986) Anaphylactic reaction to lidocaine. Arch Otolarygol Head Neck Surg 112(6):671–673
17. Anibarro B, Seoane FJ (1998) Adverse reaction to lidocaine. Allergy 53(7):717–718
18. Ovrebø KK, Grong K, Vindenes H (1997) Small intestinal perforation and peritonitis after abdominal suction lipoplasty. Ann Plast Surg 38(6):642–646
19. Mallappa M, Rangaswamy M, Badiuddin MF (2007) Small intestinal perforation and peritonitis after liposuction. Aesthetic Plast Surg 31(5):589–592
20. Di Candia M, Malata CM (2011) Aesthetic and functional abdominal wall reconstruction after multiple bowel perforations secondary to liposuction. Aesthetic Plast Surg 35(2):274–277
21. Talmor M, Fahey TJ, Wise J, Hoffman LA, Barie PS (2000) Large volume liposuction complicated by retroperitoneal haemorrhage: management principles and implications for the quality improvement process. Plast Reconstr Surg 105(6):2244–2248
22. El-Ali KM, Gourlay T (2006) Assessment of the risk of systemic fat mobilization and fat embolism as a consequence of liposuction: ex vivo study. Plast Reconstr Surg 117(7):2269–2276
23. Franco FF, Tincani AJ, Meirelles LR, Kharmandayan P, Guidi MC (2011) Occurrence of fat embolism after liposuction surgery with or without lipografting: an experimental study. Ann Plast Surg 67(2):101–105
24. Wang HD, Zheng JH, Deng CL, Liu QY, Yang SL (2006) Fat embolism syndromes following liposuction. Aesthetic Plast Surg 32(5):731–736
25. Filomeno LTB, Carelli CR, Silva NCLF, Barros TEPF, Amatuzzi MM (2005) Fat embolism: a review for current orthopedics practice. Acta Ortop Bras 13(4):196–208
26. Kubota T, Ebina T, Tonosaki M, Ishihara H, Matsuki A (2003) Rapid improvement of respiratory symptoms associated with fat embolism by high-dose methylprednisolone: a case report. J Anaesth 17(3): 186–189
27. Porto da Rocha R; Porto da Rocha EL, de Souza Pinto EB, Sementilli A, Nakanishi CP (2005) Cutis marmorata resemblance after liposuction. Aesthetic Plast Surg 29(4):310–312
28. Foo CW, Tristani-Firouzi P (2011) Topical modalities for treatment and prevention of postsurgical hypertrophic scars. Facial Plast Surg Clin North Am 19(3): 551–557

New Developments in High-Definition Lipoplasty

21

Introduction

High-definition lipoplasty is an exciting progression in body contouring. It represents a new paradigm in liposuction where many of the concepts and techniques of artistry and sculpture are incorporated into the procedure. In the author's experience, the development and application of the advanced lipoplasty techniques described in this book gave him the ability to deliver to his patients the superior results they always wanted. In experienced hands, these techniques are effective, safe, and reproducible.

Hoyos began the first design of this surgery on paper over a decade ago. Over time and with several iterations, he has modified and refined the techniques, instrumentation, and protocols in order to provide better results for patients. The introduction of high-definition body sculpting has also expanded the indications for liposuction. Patients seeking treatment now are younger, more athletic, or slimmer than before. Many of these patients who previously would not have been deemed suitable candidates for liposuction may now benefit from high-definition lipoplasty to increase definition and enhance the shape of the body.

However, as the procedure evolved, it also became apparent that liposuction only was not going to be the answer for every patient. This includes patients with excessive skin laxity and abdominal wall weakness, obese patients, or those with extensive cellulite or fibrosis from previous surgery.

Mini-abdominoplasty with Definition

After childbearing, many women present with abdominal muscle diastasis, skin laxity, and striae. Liposuction alone in these patients is usually not enough to achieve a good aesthetic result. Thus, skin excision and myofascial plication should be considered. There are different options to achieve this.

Some patients are not suitable for a full abdominoplasty, but neither are they candidates for liposuction alone. Hoyos describes a "true" mini-abdominoplasty where the muscular diastasis is closed through a Pfannenstiel incision, followed by circumferential liposuction of the torso to achieve muscular definition. This approach transforms a lax abdomen into one that appears more youthful and athletic (Fig. 21.1).

New technologies like VASER that can achieve better skin retraction can help convert selected cases that were candidates for a full abdominoplasty into less extensive procedures like the mini-abdominoplasty. Using ultrasound-assisted lipoplasty, extensive liposuction over the flap to achieve definition is feasible and safe because the process is selective to adipose tissue and relatively atraumatic to the vascular supply (Fig. 21.2).

A.E. Hoyos, P.M. Prendergast, *High Definition Body Sculpting*,
DOI 10.1007/978-3-642-54891-8_21, © Springer-Verlag Berlin Heidelberg 2014

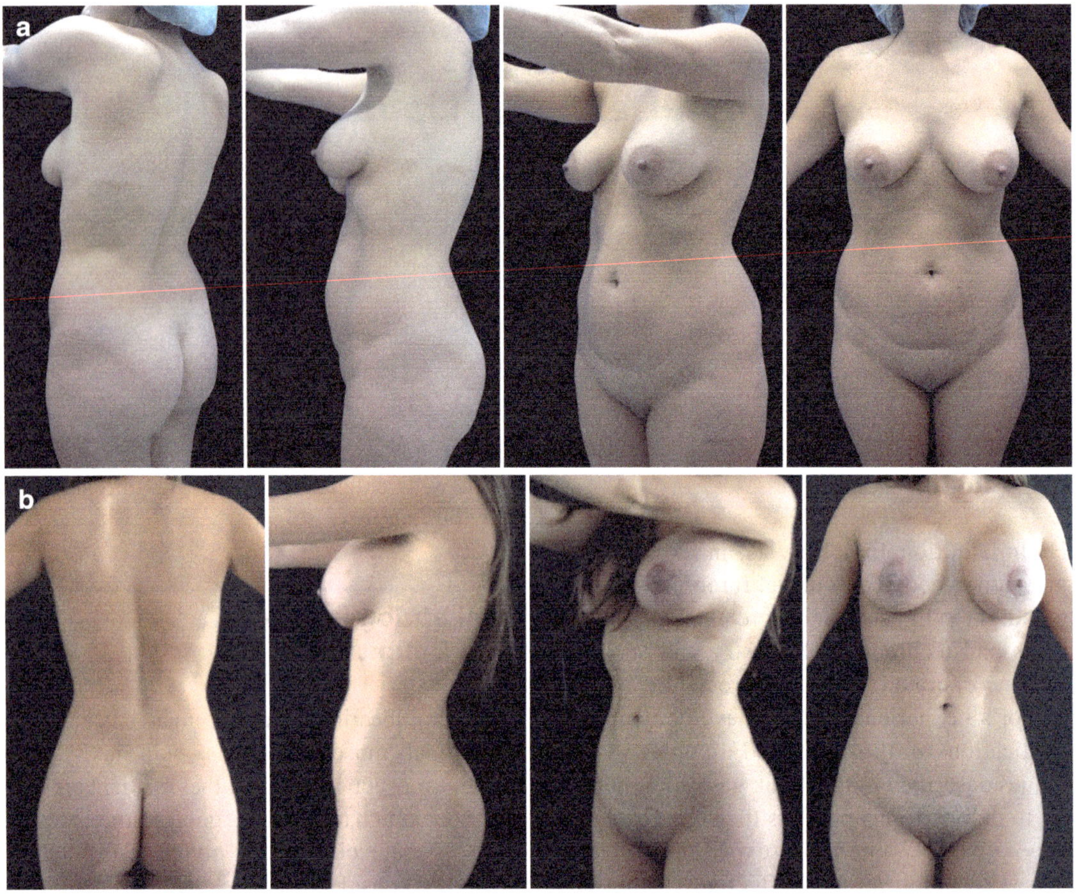

Fig. 21.1 A 30-year-old woman preoperative (**a**). One year postoperative (**b**). Mini-abdominoplasty combined with definition. Full 360° liposuction is performed, increased definition in torso and limbs, and full xiphoid to pubis closure of muscular diastasis. The scar is the same as a C-section scar

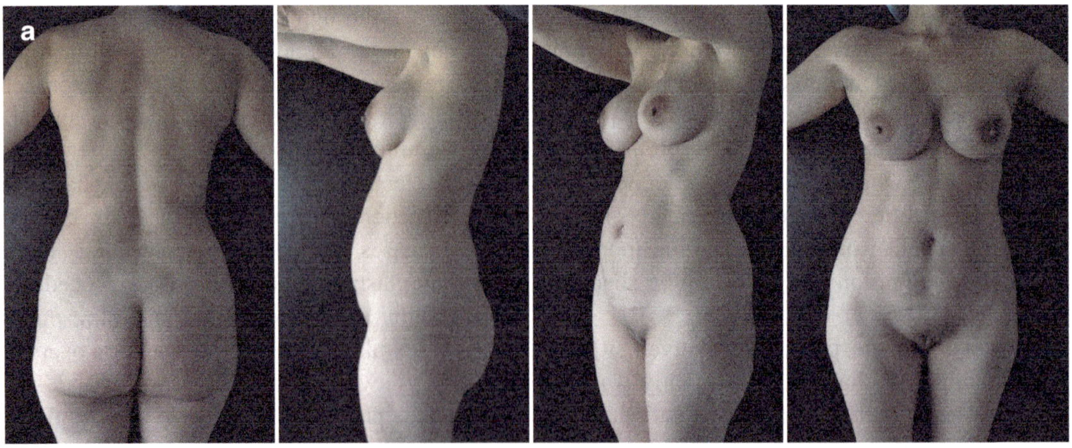

Fig. 21.2 Preoperative (**a**) and postoperative (**b**). A non-ideal candidate for mini-abdominoplasty, but the patient would not accept a large scar. Full 360° liposuction was performed, extensive VASER over the abdominal area to induce retraction, definition of the torso and limbs, and full xiphoid to pubis closure of muscular diastasis. Hiding the scar produces high satisfaction

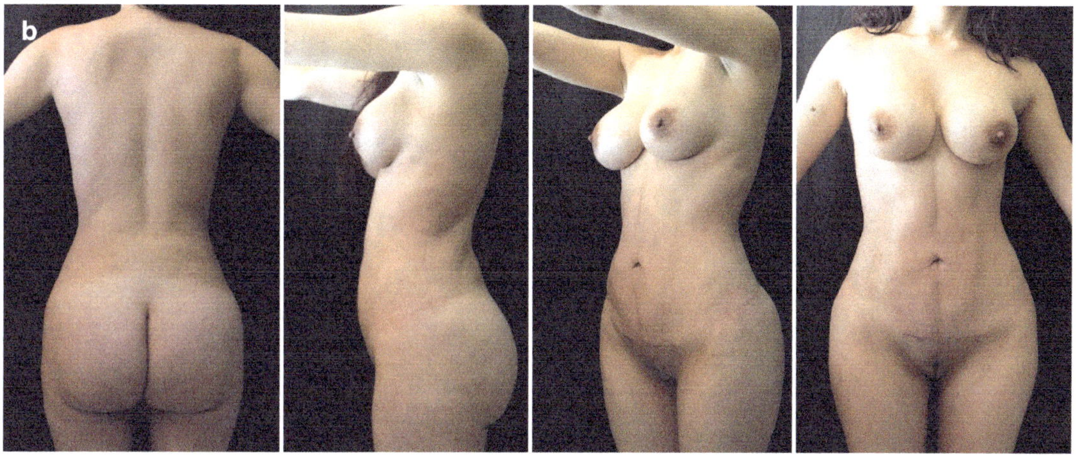

Fig. 21.2 (continued)

Full Lipoabdominoplasty with Definition

Abdominoplasty is expected to correct three main deformities: striae, extra fat, and muscular diastasis. These are common in women following multiple pregnancies or in obese patients.

The results of standard abdominoplasty are often non-ideal: The anterior abdomen can look tense, "drumlike," and overstretched; the waistline cannot be contoured as in standard liposuction; the navel looks artificial, and occasionally the visible navel scar becomes an obvious stigma of surgery. In addition, the distance between the umbilicus and the lipectomy scar might be very short and leave the patient with very limited options to conceal it.

High-definition body sculpting relies on manipulating shadow and light to reveal the underlying anatomy. The sculpting process creates convexities, concavities, and controlled grooves and irregularities in order to achieve exceptional results. The same concepts can be applied to abdominoplasty. This allows women who might previously have accepted only a flat-appearing abdomen as a result to realistically expect a beautifully athletic and toned abdomen with no visible stigmata of surgery.

Taking advantage of the fat-selective properties of the VASER technology, we perform 360° lipoplasty using the ultrasound over the flap, followed by suction using vented (VentX) cannulae to achieve definition. In our series, we report no flap necrosis, thrombotic events, or systemic complications (Fig. 21.3).

The Initial Concepts of Dynamic Definition

Consideration must be given to the dynamic nature of the muscles in the human body. The grooves created by the musculature in the upper arm, for example, are not static, but change during relaxation and contraction. Which should we mark preoperatively? The answer is *both*. By separately marking a dynamic zone and creating a tonal progression from one to the other, we can turn a picture into a movie. These efforts are made to obtain a result that is even more natural and more convincing. By adding this new dimension to high-definition body sculpting, we improve results even further and expand the indications to include nonideal patients like obese and post-bariatric surgery patients (Fig. 21.4).

Post-Bariatric Surgery Patient

After bariatric surgery or massive weight loss, patients are often resigned to expecting less-than-ideal results because of their condition. The concept of a single surgery should be changed in these patients. Staged surgeries that provide

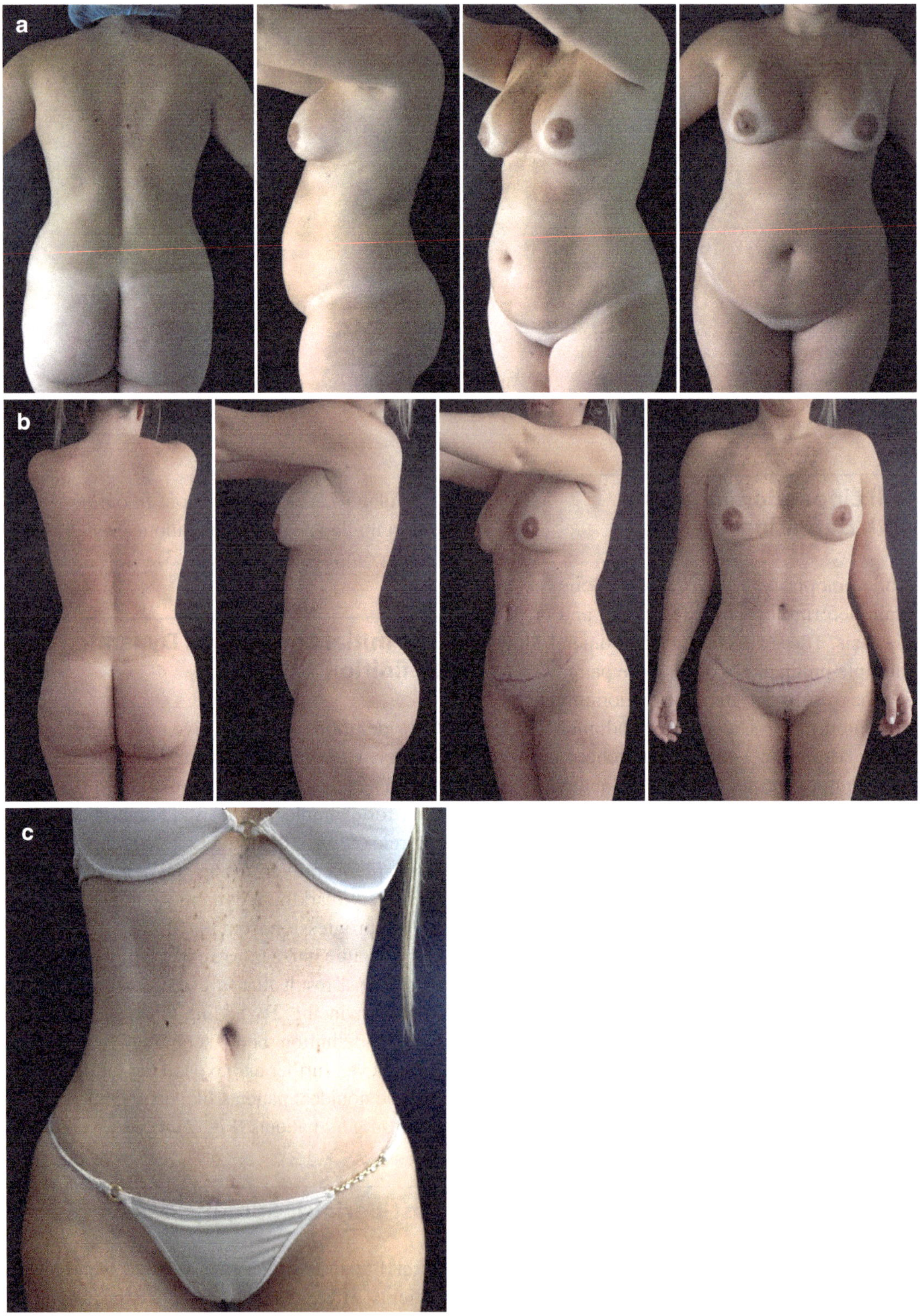

Fig. 21.3 Preoperative (**a**) and postoperative (**b**). Full lipoabdominoplasty with definition. Full 360° torso liposuction, definition over the posterior torso and limbs, slight definition over the flap area, and also a neo-umbilicus that provides a more realistic, natural aspect to the navel. (**c**) Note the natural appearance and the hidden scar beneath the underwear

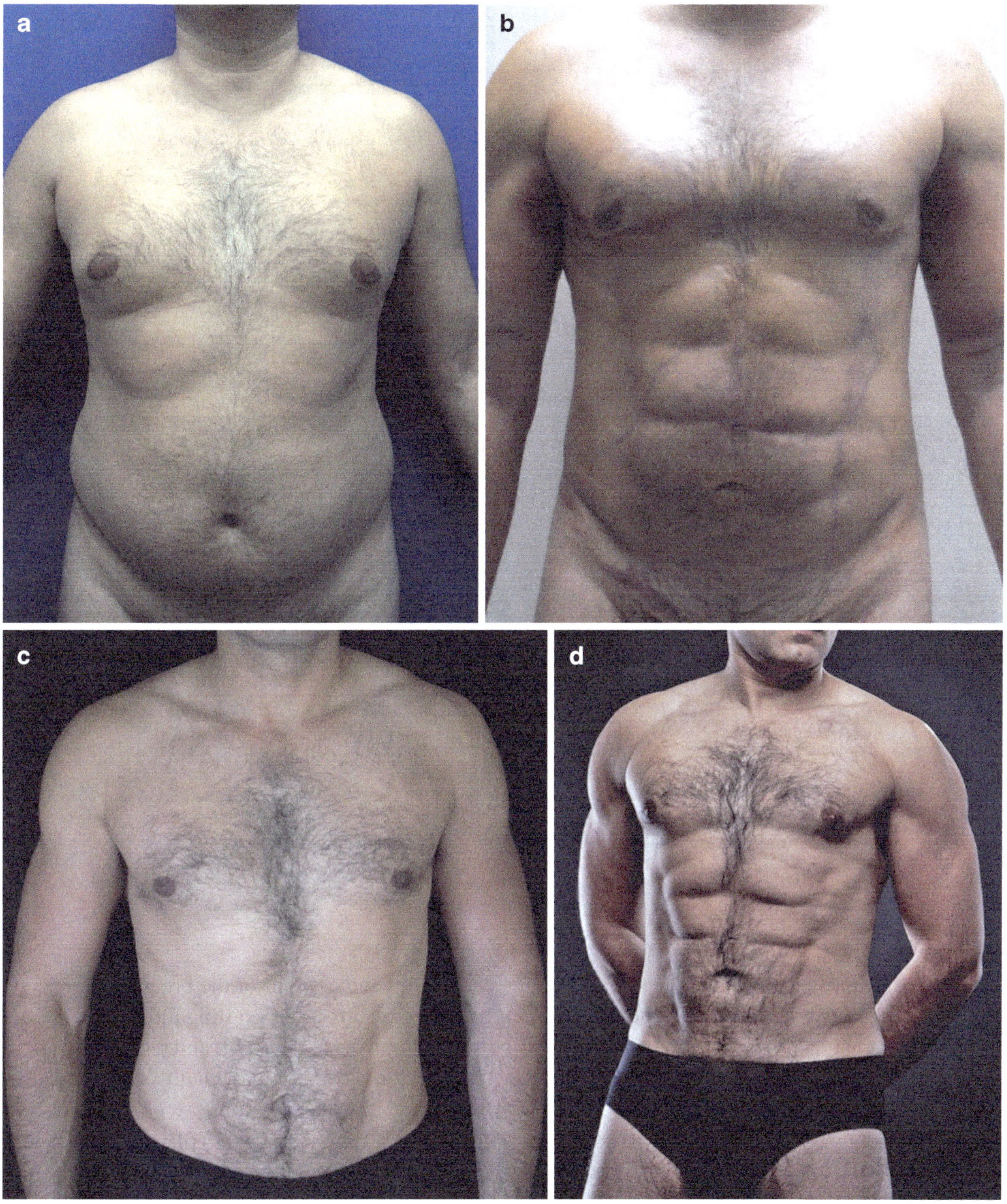

Fig. 21.4 Previously obese patient (**a**), 2 days after the procedure (**b**), 2 years after the procedure (**c**), using motion versus rest marking techniques to improve natural long-term results (**d**). In obese patients, results of non-dynamic lipoplasty tend to look unnatural and tend to dissipate over time

excellent skin retraction and change the inverted V shape common in these patients into a more aesthetically ideal form will become the new standard.

Even in these challenging cases, excellent results are possible using the principles of high-definition lipoplasty. Defining the "alpha" muscle, described by the author as the muscle that gives most of the shape to the anatomical area, is key to enhancing the upper torso in massive weight-loss male patients. Extensive superficial ultrasound

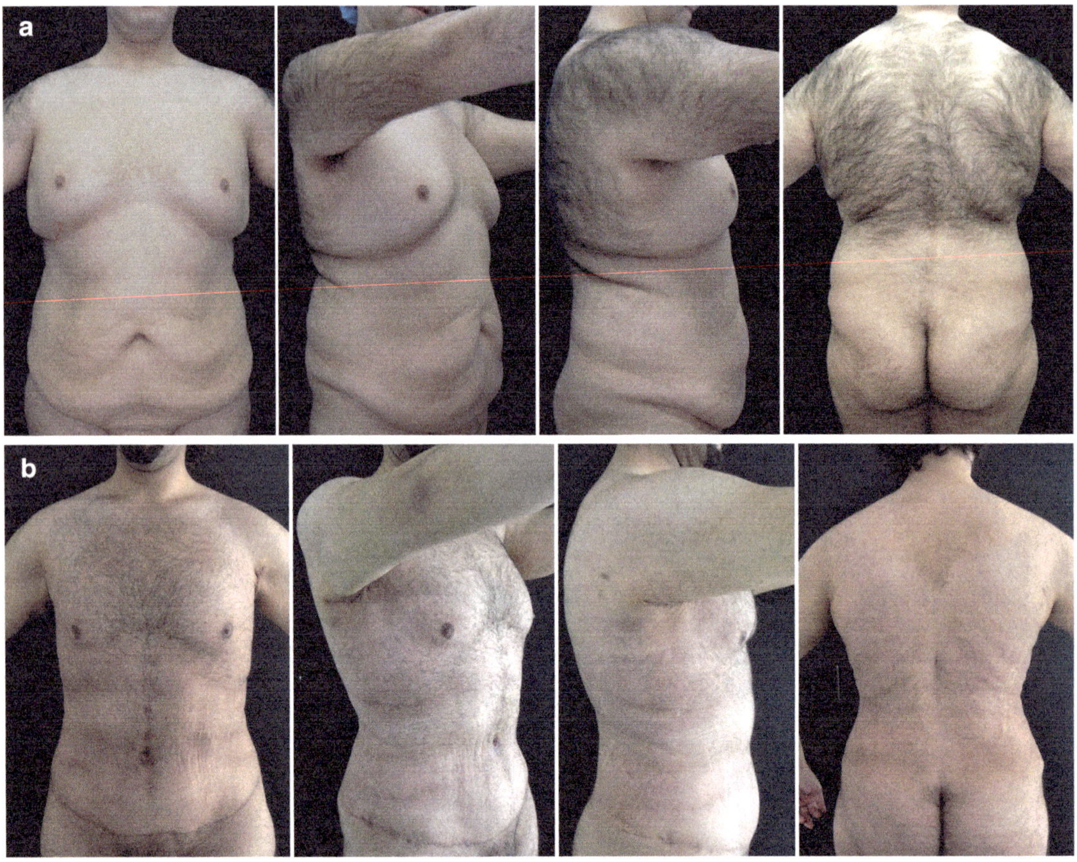

Fig. 21.5 Post massive-weight-loss patient (**a**) Preoperative and (**b**) postoperative of lipoabdominoplasty with definition

delivery and liposuction facilitate skin redraping and retraction. In women, a technique using three access points and abdominoplasty with high-definition lipoplasty restores the feminine (Fig. 21.5).

High-Definition Breast Enhancement with Enriched Fat

The use of fat grafting in the breast area has been described in Chap. 16. Enriching fat with stem cells or platelet-rich plasma aims to improve graft survival. The author uses a multilayer, multi-approach technique for breast fat grafting. Enhancing the breast with fat and creating negative spaces around the breast mass improves definition and contour of the breast and provides superior results to fat grafting alone.

Alternatives to breast lift and reduction include liposuction of the breast with VASER and/or replacing the lost volume with submuscular implants. Combining periareolar breast lift with fat grafting is another exciting possibility that may improve upon usual treatments (Fig. 21.6).

Cellulite and Secondary Fibrosis Patients

Patients who previously had failed liposuctions are eager for a correction of the deformities but often are reluctant to proceed with further surgery. The correction is difficult and often not successful. With knowledge of superficial liposuction, high-definition techniques, and selective fat grafting to camouflage some of theses deformities, the surgeon can offer these patients hope of significant improvement. Hoyos designed a new probe for VASER to treat these irregularities, called the Saturn probe. On the other hand, the surgical treatment of cellulite is also made more viable with this combination of advanced technique and specialized probes (Fig. 21.7).

Defining the Future

High-definition body sculpting is still evolving as a form of liposuction and human sculpture. With each new approach come new ideas, new

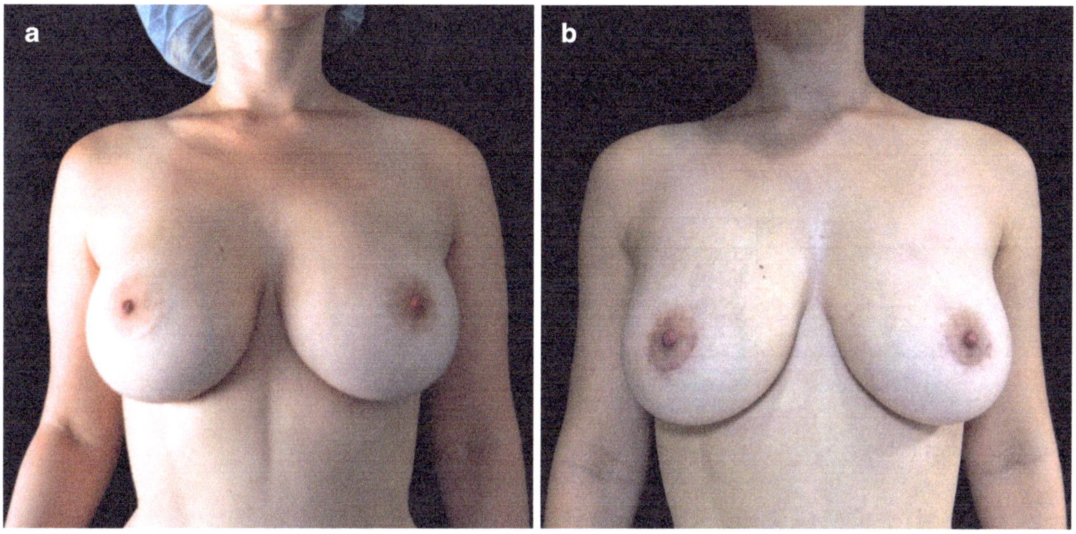

Fig. 21.6 A female patient who wanted to remove breast implants (**a**) and also have a slight reduction in breast volume but not a large breast reduction scar. Since she had large implants (400 cc), a vertical reduction scar was the main choice. Superficial VASER over the breast skin to induce retraction, implant removal, and fat-enriched grafting were performed. The result (**b**): Part of the lost volume was replaced by fat, and skin retraction resulted in a natural, appealing shape without a large reduction scar

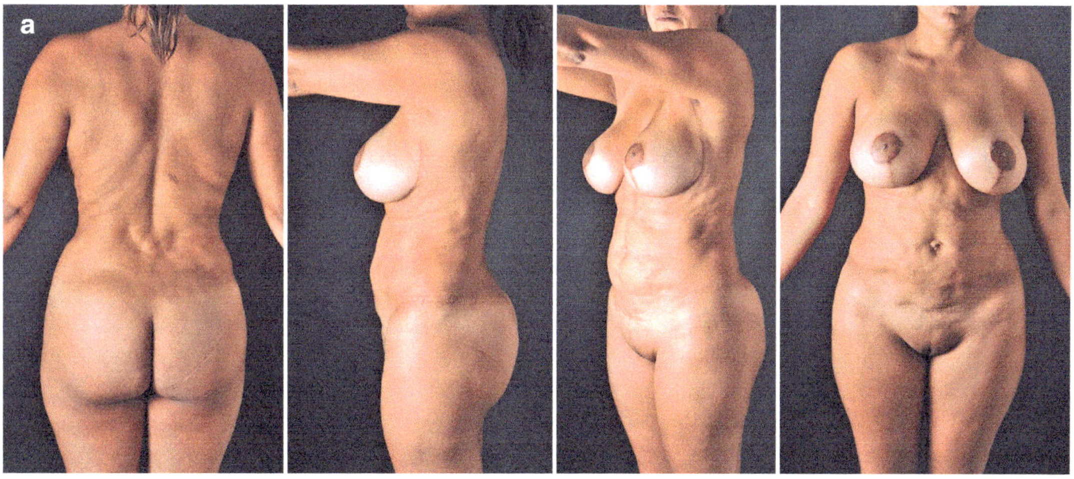

Fig. 21.7 Treatment of secondary fibrosis. Preoperative (**a**) and postoperative (**b**). Treatment of cellulite using special probes and superficial liposuction (**c**)

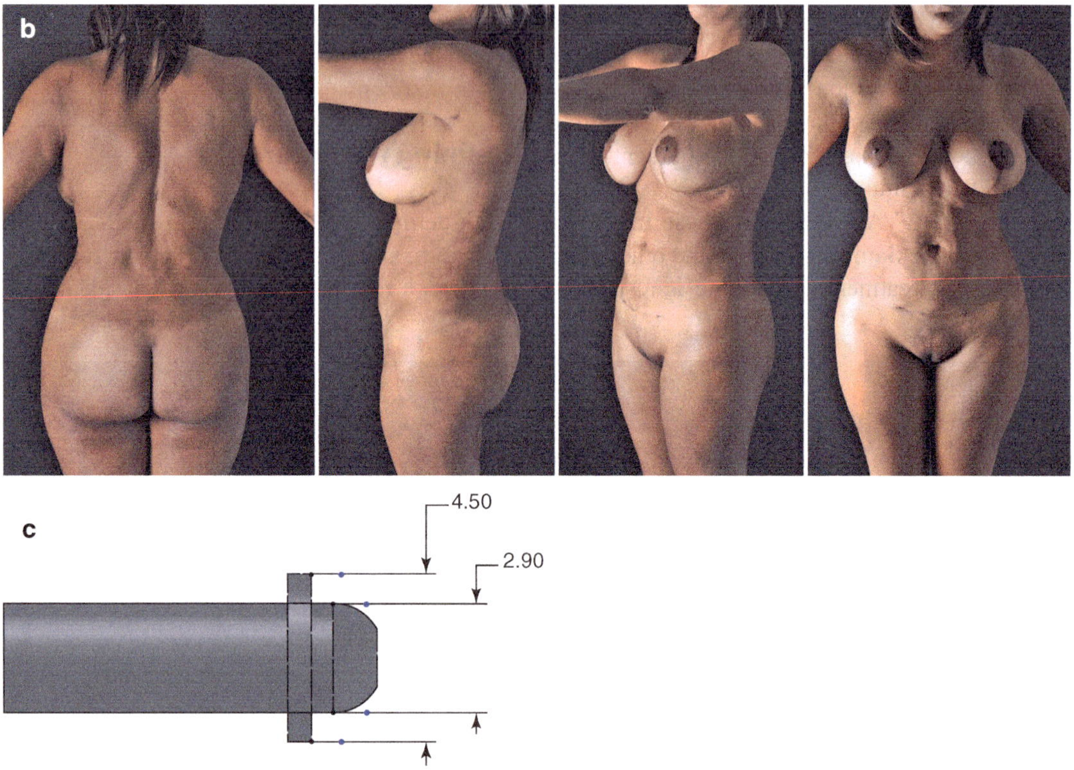

Fig. 21.7 (continued)

indications, and new therapies. The path is long, the thrill is endless, and the potential for further developments and refinements is real. Ultimately, the biggest reward is to provide happiness to our patients. To this end, the techniques we described in this book certainly deliver.

In this future of body sculpting, the only constant is human anatomy. Instrumentation, technology, and even aesthetic ideals may change. The development and popularization of high-definition lipoplasty techniques have given us some insight into what people want. There is a new standard in liposuction.

Index

A.E. Hoyos, P.M. Prendergast, *High Definition Body Sculpting*,
DOI 10.1007/978-3-642-54891-8, © Springer-Verlag Berlin Heidelberg 2014

Printed by Printforce, the Netherlands